T0380683

Technikzukünfte, Wissenschaft und Gesellschaft / Futures of Technology, Science and Society

Series Editors

Armin Grunwald, ITAS, Karlsruhe Institute of Technology, Karlsruhe, Germany

Reinhard Heil, ITAS, Karlsruhe Institute of Technology, Karlsruhe, Germany

Christopher Coenen, ITAS, Karlsruhe Institute of Technology, Karlsruhe, Germany

Martin Sand, TU Delft, Delft, The Netherlands

Diese interdisziplinäre Buchreihe ist Technikzukünften in ihren wissenschaftlichen und gesellschaftlichen Kontexten gewidmet. Der Plural „Zukünfte" ist dabei Programm. Denn erstens wird ein breites Spektrum wissenschaftlich-technischer Entwicklungen beleuchtet, und zweitens sind Debatten zu Technowissenschaften wie u.a. den Bio-, Informations-, Nano- und Neurotechnologien oder der Robotik durch eine Vielzahl von Perspektiven und Interessen bestimmt. Diese Zukünfte beeinflussen einerseits den Verlauf des Fortschritts, seine Ergebnisse und Folgen, z.B. durch Ausgestaltung der wissenschaftlichen Agenda. Andererseits sind wissenschaftlich-technische Neuerungen Anlass, neue Zukünfte mit anderen gesellschaftlichen Implikationen auszudenken. Diese Wechselseitigkeit reflektierend, befasst sich die Reihe vorrangig mit der sozialen und kulturellen Prägung von Naturwissenschaft und Technik, der verantwortlichen Gestaltung ihrer Ergebnisse in der Gesellschaft sowie mit den Auswirkungen auf unsere Bilder vom Menschen.

This interdisciplinary series of books is devoted to technology futures in their scientific and societal contexts. The use of the plural "futures" is by no means accidental: firstly, light is to be shed on a broad spectrum of developments in science and technology; secondly, debates on technoscientific fields such as biotechnology, information technology, nanotechnology, neurotechnology and robotics are influenced by a multitude of viewpoints and interests. On the one hand, these futures have an impact on the way advances are made, as well as on their results and consequences, for example by shaping the scientific agenda. On the other hand, scientific and technological innovations offer an opportunity to conceive of new futures with different implications for society. Reflecting this reciprocity, the series concentrates primarily on the way in which science and technology are influenced social and culturally, on how their results can be shaped in a responsible manner in society, and on the way they affect our images of humankind.

Madeleine Hayenhjelm ·
Christer Nordlund

The Risks and Ethics of Human Gene Editing

A Philosophical Guide to the
Arguments

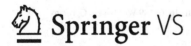 Springer VS

Madeleine Hayenhjelm
Umeå University
Umeå, Sweden

Christer Nordlund
Umeå University
Umeå, Sweden

ISSN 2524-3764   ISSN 2524-3772 (electronic)
Technikzukünfte, Wissenschaft und Gesellschaft / Futures of Technology, Science and Society
ISBN 978-3-658-46978-8   ISBN 978-3-658-46979-5 (eBook)
https://doi.org/10.1007/978-3-658-46979-5

This work was supported by Umeå University.

This Springer VS imprint is published by the registered company Springer Fachmedien Wiesbaden GmbH, part of Springer Nature.
The registered company address is: Abraham-Lincoln-Str. 46, 65189 Wiesbaden, Germany

If disposing of this product, please recycle the paper.

Preface

This book is a result of the research project "The Rise and Risks of CRISPR-Cas9: Cultural and Ethical Perspectives on the New Gene Technology," funded by the Marcus and Amalia Wallenberg Foundation (2016 and 2020) and conducted at the Department of Historical, Philosophical and Religious Studies at Umeå University, Sweden.

The idea behind the project has been to explore the ethical challenges—and the debates about these challenges—raised by the new gene-editing tool CRISPR-Cas9 (and similar gene technologies) by combining two disciplines: Moral Philosophy and Intellectual History. This has been done over the past years in a series of presentations at conferences, workshops, and seminars, in public lectures and radio interviews, and in constant conversations with scientists, policymakers, journalists, schoolteachers, and students. The present book, too, is a joint enterprise. However, it is not only due to alphabetic order that Madeleine Hayenhjelm is first author on the front cover. Although Nordlund has been project leader, Hayenhjelm is indeed the principal author of this volume.

We would like to express our gratitude to Marcus and Amalia Wallenberg Foundation for the two generous grants, to Umeå University for co-funding and hosting the project, to Kjell Asplund, Ulrika Björkstén, and Daniela Cutas for their reading and critical comments on earlier drafts, and to Cheflektor Frank Schindler and editor Britta Laufer at Springer VS for their support in the final stage of the work. Thanks are also due to all colleagues and students who have been involved in the ongoing discussion on the ethical and cultural dimensions of human germline gene editing. It is a discussion which, we predict, will continue for many years to come.

In the name of transparency, the authors would also like to declare that we have no conflicts of interest in relation to the contents of this book or its conclusions.

Umeå, Sweden   Madeleine Hayenhjelm
October 2024   Christer Nordlund

About This Book

This book is about the risks and the ethics of human germline gene editing, i.e., the possibility to make heritable changes to the DNA of early human embryos or germ cells. Is there something particularly morally problematic about editing the human germline? Is there something unique about germline editing, and, if so, does this suggest that we ought not to edit the human germline, or only in particular circumstances or for particular purposes? What would be a wise and responsible approach to editing the human germline from a moral perspective? The book has three broad aims. First, to provide an as inclusive map as possible over the current scholarly debate on the ethics of human germline gene editing in the wake of CRISPR. Second, to provide a philosophical and critical guide to the various ideas and arguments in this rich debate, including tools to analyze them. Third, to apply an ethics of risk perspective and defend a morally cautious position on human germline gene editing. *The Risks and Ethics of Human Gene Editing* is aimed at a readership of scientists, philosophers, and policymakers and points the way for future inquiry.

Contents

About the Authors

Madeleine Hayenhjelm is an Associate Professor in Philosophy at Umeå University, Sweden. Her main research interests fall broadly within the overlaps of normative theory, applied ethics, and ethics of risk, especially related to the ethics of emerging technologies. She has published on various topics related to the ethics of risk including on precaution, on responsibility and foresight, on fairness in risk distribution, on compensation and reparations, and on vulnerability and risk-taking. Hayenhjelm graduated from the Royal Institute of Technology in Stockholm and did her post-doc at UCL, London, as part of the AHRC-project on the Ethics of Risk. She is currently appointed ethics expert on the Swedish Gene Technology Advisory Board and has been a representative of Sweden on the Nordic Bioethics Committee.

Christer Nordlund is a Professor of History of Science and Ideas and the Dean of the Faculty of Arts and Humanities at Umeå University, Sweden. His main field of interest is environmental history and the history of modern life and earth sciences. Nordlund is the author of *Hormones of Life: Endocrinology, the Pharmaceutical Industry, and the Dream of a Remedy for Sterility, 1930–1970* (2011), and several articles in international journals and books. He has been a visiting scholar at Uppsala University, the University of Cambridge, the Max Planck Institute for the History of Science (MPIWG), and the Swedish Collegium for Advanced Study (SCAS). He is a member of the Royal Swedish Academy of Sciences and a Life Member of Clare Hall.

Introduction

> Gene editing forces us to grapple with the tricky issue of
> where to draw the line when manipulating human
> genetics.
>
> Jennifer Doudna and Samuel Sternberg, 2017

The recent developments in gene editing technology provides us with a power-ful tool to edit the DNA of any kind of living cell.[1] In principle, gene editing can be applied across the entire biological kingdom: from plant DNA and non-human animal DNA to human DNA. Furthermore, such edits can be done with great precision, and in a much more time-efficient way when compared with ear-lier technologies.[2] CRISPR has become a new gold standard for biomolecular research and was for this reason awarded the Nobel Prize in Chemistry in 2020.

---

[1] It has, however, been argued that the term "editing" gives the false impression of a greater degree of precision than what is currently possible and obscures the frequency of off-target modifications (Merriman, 2015; O'Keefe et al., 2015). In the earlier debate on germline alter-ations, permanent genetic alterations were referred to as "genetic modification" or "genetic manipulation," and the like. By contrast, CRISPR is most commonly described in terms of "editing" rather than modification or manipulation.

[2] CRISPR-based gene editing works as a tool that directs proteins to achieve a precise cut in the DNA—with or without adding a new set of genes to the same location—and then allow it to self-repair. Such edits consist of modifications to the double DNA strands in the form of gene knockouts, mutation repair, or incorporating new strands of DNA that only affect certain targeted cells of the individual patient. Similar kinds of modifications were possible with earlier technologies but much more time-consuming and less efficient.

© The Author(s) 2025
M. Hayenhjelm and C. Nordlund, *The Risks and Ethics of Human Gene Editing*,
Technikzukünfte, Wissenschaft und Gesellschaft / Futures of Technology, Science
and Society, https://doi.org/10.1007/978-3-658-46979-5_1

As the Royal Swedish Academy of Sciences put it in a popular presentation of the discovery: there are "almost endless examples" of how CRISPR-Cas9 could be used (Royal Swedish Academy of Sciences, 2020).

Applied to humans, this technology divides into two broad categories: *somatic* and *germline* gene editing. Somatic gene editing aims to treat or modify somatic cells in a patient, usually as part of medical treatment for genetic diseases.[3] In recent years, news of new medical applications has been frequently reported. Although such therapies are, and may continue to be, extremely expensive, it holds promise to treat several serious diseases, including hemophilia, sickle cell anemia, HIV, and even cancer, this way. The first CRISPR-based gene therapies were approved in the UK and the U.S. in 2023 for sickle cell disease and tranfusion-dependend Beta-thalassemia.

More controversially, gene editing can also be applied to the human germline, in other words, to germ cells or embryos in the very first stages of human development. Such changes, if successful, will affect every cell in the body and will also be inheritable such that the edits will be passed on to future offsprings. The possibility to edit the human germline provides an opportunity for prospective parents who are carriers of a genetic disease to have a genetically related child without passing on the risk for that disease. It also provides opportunities to prevent or eradicate severe genetic diseases on a larger scale conditional on broad screening and editing programs.

With such opportunities come all the risks attached to any kind of new but powerful technology that we do not have full knowledge about. It could fail to achieve the precise edit intended or bring about unintended mutations. It could lead to unwanted side-effects, such as cancer, in the longer term. More than that, it provides us with a tool to re-write human DNA that could be employed for all kinds of ends, including ideological, religious, political, and perfectionist ones. All this suggests that the various possibilities attached to germline gene editing also raise hard moral questions.

The prospects of human germline "modification" have been the focal point for a long-standing debate that goes all the way back to the eugenics movement. This debate predates the scientific possibility to make such changes but has regained actuality with recent developments. There are arguments from all sides in this debate. These include optimistic and hesitant medical arguments, ethical arguments of both optimistic and pessimistic kinds, visionary arguments from transhumanists, and dystopian arguments worried about fundamental losses

---

[3] Somatic gene therapy can also be used for preventive or enhancement purposes.

of values or even humanity itself. It is to this broad catalogue of arguments the current book turns and aims to provide the reader with both a map and a torch.

For a long time, the dominant view on human gene technology was that there is a moral line at the germline: We must not make inheritable edits to germ cells or embryos of future persons. The germline has been interchangeably referred to as a "boundary," "barrier," and a "red line" (see, e.g., Cwik, 2020a; Krimsky, 2015; Ranisch & Ehni, 2020; Ranisch, 2020; Evans, 2020). This previously dominant position has slowly weakened over the past decade, giving way to more cautious arguments that the germline as a moral boundary has lost its relevance (Evans, 2020, 2021; Cwik, 2020b; Ranisch & Ehni, 2020).

Human germline editing evokes the old dream of preventing some, many, or perhaps all hereditary diseases, as well as the possibility of enhancing senses and abilities, even beyond what is regarded as normal. This raises fundamental questions about the goals and risks of medical science and its impact on society. Some scientists, politicians, and ethicists have demanded a ban on such activities, while others have called for scientists to implement a self-imposed moratorium through a decisive, but possibly temporary, halt. In addition, some have argued that the current moral resistance will disappear as soon as the benefits—for medical science, health and well-being, and business—become accepted and known. Thus, it is as yet unknown how the global scientific and medical communities, politicians and policy makers, patients, and the general public will handle the potential challenges of this new gene technology. Moral arguments exist in support of both conservative and liberal positions on germline editing, along with various positions in between.

This book provides a philosophical guide to the moral questions raised by human germline gene editing: Is there something particularly morally problematic about editing the human germline? Is there something unique about germline editing, and, if so, does this suggest that we ought not to edit the human germline, or only in particular circumstances or for particular purposes? What would be a wise and responsible approach to human germline gen editing from a moral perspective?

The book has three broad aims. First, to provide a map over the current debate on human germline gene editing in the wake of CRISPR. Second, to provide a philosophical and critical guide to the various arguments in this rich debate, including tools to analyze them. Third, we apply an ethics of risk perspective and defend a morally cautious position on human germline gene editing. The ambition has been to provide an as inclusive map as possible over the various sides to this debate.

But we also take a stand. The position we defend is that the human germline can be viewed as a pragmatic moral boundary with the current epistemic shortcomings and perceived risks. It could serve as a pragmatic solution to action-guidance when there is (a) significant moral and epistemic uncertainty; (b) the risks and stakes are too high to allow for moral gambling; and (c) there is no better moral principle available that is more exact, sufficiently action-guiding, and sufficiently cautious. Should those factors change drastically, with the result that the relevant epistemic shortcomings have largely been addressed, the more serious risks are no longer viewed as irreversible, irreparable, no longer impossible to compensate for, and/or there is a more nuanced reliable moral boundary to replace the germline boundary, it will have served its purpose. This, however, still seems some way off.

The book is divided into two main parts: the first is mostly descriptive, mapping the debate, and the second is more analytical. The aim of the first part (Chaps. 1–5) is to present and disentangle the different opinions and positions for and against human germline editing that have been articulated in the scientific and ethical debate. It introduces the key scientific concepts, distinctions, and positions—as well as arguments in the broader ethical debate in the scientific literature—and provides a framework for recognizing the broader lines of argument. This part also includes an introduction to moral theory and moral reasons in preparation for the philosophical analyses conducted in the second part of the book. Instead of presenting a list of the usual normative theories, the focus here lies on highlighting the underlying kinds of moral logic that are not exclusive to any particular theory, so that these can be recognized in the various moral arguments in the chapters that follow. The second part (Chaps. 6–10) analyzes the arguments for and against human germline editing from moral philosophy perspectives and aims to answer the questions posed above. These chapters provide a theoretical introduction to the overarching line of argument set within the kinds of moral logic provided in Chap. 5. Where appropriate, current states of affairs are also historically contextualized.

Chapter 2 introduces the gene editing tool CRISPR, its benefits and its potential in the context of the renegotiation of established norms for the use of gene technology on humans. As a starting point for further analysis, three morally relevant distinctions are discussed: between somatic and germline interventions; between research and clinical application; and between therapy and enhancement. Although these frequently used distinctions are morally relevant, they are not derived from moral theory but have arisen from the scientific and public debate in which they have been ascribed an ethical role. As has been emphasized, they are not entirely definitive and somewhat controversial.

Scientists, philosophers, and other scholars have responded to these ethical challenges in different ways. Chapter 3 presents three ethical positions that have been adopted: a categorical position against human germline editing; a cautious intermediate position; and a more liberal position in favor of germline editing. While the first position advocates a ban on moral grounds, and the second argues for some kind of moratorium until scientific and other questions have been resolved, the third emphasizes the medical potential and the importance of taking advantage of scientific progress as soon as it is sufficiently safe to do so.

All the different positions on the human germline boundary share the view that heritable germline editing is *currently* not sufficiently safe to be utilized in a clinical setting. Furthermore, they also share the view that there are "ethical" aspects that must be addressed before the technology can be implemented. However, they hold somewhat different views on what these ethical aspects are, as well as what is required to address them. Chapter 4 discusses three common moral perspectives on the permissibility of germline editing. The first of these, *the Technical View*, equates ethical questions with questions about the direct risks of the intervention itself. Thus, the main concern is whether the technology works and is sufficiently safe and precise. According to the second one, *the Democratic View*, ethical questions are not only technical questions, but also pertain to values. The fact that the technology works and is safe and efficient are not adequate reasons from this perspective. Moreover, the main ethical concern is whether the technology and its consequences (even beyond individual bodies) represent a future we all find acceptable. Finally, *the Moral View* treats the ethical questions from a moral philosophy perspective. It takes safety and democratic legitimacy seriously but asks further questions: Does the technology promote what is genuinely good, or is there an aspect of it that violates fundamental moral norms or principles?

Problems linked to the Technical View can be addressed through further scientific research and regulation, and problems involving the Democratic View can be addressed through greater public engagement, debates, and dialogues. Problems associated with the Moral View, however, require philosophical analysis and reflection. This can be achieved in different ways, and Chap. 5 outlines three approaches to moral analyses. According to the first approach, moral rightness is determined by the value of the consequences; thus, the action that results in the highest net value is morally right. In the second approach, it is not only the consequences that determine the moral rightness of an action, but moral boundaries, principles, and norms that regulate what is permissible or not. The moral logic behind these first two approaches is *value maximization* and *moral permissibility*, respectively. The third approach is about *the pursuit of ideals*, which is less prominent in current moral theory but becomes relevant in this context through arguments about the desirability of various futures. These three types of moral logic give rise to different kinds of arguments and conclusions about the morality of human germline editing. They are introduced here to provide background context and tools for the analysis of and discussion about the arguments in the chapters that follow.

Chapter 6 explores human germline gene editing from the perspective of moral permissibility and takes a closer look at arguments supporting the claim that it is, in fact, categorically wrong. The chapter asks whether such interventions— provided that the technology could be considered safe on a molecular level— might violate fundamental moral norms (based on deontological concepts such as human dignity, individual and collective rights, autonomy, and informal consent). Could this lead to disastrous outcomes (such as eugenics, injustice, and loss of values)? Further, is there something inherently wrong in the use of this technology (such as "humans playing God")?

Chapter 7 focuses on consequence-based arguments for and against human germline editing. While the arguments against it appeal to safety concerns or risk, such as unintended health effects, the arguments in favor of it appeal to the potential benefits for future individuals, prospective parents, and even humanity at large. Both lines of argument are complicated by the fact that they concern the benefits and risk of harm to individuals who do not currently exist. This needs to be weighed against the alternatives to gene editing. Furthermore, from this perspective, it might be argued that there is a moral imperative not only to treat health-related problems, but also to improve humanity, thus blurring the boundaries between therapy and enhancement.

Chapter 8 takes a closer look at consequence-based arguments specifically addressing enhancement. Many of these arguments, both for and against, deal with considerably higher stakes than those discussed in the previous chapter— many of the anticipated benefits, and risks, are on a much larger scale. On the one hand, there are hopes of taking control of evolution, dreams of perfecting humankind and reaching a posthuman Utopia, and visions of saving humanity from natural disasters, while on the other hand, there are fears about jeopardizing the existence of humanity itself. Even though these arguments are much more speculative, they raise some difficult questions about the kind of future we value, who we might want to be in that future, and who would and would not truly benefit from such interventions.

Is there something particularly morally problematic about human germline gene editing, to the extent that it would warrant another moral approach than weighing the risks against the benefits, or asking whether it violates any moral principles or norms? Given the stakes and risks involved, do we need to place this kind of intervention in a special risk category? Chapter 9 discusses these questions and supports the notion that there might be grounds for deeper concerns. If this is the case, then we might not be able to assess the morality of germline editing merely by weighing up the pros and cons. This need not imply that there is a categorical argument against all forms of human germline editing, but it is something that requires serious caution.

In Chap. 10, we turn to the question of whether the germline could be viewed as a moral boundary—a red line. Without the support of convincing categorical objections, the germline does not seem to imply a moral threshold of impermissibility. Yet, the problems pointed out in Chap. 8 and the risks and lingering concerns raised in Chap. 9 suggest that the moral question of human germline editing goes beyond what can simply be determined by weighing up the anticipated benefits and risks. We argue that a sufficiently precautionary approach would need to take three dimensions of risk into account: risk of harm, epistemic risk, and risk of making irreparable moral mistakes. Until these risks have been sufficiently addressed, human germline editing should be treated with great caution. The germline could thus, for now, be regarded as a kind of *locum tenens* moral principle.

A New Pair of Scissors and Moral Alarm Bells

Between 2011 and 2013, a series of scientific articles were published that laid the foundation for a new kind of gene editing technology in a laboratory setting (Deltcheva et al., 2011; Gasiunas et al., 2012; Jinek et al., 2012, 2013; Cong et al., 2013). Several research groups, notably Emmanuelle Charpentier's team at Umeå University, and Jennifer Doudna's at the University of California, Berkeley, were instrumental in the development of knowledge that eventually resulted in the breakthrough of the CRISPR-Cas9 system, soon known to the general public as "gene scissors."[1]

At that point, other gene editing technologies, such as zinc fingers (ZFNs) and transcription activator-like effector nucleases (TALENS), had already been in use for several years. Prior to that, recombinant DNA technologies had been used to modify genes since the 1970s. Yet, according to the scientists involved, CRISPR-

---

[1] CRISPR-Cas9 is an abbreviation of Clustered Regularly Interspaced Short Palindromic Repeats-Associated Protein 9. The discovery did not occur in a vacuum, of course. According to Lander's somewhat controversial paper on the history of the science of CRISPR, research on the phenomenon can be traced back to work carried out by the microbiologist Francisco Mojica and collaborators at the University of Alicante in the early 1990s (Lander, 2016). It was also Mojica who coined the name CRISPR in 2001. A detailed account of this history and the scientific development up to 2016 is presented in Kozubek (2016). For many years after its discovery, a harsh patent dispute about the innovation of CRISPR-Cas9 took place in the US. We are well aware of this dispute, and of gene technology's economic dimension, but this fight over "biotech's big breakthrough" (*Scientific American*, 2016) will not be captured in the present book.

© The Author(s) 2025

M. Hayenhjelm and C. Nordlund, *The Risks and Ethics of Human Gene Editing*, Technikzukünfte, Wissenschaft und Gesellschaft / Futures of Technology, Science and Society, https://doi.org/10.1007/978-3-658-46979-5_2

Cas9 offered a much more efficient way to conduct gene therapy (Schultz-Bergin, 2018, p. 221; Ledford, 2015, p. 21). Qiu (2016, p. 309) writes, "With CRISPR-Cas9, we can more easily and precisely target DNA in cells than ZENs [sic] and TALENs. So far CRISPR-Cas9 is the most effective, inexpensive and easiest method to make precise gene manipulation possible to perform in all living cells." Compared to technologies such as zinc fingers and TALENs, CRISPR also requires less expert knowledge and fewer skills. Whereas the older technologies required particular proteins to be grown for each modification sought, CRISPR can use one for many changes (Doudna & Charpentier, 2014, cited in Schultz-Bergin, 2018). In the words of Sternberg and Doudna (2015, p. 568), "What had once been laborious and time-consuming was now facile and rapidly achievable."

Since its discovery, CRISPR technology has been hailed as the "go to" technology in many areas of molecular life science and biotechnology (Mariscal & Petropanagos, 2016). Within a couple of years, CRISPR-based genome editing was being used for research on a number of biological problems and tested on a variety of model organisms, from yeast to mice. In 2014, scientists in China employed CRISPR in primates, creating genetically edited monkey embryos (Niu et al., 2014). In addition to CRISPR-Cas9, other related "gene scissors," such as CRISPR-Cas12, CRISPR-Cas13 and CRISPR Prime, have been developed as well. However, given its versatility and ease of use, and thus potentially far-reaching effects, the technology has been called a disruptor (Ledford, 2015), a biological—and possibly an ethical—game-changer (Schultz-Bergin, 2018), and a revolutionary technology whose consequences are difficult or even impossible to foresee (Zhang & Zhou, 2014; Mariscal & Petropanagos, 2016). At the same time, the prospect of germline editing has also challenged the previous ethical consensus in the scientific community. Three sets of events illustrate how CRISPR technologies came to be viewed as an urgent ethical challenge.

2.1   Three Decisive Events

In April 2015, human genome editing went from being merely hypothetical to an actual possibility. A research team led by Junjiu Huang at Sun Yat-sen University set out and in fact managed to edit the human germline of non-viable embryos—albeit with serious concerns about off-target mutations and so-called mosaicism (Liang et al., 2015). Questions about the ethics of CRISPR had in fact been raised beforehand. One month before publication, a group of scientists, bioethicists, a filmmaker, and an administrator from the University of California, Berkely, met for a one-day conference in Napa Valley, California, to discuss ethical issues raised by the new technique, notably regarding the modification of the human germline (Doudna, 2015). The crossing of this boundary, even though it had still only taken place in the laboratory, caused extraordinarily strong reactions within the scientific community and the media. According to *The Economist* (May 2015), Huang's group had crossed "a red line."

All of this made the moral issues surrounding gene technology much more urgent. Concerned scientists and science writers feared germline gene editing would move into the clinic too soon, causing a public backlash and resulting in stronger regulations for basic life science research. The standard view within bioethics had been that we ought not to cross the human germline boundary—at least not until it was sufficiently safe, and possibly never. Not yet, because it *was* not currently safe, and possibly never, because there might be categorical arguments against germline editing that may imply there was something inherently wrong with such interventions.[2]

Against this background, some researchers called for a moratorium (Lanphier et al., 2015) until both technical and ethical issues had been properly addressed. Other researchers argued that the scientific community had to have transparent discussions about this topic, and that the general public should be involved in the debate (Baltimore et al., 2015). At the same time, the US National Institutes of Health (NIH) felt it necessary to reaffirm its ban on research that involved gene editing of human embryos (Reardon, 2015b). The general view seemed to be that it was still too uncertain and risky to edit the human germline , and that the ethical implications were not yet fully known.

However, with broad agreement that ethical issues had to be considered, and as safety issues meant germline editing was off-limits at that time, opinions were divided between those who viewed it as a categorically bad idea, those who saw it as a significant and promising tool for medical—and possibly non-medical—progress in principle, and those who wanted to withhold judgment until further information and a general consensus about such technology was available. Sugarman (2015, p. 1) states the following regarding the 2015 events: "Although these experiments were performed in nonviable, triploid embryos that were neither intended nor suitable for clinical use, the work nonetheless demonstrates

---

[2] The fact that both *Nature* and *Science* rejected the (Liang et al., 2015) paper based on ethical objections before it was published in *Protein & Cell*, a journal associated with China's Ministry of Education, gave rise to the idea among (mainly Western) scientists that "everything" was possible in China. Yet, according to Jiang and Stevens (2015), the experiment had, indeed, undergone ethical review at Sun Yat-sen University before it was conducted. In China, the results were also celebrated as being of fundamental scientific value, regardless of future applications.

how the prospect of manipulating the human germline elicits hopes and fears and triggers moral debates."

Since then, there have been a number of conferences and seminars on the scientific and ethical challenges and policy implications of CRISPR and human gene editing. Notable among the first ones are the Hinxton Group meeting in Manchester, September 2015 (Mathews et al., 2015), and the first International Summit on Human Gene Editing in Washington, organized by the US National Academy of Sciences and the US National Academy of Medicine, together with the Chinese Academy of Sciences and the UK Royal Society, in December of the same year (NASEM, 2015; Reardon, 2015a). The aim of the Washington summit was to facilitate exchange among experts from across the academic world and initiate a global discussion, rather than to draw any final "red lines."

Subsequently, in 2017 and in 2018, two influential policy reports were published on germline editing from the US and the UK, respectively—the National Academies of Sciences, Engineering and Medicine (NASEM) report (2017) and the Nuffield Council on Bioethics report, *Genome editing and human reproduction* (2018). These reports were widely read *as opening the ethical door* to germline editing, which had previously been shut. The NASEM report was viewed as giving human germline editing the "yellow light," while the Nuffield Council report concluded, "We can, indeed, envisage circumstances in which heritable genome editing interventions should be permitted" (Nuffield, 2018, p. 154). This was in sharp contrast to the earlier position expressed by UNESCO (1997), which viewed the human germline as a shared heritage, and the so-called Oviedo Convention (Council of Europe, 1997).[3] Others argued that the new reports did no such thing really, as they strongly advocated democratic dialogue, and any recommendation would necessarily be tentative before an agreement was achieved (Juengst, 2017).

In any case, it was widely claimed in the media that the Nuffield Council report on human germline editing had indeed opened the door to "designer babies."[4] Similarly, the German Research Foundation had already claimed in

---

[3] "Convention for the Protection of Human Rights and Dignity of the Human Being with regard to the Application of Biology and Medicine: Convention on Human Rights and Biomedicine."

[4] See, e.g., the following British headlines for 17 July 2018: "Genetically modified babies given go ahead by UK ethics body," *The Guardian* (Ian Sample); "Designer babies: Picking traits for non-medical reasons could be 'morally permissible', says UK ethics group," *The Independent* (Alex Matthews-King); "Editing human embryos 'morally permissible,'" *BBC News*; "Designer babies on horizon as ethics council gives green light to genetically edited embryos," *The Telegraph*.

2015 that not all forms of germline editing were morally problematic (Wirth, 2018, p. 130). This has been described as a slight shift in the view on germline editing, partly in light of the NASEM report (Braun et al., 2018, p. 5; Ranisch & Ehni, 2020, p. 3; Baylis, 2019, p. 135 f.).[5] Ranisch & Ehni (2020, p. 3) describe 2015 as the "peak" of the moral discussion and state that, since then, "most quandaries appear to have evaporated." According to them, the moral focus has changed from the question of "whether GGE [germline gene editing] could ever be ethically justified" to "under what conditions GGE may be used and eventually brought into clinical practice" (Ranisch & Ehni, 2020, p. 3).

In November 2018, shock waves ran through the scientific community when He Jiankui, a US-trained researcher at the Southern University of Science and Technology in China, claimed that he had (in his private IVF practice) genetically edited the embryos of two twin girls with the aim of making them immune to HIV (Normile, 2018; see also Greely, 2019; Baylis, 2019, p. 139 ff.). Jiankui announced the news about the babies, born one month earlier, at the Second International Summit on Human Genome Editing in Hong Kong. Apparently, he thought he had managed to do good in the service of science and medicine, but his audience did not agree. The conference's organizing committee concluded the following:

> At this summit we heard an unexpected and deeply disturbing claim that human embryos had been edited and implanted, resulting in a pregnancy and the birth of twins. We recommend an independent assessment to verify this claim and to ascertain whether the claimed DNA modifications have occurred. Even if the modifications are verified, the procedure was irresponsible and failed to conform with international norms. Its flaws include an inadequate medical indication, a poorly designed study protocol, a failure to meet ethical standards for protecting the welfare of research subjects, and a lack of transparency in the development, review, and conduct of the clinical procedures. (Baltimore et al., 2018)

Jiankui's clinical experiment not only sparked intense reactions in the scientific community (*The Guardian*, 27 November 2018; Baltimore et al., 2018), but also raised questions about its legality in China and its scientific rigor (see Southern University of Science and Technology 2018 and Yong's piece in *The Atlantic* 2018). Baltimore, one of the authors behind the call for a moratorium on germline

---

[5] Braun et al. (2018, p. 5) write, "However, the initial broad consensus on a moratorium—backed by the Oviedo Convention as well as by nearly all scientific and political institutions—has recently come under pressure in light of new developments (Ma et al., 2017) and institutional statements." Harris (2015, p. 31) describes the "consensus against germline interventions per se" as crumbling after the mitochondrial DNA debate.

edits (Baltimore et al., 2015), called the action "irresponsible," and a member of the audience at the summit said Jiankui had crossed a "red line" (*The Guardian*, 28 November 2018). Most of the criticism seemed to come down to concerns that this kind of intervention had been performed far too prematurely, that it was not currently safe, that too many uncertainties remained, that the choice of genes to edit was a questionable one, given that alternative treatments existed, and that it was done contrary to the moral consensus within the scientific community *not* to edit the human germline at this time.

After the public announcement, Jiankui's intervention was universally condemned, including by his own university (Southern University of Science and Technology, 2018). In a particularly damning letter to the editor for *Nature Biotechnology*, Krimsky (2019) listed no fewer than ten ethical violations Jiankui was supposedly guilty of, concluding that "the ethical infractions in this work are among the most egregious that have been recorded in modern medical history since the Second World War" and "there is every reason for researchers across the world to be embarrassed and for the scientific community to speak of this work as 'reckless'" (Krimsky, 2019, p. 20). In December 2019, Jiankui and his collaborators were fined and sentenced to prison—Jiankui for three years and his collaborators for a shorter time, for "illegal medical practice" (Cyranoski, 2020).[6] Later, a second pregnancy and a third genetically edited child from the same clinical project were confirmed by Chinese authorities and covered by the *Futurism* website (Houser, 2020).

2.2   The Moral Debate: Three Morally Relevant Distinctions

Three conceptual distinctions, or rather conceptual pairs, have provided much of the moral landscape in the literature on human gene editing and the recent CRISPR debate. These comprise the distinction between somatic and germline gene editing; between therapy and enhancement; and between gene editing "in the laboratory" and "in the clinic." Although the exact choice of wording differs, the core of the distinctions remains largely the same—these pairs are ubiquitous. Thus, throughout the literature, there is a recognized, potentially morally important, difference between (a) non-heritable edits of somatic cells and the heritable

---

[6] A detailed account of Jiankui's genetic intervention and its ethical consequences is presented in Greely (2021).

edits of germ cells; (b) between gene editing aimed at treating or preventing disease and gene editing aimed at improving the genetic prospects of an individual or a whole population; and (c) between gene editing limited to research and gene editing that is brought to the clinic.

All three conceptual pairs have been used in a moral capacity, with the first element of the pair understood to be less morally controversial or problematic than the second. Thus, somatic gene editing is considered to be less controversial than germline gene editing; gene editing limited to the treatment and prevention of disease is less contentious than gene editing seeking to improve the genetic prospects of a person or a whole population beyond what they would normally be born with; and gene editing limited to basic research is less divisive than gene editing in the clinic.

However, these conceptual pairs can also be combined.[7] The combined category of somatic therapy with the aim of treating severe genetic disease is thus generally seen as being far less controversial than clinically applied gene editing of the germline with the aim to perfect or improve upon a future person or population. In this simple way, all three distinctions agree on the least controversial and most controversial uses of the technology in ways that largely overlap with the general debate. The first distinction and the third distinction have also served as outright moral barriers: gene editing may be morally permissible when applied to somatic cells but not if applied to the germline, or germline gene editing may be morally permissible but not beyond what could be thought of as therapy or treatment.

We can now place the three key events mentioned above against these categories and distinctions. The 2015 event of the first CRISPR-gene edited (non-viable) human embryos in China crossed the germline boundary, but not the research/clinic boundary and not the enhancement boundary. The cautious shift in parts of the debate and policy contributions was a softened approach to viewing the germline as a boundary, while keeping the enhancement boundary in place. The genetically edited twin sisters born in China in 2018 crossed both the germline boundary and the research/clinic boundary. It has also been argued that it was not a definitive case of treatment, in that the aim was to achieve immunity for HIV.

---

[7] These six aspects combined thus give us eight different kinds of genetic interventions: (a) somatic gene editing research for medical purposes; (b) somatic gene editing applications for medical purposes; (c) somatic research for non-medical purposes; (d) somatic applications for non-medical purposes; (e) germline gene editing research for medical purposes; (f) germline gene editing applied for medical purposes; (g) germline gene editing research for non-medical purposes; and (h) germline gene editing for non-medical purposes.

We will now take a closer look at each of these three conceptual pairs, which have been so prominent in the debate.

2.2.1 Somatic Versus Germline Gene Editing

The central distinction in this book is between *somatic* gene editing and *germline* gene editing in humans.[8] This distinction has been paramount in legal and policy documents and has formed a crucial moral framework in the scientific community: As long as we only edit somatic cells, we are erring on the safe side of justified medical interventions. Descriptively, the distinction seems fairly definitive in that it draws the line between somatic cells and germline cells (eggs, sperm, zygotes, and embryos). However, this distinction may not be quite as clear-cut as often presumed (Beriain, 2019a, b). The main difference between the two kinds of gene editing is that of *inheritability*: Somatic gene therapy treats only the patient in question, while germline gene editing treats a developing person in a way that means the genetic changes are potentially passed on to all their future offspring. In fact, germline editing is often defined in terms of heritability.[9] For instance, the German *Act for Protection of Embryos* of 1990 (Sect. 8, §3) defines germline cells in the following way: "Germ line cells for the purposes of

---

[8] Although this distinction was formed already around 1970, Krimsky (2015) mention that it was highlighted in the statement of the Chair of the US President's Commission for the Study of Ethical Problems in Medicine and Biomedical and Behavioral Research Report of 1982, *Splicing Life: The Social and Ethical Issues of Genetic Engineering with Human Beings* (United States President's Commission, 1982). This report, according to Krimsky, distinguished between genetic engineering of somatic cells and zygotes, and argued that the latter required ethical attention and consideration in that "such interventions differ from prior medical interventions that have not altered the genes passed onto patients' offspring." (United States President's Commission 1982, cited in Krimsky 2015, p. 258). Krimsky continues: "This document set the stage for over 30 years of policy on human genetic engineering. During that period there was an implicit consensus within the scientific and regulatory communities that somatic cell gene therapy was acceptable medical experimentation once it was approved by federal authorities and ethics committees, but that genetically modifying the germ cells was out of bounds. It was a kind of Maginot Line that was widely publicized in science magazines and the media to reduce public concerns about eugenics. And by and large it worked" (Krimsky, 2015, p. 258).

[9] De Miguel Beriain (2019b) challenges the conception that germline editing must be performed on a not-yet-existing person in contrast to somatic gene therapy. He argues that: "Germline modification can be performed on both a non-existing or an existing person. I could perfectly well receive a therapy that changes my germline (not to mention a therapy that is not intended to produce such a result but provokes it as a side effect) even though I am an existing person. Of course, if I have descendants, they will suffer the consequences

this Act, are all cells that, in one cell-line, lead from the fertilized egg cell to the egg and sperm cells of the resultant human being and, further, the egg cell from capture or penetration of the sperm cell until the ending of fertilization by fusion of the nuclei" (translated and modified by Rixen, 2018, p. 24). Or, to take another example: "Human Germline Genetic Modification refers to techniques that would attempt to create a permanent inheritable (i.e., passed from one generation to the next) genetic change in offspring and future descendants by altering the genetic makeup of the human germline, meaning eggs, sperm, the cells that give rise to eggs and sperm, or early human embryos" (Baruch et al., 2005, p. 9).

Morally, this distinction highlights three potentially significant differences, the most important being one of *risk and uncertainty*.[10] This is a function of two parameters that amplify each other: On the one hand, germline editing is a pervasive technology (in that ideally all cells are affected) and on the other, many of the consequences are hard to predict (since genes could interact with each other and with the environment). This means that as soon as we cross over to germ cells, there is a chance that we will impose unpredicted and irreversible risks on many individuals (cf. Birnbacher, 2018).

Secondly, from a medical ethics perspective, what we may and may not do to a patient comes down to *consent*. Whereas an adult or an existing child can consent to somatic gene therapy directly or by parental consent, edits performed on embryos or germ cells will only affect persons that do not currently exist and thus cannot consent. Furthermore, it is hard to be fully informed about risks that are not currently known. These concerns are, however, more about moral pragmatism; lack of consent becomes a problem because safety cannot be ensured and because the outcome value may not be in the person's best interest.[11]

Thirdly, germline editing evokes connotations of *the eugenics programs* of the past in a way that somatic treatment does not. In this regard, Krimsky (2015, p. 241) comments on the prospects of eradicating a disease by removing an unwanted gene and replacing it with a normal one of the same kind: "[b]y most accounts, this is a form of eugenics or cleansing of the genome of 'bad genes'." Thus, as long as we use gene therapy in the aid of single patients, we are squarely in the domain of medicine, but once we seek to edit and alter the genome of future generations not yet born, we seem to embark on a path of eugenics. "Eugenics

---

of such an intervention, but it will not be them but me, in whom the modification will have taken place." (De Miguel Beriain, 2019b, p. 1257).

[10] However, somatic gene editing is of course not without risk either. See, e.g., Cavaliere (2019, p. 3 f.).

[11] Häyry identifies the ethical concerns underlying the distinction with the concern about consent and potentially long-term risks and epistemic gaps (Häyry, 2010, p. 17).

is the self-direction of human evolution," stated the logo of the second International Congress of Eugenics in 1921.[12] Hence, systemic and deliberate attempts to shape the genes of future generations could be viewed as a case of eugenics per definition. On this view, any attempt to alter the germline is a case of eugenics. For this reason, Krimsky (2015, p. 241) writes, some scientists were unhappy about the somatic/germline distinction and instead wanted to replace it with the therapy/enhancement distinction to draw the line elsewhere: between good, medically motivated eugenics, and the problematic cases of eugenics with the aim of "perfecting mankind." Others view such concerns as mere guilt by association. The objection to eugenics did not arise with current gene editing technology, but in the early days of gene therapy and bioethics—notably in relation to cloning and recombinant DNA—where spontaneous human reproduction is replaced by cloning and non-human genes are transferred to the human genome.[13]

Over the years, the human germline has served as something of a "red line," a moral boundary not to be crossed by scientists (Ranish & Ehni, 2020, p. 3).[14] Opinions have been divided on whether the moral boundary is merely a temporary one on precautionary grounds, or a moral boundary on categorical grounds. In either case, germline editing was until relatively recently considered morally

---

[12] The striving for the improvement of human nature or human abilities is ancient, but the term "eugenics" was coined in 1883 by Francis Galton. In the first half of the of the twentieth century, there were three different approaches to eugenics: (a) "negative eugenics" sought to prevent undesirable individuals from being born through birth control and sterilization; (b) "positive eugenics" aimed to produce individuals with better-than-average characteristics; and (c) hormone therapy was concerned with remaking, improving, and refining the human material which was already at hand (Nordlund, 2007, p. 100).

[13] Both concerns, however, lean towards a potential fourth moral boundary between a naturally evolved human and "fabricated" one. Theologian Ramsey, in his book entitled *Fabricated Man* (1970), describes, with concern, a future development where humanity as a species dies and is replaced by a new improved and more desired species as a result of a gained control over evolution (p. 151 f.). Similar concerns are expressed by Annas and colleagues in their proposed treaty against cloning and inheritable alterations: "Cloning and inheritable genetic alterations can be seen as crimes against humanity of a unique sort: they are techniques that can alter the essence of humanity itself (and thus threaten to change the foundation of human rights) by taking human evolution into our own hands and directing it toward the development of a new species sometimes termed the 'posthuman.'" (Annas et al., 2002, p. 153) The same development is echoed by the transhumanist but with the aim of achieving precisely the posthuman to succeed the current model (see e.g. Bostrom, 2008c).

[14] Krimsky also describes it as "a kind of Maginot Line" (2015, p. 238). Birnbacher asks whether the crossing of the germline in the case of mitochondrial DNA transfer constitutes "crossing of the Rubicon" (Birnbacher, 2018, p. 54).

off-limits and it is currently illegal in many countries (Boggio et al., 2021; Lander et al., 2019; Krimsky, 2015). In Europe, Article 13 of the Oviedo Convention (Council of Europe, 1997), a binding convention signed by 49 member states, bans inheritable intervention in the human germline and all interventions for non-therapeutic purposes. Additionally, the updated EU regulation on clinical trials, "bans all 27 EU member states from conducting gene therapy trials that can result in modifications to the research subject's germline," according to Boggio et al. (2021, p. 204; Regulation (EU) 536/2014). However, although clinical applications of germline gene editing are legally off bounds in most countries, the overall legal landscape is far from unified or even internally consistent. In their comparative overview of national regulations in 18 nations, conducted by Boggio et al. (2021), they found the regulatory landscape to be both "fragmented" and "outdated" (Boggio et al., 2021, p. 202, p. 221).

The strict view that the moral boundary should never be crossed has slowly lost ground. As far back as 1995, Peters wrote "In the 70s and 80s there was a strong taboo against the then hypothetical prospects of germline interventions. However, in the 90s this began to erode." (Peters, 1995, p. 381, n4.) His reference is the work by Fletcher and Anderson (1992) who argue for this point. According to Sagoff (2005, p. 71), "By the 1990s, scholars had thoroughly criticized the assumptions—and the underlying metaphors—that encouraged the anxieties and expectations commonplace 20 years earlier. These commentators explicitly attacked the idea that genetic technology differed in kind from other medical interventions." The idea was that such special concern about the germline was a form of "genetic exceptionalism" (Sagoff, 2005, p. 71). At the same time, many of the vivid metaphors of "Prometheus," "Frankenstein," "GMO man," "designer babies," "Pandora's box," and so on are back in public discourse on gene technology due to the CRISPR breakthrough.

In any case, the hardline positions of the Oviedo Convention and the UNESCO documents of the 1990s are no longer dominant. More recent policy and opinion documents are divided on the matter, and some cautiously open the door to the brave new world—on condition that it is safe, medically motivated, accepted by the public, and has broad ethical support (see, e.g., Ormond et al., 2017; NASEM, 2017; Nuffield Council on Bioethics, 2018). However, that need not necessarily undermine the moral relevance of the distinction. The somatic/germline distinction is still relevant in terms of caution, and it is important for advocates of a moratorium, especially as a means not to jeopardize promising research and development of somatic gene therapy. Lanphier et al. (2015) conclude the importance of the distinction with the following statement:

Key to all discussion and future research is making a clear distinction between genome editing in somatic cells and germ cells. A voluntary moratorium in the scientific community could be an effective way to discourage human germline modification and raise public awareness of the difference between these two techniques. (Lanphier et al., 2015, p. 411)

This is also the role that Krimsky (2015, p. 240 f.) describes: By stressing the difference between somatic gene therapy and germline gene therapy, a general skepticism towards human gene therapy—based on its association with eugenics—could be avoided by highlighting that only germline editing would warrant such an association. Some scientists, however, argue that the distinction would be better if it were replaced by one between general therapy and enhancement, and that even germline editing, provided it was limited to therapeutic purposes of treatment and prevention of disease, would not really constitute eugenics, as long as it did not cross over into projects of human perfection.

2.2.2 Therapy Versus Enhancement

A second distinction, between *therapy* and *enhancement*, also plays a key role in the debate.[15] At least until the Second World War, it was common in Europe and the US to think that an "improvement" of human biological heredity would be beneficial for society (Roll-Hansen, 2017, p. 182). Visions about the possibility of creating "perfect" human beings through medical interventions were articulated in the 1930s, although, at that time, hormone therapy rather than gene therapy was the preferred biotechnology (Nordlund, 2007; Beccalossi, 2020). In the public discourse and popular culture, statements about the possibilities of human enhancement, mental and physical, have also received significant attention throughout the last century (Turney, 1998). According to Comfort (2012), medical genetics, notably in the US, has always been driven by two goals in addition to knowledge production: relief of suffering and improvement in human heredity.

Yet, most actors in the current scientific and ethical debates on gene editing tend to support a distinction between therapy and enhancement. Cwik (2019, p. 695 f.), for instance, describes this centrality in the following way: "Most statements on the use of gene editing in human beings so far from professional

---

[15] See Resnik and Langer (2001, p. 1450) for historical background on the distinction from the 1980s to 1990s.

organizations, ethics boards, and advisory panels— including the recent exhaustive report by the United States National Academies of Science, Engineering and Medicine—have called for drawing the line at 'therapeutic' uses and forbidding 'enhancement' with gene editing, thus reaffirming the centrality of the distinction."

However, the distinction has less definitive descriptive underpinnings. What counts as treatment as opposed to enhancement is not clear, but depends on how concepts such as "normal," "human," and "health" are defined (Resnik & Langer, 2001). The key problem is that any notion of "enhancement" must operate in relation to some kind of baseline, some notion of what is a "normal, healthy, human being" (Resnik & Langer, 2001, p. 1451). Resnik and Langer (2001) conclude that "the boundaries between therapy, prevention, and enhancement are not clear in genetic medicine" (p. 1450). Such terms could be defined in various ways, which makes the distinction particularly prone to arbitrariness.

On the one hand, nearly all of the serious categorical objections towards germline editing, aside from concerns about risks of harm (resulting from off-target risks, mosaicism, etc.), seem to be based on concerns about enhancement: fear of eugenics, perfectionism, designer babies, dissolution of human nature, violation of what is natural, and so on. By contrast, germline gene editing with the aim of removing severe genetic diseases that are difficult to treat, such as sickle cell anemia and Huntington's disease, is not controversial in itself, aside from the risks (to the patients) and "slippery slope" concerns that this will open the door to eugenics, designer babies, and so on. Therefore, it makes a sense to narrow the class of objectionable germline edits from all kinds of germline edits to only those that aim at enhancement or non-medical intervention. Even so, this position has been challenged from the disability community including those born with severe genetic diesease (Sufian & Garland-Thomson, 2021).

That said, the category of enhancement does not constitute a morally unified class with a similar degree of controversy. Some kinds of interventions may not offer any treatment to any ailments or disease, but rather correct a deviation from what is considered "normal" and of little or no medical importance (such as correcting for height). These kinds of interventions to reach something "normal" do not seem to belong to the same moral class as deliberate attempts to "perfect" mankind and improve for example memory or muscle strength and create some perfect "master class." Resnik and Langer (2001) echo this: "Most people can think of some obvious cases of morally 'suspect' genetic enhancement, ..., but borderline cases are difficult to classify" (p. 1451).

Another line could thus be drawn between enhancements that aim to achieve "normal standards of health" for embryos that otherwise would fall short of what is considered normal and enhancements that aim for some kind of excellence beyond the "normal." Enhancement with the aim of achieving "normality" for more persons born would then constitute enhancement but would not alter human nature as such. However, even if enhancement is limited to achieving "normality" rather than "excellence," it still raises concerns about how this would affect over-all tolerance for the genetic differences. It could put pressure on parents to edit children to be not perfect but "perfectly normal" (see Garland-Thomson 2019 for a related discussion). In any case, it is not clear how exactly such normality aiming enhancement differs from the old negative eugenics.

The distinction between therapy and enhancement is perhaps the least defini-tive of the three, since what constitutes disease, health, and enhancement will depend on how those concepts are understood and interpreted, which to a high degree is context dependent. Thus, although most controversy around germline editing seems to arise at the far end of enhancement and considerably less around somatic treatment of disease, it is not clear that the therapy/enhancement distinc-tion can provide a reliable guide on where the line ought to be drawn between these two ends.

2.2.3 Research Versus Clinical Application

There is also a third distinction: between germline gene editing "in the labo-ratory" and germline gene editing "in the clinic." Though worded in different ways, essentially a line is drawn between germline editing as an applied practice in the clinic (as part of clinical studies or as part of future practice after clin-ical trials) and germline editing limited to a research context and, presumably, only basic research and possibly also preclinical studies on animals. Research on the germline that remains "in the lab" would then not involve any patients, as opposed to research and application "in the clinic," where a genetically edited embryo could be transferred to a uterus and carried to term. Like the other two distinctions discussed in the previous sections, this distinction has been given moral significance, although it plays a less prominent role in the debate than the others.

This distinction seems to make sense both descriptively and normatively. Descriptively, there is an obvious difference between research that remains in the laboratory context and effectively "stays out of the womb" and edited embryos that are transferred to a womb and carried to term. It thus seems sufficiently definitive as a distinction and sufficiently action-guiding if understood norma-tively. Normatively, it also makes sense to distinguish between research and application: As long as an embryo is not transferred to a uterus, no one suffers any risks as a consequence of having their genome edited. Furthermore, there will be no cause for concern about "designer babies" or social injustice.

If germline editing never leaves the laboratory, it is hard to see how any person could be harmed. Therefore, some argue that whereas we ought to permit research on the germline, we ought not to take it to the clinic. Mertes and Pennings (2015) write, "As long as the embryos are not transferred and will thus not grow into a person, it is very difficult to find a solid argument why gene editing should be excluded as research methodology." Along the same lines, the European Society for Human Genetics (ESHG) and the European Society for Human Reproductive Embryology (ESHRE), issued the recommendation that "both basic and pre-clinical research regarding GLGE [Germline Gene Editing] can be justified, with conditions" but "clinical GLGE would be totally immature" (de Wert, Heindryckx, et al. 2018; de Wert, Pennings, et al. 2018). Moreover, such research falls well within existing ethical and regulatory boundaries. The National Academies of Science, Engineering and Medicine make the following point: "Laboratory research involving human genome editing—that is, research that does not involve contact with patients—follows regulatory pathways that are the same as those for other basic laboratory in vitro research with human tissues, and raises issues already managed under existing ethical norms and regulatory regimes" (NASEM, 2017, p. 185). Such research could also provide important information about germline editing, should it be approved at a later stage.

Ormond et al. (2017) consider it "inappropriate" to perform germline gene editing that culminates in human pregnancy at present, while also claiming that currently "there is no reason to prohibit in vitro germline genome editing on human embryos and gametes, with appropriate oversight and consent from donors, to facilitate research on the possible future clinical applications of gene editing." To take the last step in clinical application, however, would, according to them, require "compelling medical rationale," an evidence base in support of clinical use, and the solicitation and consideration of ethical and social values (Ormond et al., 2017). The distinction could thus support either a morally restrictive position on germline applications or a temporary measure of precaution to ensure that the technology is sufficiently safe, morally acceptable, and medically motivated before proceeding.

Some are even more optimistic about future applications as a result of such research. According to Sykora and Caplan (2017a, p. 1871), "Although they are not yet sufficiently safe to be used in clinical trials, research has made rapid progress in improving efficiency and precision of the CRISPR technology. With further improvements, gene editing technology therefore has the potential for

safely modifying the human germline for prophylactic and therapeutic purposes".
On this view, basic and clinical research are necessary steps to ensure that future
applications are sufficiently researched before they move to the clinic.

Others express further caution against germline editing in research. While
some view research as either unproblematic and valuable, or even important as
a prerequisite for a future move to the clinic, others argue for a halt to germline
research while more information is gathered. And some might be opposed to
research simply because they suspect that it eventually will result in a "slippery slope" that slides to actual use. Of the two *Nature* and *Science* statements
of 2015, Lanphier et al. (2015) want to draw a line against human germline
editing both in the laboratory and the clinic so as not to risk a public backlash and thereby jeopardize promising somatic gene therapy research. Baltimore
et al. (2015), by contrast, encourage gene editing research on the germline to
better "understand and manage risks" and investigate the safety and efficacy of
the technology (Baltimore et al., 2015, p. 37). In fact, one of their recommendations is to "[e]ncourage and support transparent research to evaluate the efficacy
and specificity of CRISPR-Cas9 genome engineering technology in human and
nonhuman model systems relevant to its potential applications for germline gene
therapy" (Baltimore et al., 2015, p. 38).

However, much of the motivation for the scientific project stems from the
anticipated benefits of clinical applications. It cannot prevent severe genetic disease unless it is, at some point, clinically applied. Thus, Baltimore et al. (2015)
argue that there is a need for both research and risk management, as well as
a broad ethical conversation to ensure translational pathways to responsible use
(Baltimore et al., 2015, p. 37). The hope is that once germline editing is sufficiently safe, it can be brought to the clinic, and that a moratorium on clinical
applications will provide a "safe space" for research and can serve as a safeguard
against different kinds of concerns.

2.3   Vague Distinctions and Porous Moral Boundaries

The three distinctions discussed above are not derived from moral theory but are
descriptive distinctions that have arisen from science and play an ethical role.
Theoretically, they are not as strict as one would want, since all the distinctions
have gray areas that make it difficult to base criteria of rightness or wrongness upon any of them. In this section, we will take brief look at some of these
gray areas.

The first distinction, between the editing of somatic gene cells and germ cells, seems definitive. One can see how the moral accuracy of tracing a line between the permissible and impermissible could be questioned, but the descriptive line between somatic cells and germ cells seems indisputable. Likewise, the moral relevance of the distinction seems straightforward in that germ cell edits are heritable and somatic edits are not. However, neither of these seemingly definitive categories are as straightforward as that.

The somatic/germline distinction, at least as a morally decisive distinction, is complicated by the case of mitochondrial DNA transfer. These are clear cases of germ cell intervention, which are thus heritable. There is no doubt that when the first mitochondrial DNA transfers occurred, they were framed as crossing the germline (Krimsky, 2015), yet the case does not seem to belong to the same morally controversial category of germline edits discussed here. The main difference is that when we discuss edits to the germline in order to prevent sickle cell anemia, Huntington's disease, and the like, we are talking about edits to the nuclear DNA, where most genetic information is located. Mitochondrial DNA, by contrast, only serves as the energy supplier of the cell. Thus, the scope of risks is limited to this function alone, although diseases that affect the function of the mitochondria can be severe. It has thus been regarded as relatively uncontroversial, morally, to prevent such a disease, while there is little risk of severe side effects due to the multifunctionality of genes.

However, if mitochondrial DNA is a definitive case of germline intervention, and it is morally different from the germline gene edits in a way that does not correspond to the somatic/germline distinction, then this significantly weakens the force of the distinction as a moral boundary. The distinction between somatic and germline gene editing as a moral boundary would need either to treat the much less controversial gene edits of mitochondrial DNA as morally equivalent to edits of nuclear DNA, or allow for exceptions and thus make the distinction more of a moral approximation than a moral boundary or red line.[16] This could, of course, be remedied by specifying that any moral distinction between germline editing and somatic gene editing refers only to germline editing of the cell *nucleus.*

The main driver of the moral implications generated by the distinction seems to rest on the moral significance of heritable versus non-heritable alterations to human DNA. Germline edits are different to somatic gene edits as the former

---

[16] Mitochondrial DNA transfer raises controversial moral issues in itself, but not the same as those associated with germline gene editing of nuclear DNA. In particular, the donation of mitochondrial DNA allows for a child to be born with the DNA from three parents: nuclear DNA from a biological mother and father, and mitochondrial DNA transfer from an additional woman.

introduce heritable alterations but the latter do not. What makes germline editing morally problematic is the fact that any alterations made will be passed on. Again, on this distinction, mitochondrial DNA belongs to the germline side of the distinction. Such interventions are heritable in the same way as other germline edits, but they are limited to the mitochondrial DNA (see, e.g., Birnbacher, 2018, p. 54). Yet, such edits do not seem to be equally morally problematic, given their limited scope. There is no room here to explain this difference in moral significance, if indeed there is one, if heritability is what determines moral significance.

More worryingly, somatic interventions *could* have heritable side effects. Thus, the somatic/germline distinction would fail to accurately draw a line between heritable interventions and non-heritable ones. Häyry (2010, p. 17) comments, "The line is not impermeable, though, as genes inserted to other parts of the body can travel to reproductive tissues." He adds, "This is potentially embarrassing for legislators, because many governments have allowed trials on somatic cells while making a point of banning germ-line therapies as unethical" (Häyry, 2010, p. 17). Again, the line seems to be more tentative, roughly sketching out a difference, rather than constituting a hard red line. In fairness, in the somatic case these heritable effects are generally incidental consequences rather than direct ones, and they are the exception rather than the rule. The distinction could thus be viewed as *roughly* drawing the line in the right place. However, the case for the somatic/germline boundary as a firm moral boundary is obviously weakened.

Moreover, if heritability is what is morally significant, then this does not single out germline editing. Heritability across generations is not limited to genetic inheritance, but also includes such things as epigenetic inheritance due to environmental and nutritional factors, as Lewens (2020) points out. Heritance imposed on future generations would then fall into the same moral category as germline editing, if heritability alone is of significance.

Morally speaking, the therapy/enhancement boundary may seem to be a better option, drawing a more accurate moral line. Beriain (2019b) argues that the therapy/enhancement distinction is preferable to the somatic/germline distinction, given the weaknesses of the latter. He challenges especially the idea that germline editing treats a "patient that does not yet exist" (Walton, 2016, p. 1527). According to De Miguel Beriain (2019a), germ cells can be altered in an existing person as part of therapy:

> Germline modification can be performed on both a non-existing or an existing person. I could perfectly well receive a therapy that changes my germline (not to mention a therapy that is not intended to produce such a result, but provokes it as a side effect) even though I am an existing person. Of course, if I have descendants, they will suffer

the consequences of such an intervention, but it will not be them but me, in whom the modification will have taken place. (De Miguel Beriain, 2019a, p. 1257)

In other words, if what we want to do is draw a line between experiments on embryos or germ cells before they are transferred to a uterus and develop into a person later born with those edits, and those that are offered to a patient to cure genetic illness, the germline/somatic cell distinction may not be descriptively accurate. If germline editing is made more problematic than somatic editing because we, in the case of the former, alter the DNA of a future person who will be born with those changes, then this concern may not descriptively overlap with those categories.

Unfortunately, the therapy/enhancement distinction is not more definitive than the somatic/germline one—if anything, it seems less definitive. Undoubtedly, definitive examples exist for both categories: Some germline interventions are plainly cases of medical prevention, while other germline interventions are clear examples of enhancement. It is also the case that more serious concerns about germline editing are typically based on concerns about enhancement. Nevertheless, advocates for human enhancement sometimes downplay the difference and argue that every therapy is a kind of enhancement and that aging is a disease, and thus that aiming for immortality constitutes therapy. As we shall see, it is not clear that germline editing could constitute therapy at all, in that there is no patient and no condition to treat. Rather, germline editing operates at the level of prevention. Sometimes, the disease prevented is one that would certainly have affected the person, and sometimes the prevention is directed at a disease that merely *could* have materialized, with some probability. Sometimes it merely increases the odds of preventing certain kinds of disease. It is unclear where germline editing as "treatment" ends and germline editing as "enhancement of health" begins.

Furthermore, it is unclear where "enhancement of health" ends and "enhancement for social advantage and privilege" begins. One could use the notion of therapy very broadly to include all kinds of probabilistic improvements related to health prospects. Certain improvements would more easily fall into the category of therapy, while others would look very much like they had provided a person with a different set of odds and prospects than they would otherwise have had. Alternatively, one could distinguish between different kinds of enhancement based on some concept of normalcy or statistical average. Thus, enhancement that ensured such an average was reached would be different from enhancement aimed at going beyond what was currently considered normal. All of this suggests that there is more than one way to draw a moral distinction between therapy and enhancement.

The moral line could be established so that only the prevention of certain or near-certain probability of genetic disease is considered "therapy," while anything beyond that is considered "enhancement." Alternatively, it could be drawn such that all edits limited to leveling up to "normal" genetic health prospects would be considered therapy and anything beyond that enhancement. However, if "normalcy" is defined statistically, then such "normality" could, of course, be pushed forward by such interventions if they were to become a widespread practice and affect the average. Additionally, a moral line could be drawn between improvements of distinctly "human capacities" and interventions that seek to go beyond these.

If "enhancement" can refer to anything from lowering the odds for contracting disease to experiments aimed at transcending the boundaries of what it means to be human, then it is clear that it cannot be very action-guiding. Still, many of the more serious moral concerns about germline editing all seem to cluster around the far end of enhancement.

The third distinction between "the laboratory" and "the clinic," at first glance, seems to helpfully draw a morally significant line between research and controversial applications in the clinic. It seems straightforward: We distinguish between germline research in the context of science and germlines edited for the purpose of being transferred to a uterus. For instance, the German *Act for Protection of Embryos* (1990) clearly makes any artificial alteration to the human germline not only illegal but also punishable, while allowing for certain exceptions, including "an artificial alteration of the genetic information of a germ cell situated outside the body, if any use of it for fertilization has been ruled out" (Sect. 4, § 5). Here, germline alterations are possible if it is both "outside the body" (i.e., "in the laboratory") and it cannot be used for fertilization; that is, its alterations will also "stay in the laboratory" and will not be passed on. It thus seems that there is a clear line to be drawn between altered germ cells that are transferred to a uterus, or in other ways develop into a person, and those that are not. In this respect, the distinction could be action-guiding and make moral sense in that it would effectively prevent any harmful consequences that could result from individuals being born with an edited germline.

The problem is that the middle ground between these two outcomes can be established in different ways. Thus, even if we have, at one end, basic research in the lab, and clinical applications at the other end, we have preclinical studies, clinical studies, and innovative methods (before a clinical phase 3 study has been conducted) between those two poles. Furthermore, research can be conducted with the aim of increasing knowledge (about genetic development) or developing treatment. In any case, any developed medical gene therapy will have been preceded by genetic research, and to know that it is sufficiently safe, it would have needed to pass through various stages of medical research, including basic, preclinical, translational, and clinical research. For instance, Birnbacher (2018, p. 56), speculates that perhaps the study on non-viable embryos done in China in 2015 (Liang et al., 2015), which caused significant controversy on the grounds that it seemed to accelerate germline gene editing, might not actually have been illegal under German law (*Act for Protection of Embryos*, 1990), even though it is considered to be particularly strict. Here, one could argue that if one is concerned about clinical applications of germline gene editing, then any step towards this end is also a reason for concern. From this perspective, it would make sense to draw the line before it is applied to actual embryos, viable or not. Others have expressed a concern that drawing too sharp a line between basic research into germline gene editing and clinical research might have negative effects on other kinds of genetic research, including research on early human development and somatic gene therapy (Birnbacher, 2018, p. 56). Others have pointed out that the line between research aimed at therapy and research aimed at knowledge is far from clear, thus blurring the boundary between research and clinical innovation (Neuhaus, 2018).

As we have seen above, part of the moral appeal of the laboratory/clinic distinction, or a distinction between research and application, is that it implies the existence of a "safe" space where only research is conducted and no moral concerns arise. However, this would only work if research was limited to basic research and models, and never aspired to more knowledge than could be achieved in this way. In essence, any appeal to the research/application distinction seems largely to appeal for more time: It makes sense as a temporal boundary— we must not move to the clinic too quickly, before and until it is better known, safer, and so forth. In that sense, more research could simply provide the next step towards germline editing in the clinic, avoiding the risks and public backlash by insisting on maintaining the boundary while more clarity is obtained. However, that would only hold as long as the boundary is never crossed. Instead, most advocates for a division between germline editing in the laboratory and the clinic seem more inclined towards a temporary division at this point, such that what we can currently do morally remains on this side of the laboratory/clinic boundary. Often the rationale for this is that it is not sufficiently safe and that we do not yet have public consensus for germline editing as a practice. Therefore, it makes sense not to edit the germline—for now—and instead focus on basic research to, on the one hand, make it safe and learn more, and on the other, gain public trust and reach some societal consensus about what we ought to do. This makes sense, but it avoids the question of where the proper moral line should be drawn, as opposed to where the precautionary line should be under current circumstances. If the line is temporary, it is hard to see how it can both be upheld and allow for the kind of research necessary to learn what is safe and what is not. Without clinical trials and follow-up studies over multiple generations, we will not know what is possible and what the possible side effects are.

In a way, it is hard not to view the laboratory/clinic distinction as little more than a sensible notion that we ought not to proceed to the next step until we have passed the preceding one successfully. Occasionally, it is also suggested that there is no point in discussing the moral aspects of various practices until we know what is medically and scientifically possible.

Of the three distinctions, it is predominantly the first two, between somatic and germline gene editing, and between therapy and enhancement, that have been proposed as candidate moral boundaries and a barrier against slippery slopes (see, e.g., Evans, 2020). If the slippery slope is the main driver of moral concern, then both of these seem to offer some kind of protection against designer babies and genetic injustice, while allowing for somatic therapy and/or germline edits to prevent disease. The laboratory/clinic distinction is driven more by a concern about risk: As long as germline editing is limited to research, no one will come to harm while knowledge could still be pursued. However, it does not provide any clear moral guidance that could be applied, should germline gene editing be deemed sufficiently safe to move out of the laboratory and into the clinic.

2.4   "No One Knows What the Rules Are"

A number of aspects thus make the moral boundaries of human germline gene editing unclear. First, most of the bioethical arguments (and legislation) regarding gene technology predates CRISPR and gene edits and were primarily articulated with recombinant DNA and cloning in mind, rather than edits of the germline. The same seems to hold for regulation; Boggio et al. (2021, p. 221) found that most legal frameworks predated the CRISPR breakthrough. The earlier debate treated germline interventions merely as a theoretical possibility. Thus, some believe that public opinion will change in much the same way that it did with IVF and "test tube babies," which won public support once the benefits were obvious. Others view the basic moral sentiments of the Oviedo Convention as still holding and perfectly relevant with regard to the newest forms of gene editing. Notably, Emmanuelle Charpentier, one of the key scientists behind the CRISPR-Cas9 breakthrough, has expressed her general support for the Oviedo Convention (Bosley et al., 2015). In one sense, the current debate follows the same lines as the earlier one. Already in 2006, Resnik and Vorhaus (2006, p. e2) observed that the debate was largely divided between "those who think that genetic modification should proceed under some type of regulatory scheme, and those who think that the best solution is to ban genetic modification entirely."

The possible addition is that the consensus seems to be in favor of a moratorium for now, until we have a sufficient understanding of the medical, social, economic, political, and biological consequences and we can sufficiently regulate and oversee its application. Even if the arguments are largely similar, it is far from clear to what extent they apply equally to the CRISPR case and whether there might be new arguments not yet posed.[17] However, what such a moratorium entails would again depend on how terms are defined and on what grounds lines are drawn. In the current legal landscape, it is for example not always clear what falls into the category of permissible research and what does not in national regulation (Boggio et al., 2021).

Yet, even if the technology and the epistemic gaps are significant, the interests (including financial ones), stakes, and rapid development (not least with recent events in mind) add a sense of urgency to the ethical aspects: that is, before we have had time to analyze and discuss its implications properly (Mariscal & Petropanagos, 2016). There is a sense that reliable rules are absent as moral uncertainty abounds. Some even seem to imply that urgent moral issues simply arise from the fact that there are no clear moral standards (professional ethics rules) or legislation to follow—and that oversight and regulation are critical. Thus, on the one hand, the debate seems very familiar and far from new, while on the other, "no one knows what the rules are" and addressing the relevant ethical concerns is imperative.

---

[17] Most comparisons in the ethical debate are between germline edits and somatic edits on the one hand, and germline edits and PDT (prediagnostic therapy with selective abortion) on the other. However, in the ethical case, we also need to consider to what degree arguments originally posed with cloning and recombinant DNA in mind apply to CRISPR: Is there a moral difference between transgenic interventions and edits to existing genes?

Positions on the Germline Boundary: Stop, Wait, or Go?

3

Three positions dominate the debate over the possibility of editing the human germline: a categorical position against germline editing, a cautious intermediate position calling for a moratorium, and a more liberal position stressing the benefits and urging research to continue and progress when safe.[1] We could divide these in the following way:

1. *A categorical ban*: Ban all human germline editing.
2. *A moratorium*: Introduce and uphold a moratorium on germline editing in the clinic until relevant issues of safety and ethics have been sufficiently addressed.

---

[1] There seems to be broad agreement that there are, roughly speaking, three dominant positions. However, how these are divided and named differ. Ormond et al. (2017, p. 169) divide the dominant positions into "restrictive," "intermediate," and "permissive." Others talk about red, green, and/or yellow lights (e.g., Peters, 2017; Kaiser, 2017). Peters, however, identifies yellow as "proceed with caution" and green as "proceed with speed." He also identifies yellow with the precautionary principle, which is odd, given that it would most likely speak against germline edits under the current levels of risk and uncertainty. De Lecuona et al. (2017) describe various positions ranging from "demanding a moratorium that would paralyze this kind of research to authorizing certain uses of gene editing in humans, passing through a gradualist paradigm." (p. 673 f.). The outlier here is Evitt et al. (2015), who suggest that there are four dominant regulatory approaches: "[i]nternational ban, temporary moratorium, regulation, and laissez-faire" (p. 26). This is in line with the earlier debate on regulation that predates CRISPR. Resnik and Vorhaus (2006) divide the then dominant positions on regulation into the following three: no legislation (laissez-faire); proceed "under some type of regulatory scheme"; or ban genetic modification entirely (p. 1). It is hard to see anyone advocating no regulation in the current debate.

© The Author(s) 2025
M. Hayenhjelm and C. Nordlund, *The Risks and Ethics of Human Gene Editing*,
Technikzukünfte, Wissenschaft und Gesellschaft / Futures of Technology, Science
and Society, https://doi.org/10.1007/978-3-658-46979-5_3

3. *Proceed when safe*: Aim to proceed with both research and clinical applications once sufficiently safe from a medical perspective.[2]

The first position advocates a categorical ban on germline editing largely based on the grounds of ethics and risk. The ethical considerations and the risks involved are seen as something not likely to ever be overcome. The second position advocates for a more partial or temporary ban in the form of a self-imposed moratorium within the scientific community, modeled on the Asilomar moratorium on recombinant DNA from the 1970s. This would allow for basic research to proceed and the ethical aspects to be widely debated before any final moral conclusion can be drawn either way. Here, the morality of germline editing is undecided. Until we know more and the technology is safer, and until there is broad consensus that this is the correct path forward, we ought to wait before proceeding. The third is largely optimistic about the technology's potential and the good it could achieve. The only reason not to proceed is safety. As soon as the technology is sufficiently safe, there is no principled reason not to proceed—unless a new, even better, technology would replace it.

The categorical position remained dominant for almost 30 years (Krimsky, 2015, p. 237) and still dominates legislation around the world (cf. Council of Europe, 1997; UNESCO, 1997; the German *Act for Protection of Embryos*, 1990). Such a position, however, has fewer proponents among the more recent commenters on CRISPR (*pace* Lanphier et al., 2015) in contrast to earlier biotechnologies, such as cloning and recombinant DNA. By contrast, the moratorium position, or more broadly, a "wait until safe" position in combination with some notion of requirements, regulations and/or restrictions, seems to be dominant

---

[2] Of course, this is not the only way in which we could divide the various positions. However, the tension is clear between those who advocate a ban and those who see possible ways forward (under appropriate oversight and regulation and when sufficiently safe). Resnik and Vorhaus made the following point about the debate on gene editing in 2006: "Most of the current debate is between those who think that genetic modification should proceed under some type of regulatory scheme, and those who think that the best solution is to ban genetic modification entirely. Those who favor regulation see nothing inherently wrong with genetic modification: the morality of the genetic modification depends on an adequate understanding and evaluation of the medical, social, economic, political, and biological consequences. Society should take appropriate steps to control genetic modification in order to maximize its benefits and minimize its harms" (Resnik & Vorhaus, 2006, p. e2). The main difference here seems to be that instead of debating the moral permissibility of hypothetical human germline gene edits, as categorically impermissible or permissible when sufficiently safe, the advent of recent events have prompted a third position: to, in any case, ensure that we do nothing hastily, in order to avoid things going wrong or backfiring by acting too quickly, or before we have agreed on its safety and moral acceptability.

within the scientific community (Baltimore et al., 2015). Both these positions advocate a ban on germline editing, at least for clinical research and application. The former is a permanent ban, the latter one that could be lifted or revisited later. The third position is largely optimistic, either because medical and ethical reasons are thought to weigh in favor of germline gene editing, or because it is deemed to be part of an inevitable development. Either way, the ethical issues about germline gene editing are more about how and when to make use of it to ensure safety, not whether or not we should make use of it at all. This broad category includes those who view germline editing as a somewhat deterministic given that needs to be sufficiently regulated and researched to make it safe (Evitt et al., 2015; Brokowski & Adli, 2018) and those who largely see the benefits as significant enough for further research, development, and hopefully application (Gyngell et al., 2017; Savulescu & Gyngell, 2015), or as a potential tool for enhancement and maintaining population health (Powell, 2015).

Thus, these three positions should be regarded as points along a continuum. Metaphorically, the first position involves locking the door and throwing away the key; the second, locking the door but keeping the key; and the third, closing the door without locking it.

3.1 A Categorical Ban

The *categorical ban on germline editing* is largely based on the somatic/germline distinction above: it would impose a ban on all human germline editing, typically in both research and the clinic, but not on somatic gene therapy (see, e.g., Norman, 1983). For a long time, the dominant view was that germline editing was morally off-limits (Krimsky, 2015, p. 238). This has also been the view expressed in public documents such as the Council of Europe's Oviedo Convention (1997) and UNESCO's Universal Declaration on the Human Genome and Human Rights issued in the same year. The German *Act for Protection of Embryos* (1990) takes a similar stand. The position has been very influential, particularly as a reaction to scientific racism, the eugenics programs of the Nazis, and the commitment to never again repeat that history. In fact, eugenics, we might recall, was defined as "the self-direction of human development" during the first half of the twentieth century.

In Europe, Article 13 of the Oviedo Convention (Council of Europe, 1997) bans any intervention in the human germline in embryos or germ cells. It states, "Interventions seeking to modify the human genome may only be undertaken for preventive, diagnostic or therapeutic purposes and only if its aim is not to introduce any modification in the genome of any descendants." (Council of Europe, 1997, Article 13). The rationale behind this boundary was based on concerns about human dignity and human rights.

Another document from the same year as the Oviedo Convention is the Universal Declaration on the Human Genome and Human Rights issued by UNESCO. It states, "The human genome underlies the fundamental unity of all members of the human family, as well as the recognition of their inherent dignity and diversity. In a symbolic sense, it is the heritage of humanity" (Universal Declaration on the Human Genome and Human Rights, 11 November 1997, Part A, Article 1).

Sugarman comments, "After all, deliberately manipulating the human germline has generally been viewed as unacceptable, and it is prohibited in many parts of the world" (Sugarman, 2015, p. 1). Eric S. Lander, former Director of the Whitehead Institute's Center for Genome Research and Founding Director of the Broad Institute of MIT and Harvard, has supported a ban on modifying the human germline, based on an argument that humanity should remain on this side of the boundary between "the world of the born" and "the world of the made." He is concerned that if we cross the threshold and begin to view humanity as a product of manufacture rather than one of nature, we will never return (cited in Sagoff, 2005, p. 67).

Much of the current legislation has its roots in the older bioethical debates and was formed in response to cloning and recombinant DNA. In most countries, germline editing is also illegal (Lander et al., 2019; Simonstein, 2019; Braun et al., 2018, p. 4 f.; and Rixen, 2018 for international legal comparison).[3] However, this position has weakened over time. In a statement by the European Group on Ethics in Science and New Technologies (EGE) under the European Council (EGE, 2016), they reaffirm the boundary against germline editing, but more in the form of a moratorium than a categorical ban, and leave the broader issue open, depending on whether both safety and precision, as well as public consensus, could be achieved. They observe the following:

> Germline gene modification is still in its infancy and there are many significant technical hurdles to be overcome before clinical applications become a viable reality. The

---

[3] See, e.g., German *Act for Protection of Embryos* (Embryonenschutzgesetz—ESchG) 1990, Article 5, para. 1, ESchG9, in Braun et al. (2018), p. 4. Note: research and mtDNA transfer is permitted in the UK on a case-by-case basis.

question of whether, if ever, germline engineering of human embryos would be precise enough to guarantee a successful outcome and would be acceptable to the public is still an open one. (EGE, 2016)

Instead, they turn the focus to the issue of germline editing *research*, rather than clinical application:

> The more pressing question for policy makers at this moment is whether germline genome editing technology research should be suspended, under which conditions it could proceed, and in this respect varying views have been articulated. The EGE is of the view that this question warrants careful consideration, given the profound potential consequences of this research for humanity. (EGE, 2016)

In all, the broader conversation seems to have moved on from talk of a ban, prohibition, and a red line, to that of a moratorium and ethical and technical challenges to resolve, leaving the matter open for debate.

3.2   A Call for a Moratorium

A *moratorium* on germline editing involves a voluntary self-imposed temporary "ban" on germline editing initiated by the scientific community.[4] Such a moratorium need not prohibit germline research in a preclinical sense, but could limit clinical research and application only—in fact, the reference to a moratorium on germline editing is used in both a narrow sense (against clinical application only) and a broader sense (against both preclinical research on the germline as well as clinical applications).

A moratorium would serve as a ban that could ultimately be lifted, should it at that time be thought to be sufficiently safe and medically and ethically justified. Only once it is considered safe and ethically sound should germline editing

---

[4] Guttinger (2018, p. 1084) argues that a moratorium is essentially both a temporary and partial ban. "The ban is partial because it still allows researchers to edit the genomes of humans (if somatic cells are targeted) and because it still allows for germline editing in non-human organisms. It is temporary because it can be revised should research demonstrate it to be sufficiently safe. The ban is also temporary as the researchers suggest that it could be revised at some point, depending on the results of further research into the safety and efficacy issues that surround the technology. This (potentially) temporary nature of the ban is crucial as it ensures that the further development/use of the technology is still an option, meaning the ban can still be part of a 'way forward'" (Guttinger, 2018, p. 1084).

proceed. This means that there is a self-imposed ban for now, but the final question about whether to bring germline editing to the clinic or not remains open. This is essentially the position advocated by Lanphier et al. (2015), the European Group on Ethics in Science and New Technologies (EGE, 2016), Lander et al. (2019), Mertes & Pennings (2015), Wolinetz & Collins (2019), and others (see Brokowski, 2018 for overview). The broader view, that it is currently not safe and that we currently ought not to edit the germline, is—as we shall see (Sect. 3.4)—the majority position (Brokowski, 2018). In their consensus statement, the Organizing Committee for the International Summit on Human Gene Editing wrote the following:

> It would be irresponsible to proceed with any clinical use of germline editing unless and until (i) the relevant safety and efficacy issues have been resolved, based on appropriate understanding and balancing of risks, potential benefits, and alternatives, and (ii) there is broad societal consensus about the appropriateness of the proposed application. Moreover, any clinical use should proceed only under appropriate regulatory oversight. At present, these criteria have not been met for any proposed clinical use: the safety issues have not yet been adequately explored; the cases of most compelling benefit are limited; and many nations have legislative or regulatory bans on germline modification. However, as scientific knowledge advances and societal views evolve, the clinical use of germline editing should be revisited on a regular basis. (Thrasher et al. 2016)

A raw model for this position was the call for a moratorium on recombinant DNA experimentation that was put forward after a conference in Asilomar in 1975. As mentioned above, a similar meeting on CRISPR was held in Napa Valley in 2015. Following the Napa meeting, two influential statement pieces in *Nature* and *Science* (Baltimore et al., 2015; Lanphier et al., 2015) sparked the conversation about a moratorium on germline editing. However, there were some subtle differences between the two papers. The titles provide a clue in this regard: Baltimore et al. (2015) called for "a prudent path forward," while Lanphier et al. (2015) simply requested to "not edit the human germline." Crucially, there is a difference when it comes to how research on germline gene editing is viewed. Where Lanphier et al. assume a stronger position on a moratorium on germline gene editing, including germline gene research, Baltimore et al. want to see a moratorium on germline editing in the clinic, while crucial germline research is pursued.

The prudent path forward, advocated by Baltimore et al., would prohibit all clinical applications of germline editing while continuing research and building trust. Many have noted the parallels between this position and the Asilomar Conference: scientists regulating themselves through voluntary restrictions to ensure that all potential risks are contained in the research setting and the research is made public. Baltimore et al. (2015) raise concerns about unintended outcomes and epistemic shortcomings. They suggest that more research is needed to understand and manage the risks associated with the technique. Any clinical application must wait until more details are known. "At present, the potential safety and efficacy issues arising from the technology must be thoroughly investigated and understood before any attempts at human engineering are sanctioned, if ever, for clinical testing" (Baltimore et al., 2015, p. 37). Mertes and Pennings (2015) hold a similar position. They support "a moratorium on any clinical applications of germline editing, while permitting the genetic modification of human embryos for research purposes, as also suggested by Baltimore et al. (2015). … such research protocols would have to obtain the approval of ethical committees, who would essentially be the gatekeepers." (p. 52) Thus, the notion of a moratorium in this regard is one that leans heavily on the research/application distinction discussed in the previous chapter (Sect. 2.2.3): We should not edit the germline in the clinic, but we should pursue basic research to improve our knowledge on the matter.

By contrast, the position advocated by Lanphier et al. (2015) is more restrictive. Rather than leaning towards the research/application distinction, their position tends more towards the somatic/germline distinction. The fear is that, should we begin to explore germline gene editing without it being sufficiently safe and without broad public support, it could create an eventual backlash against human gene editing as a whole. The concern is that, aside from the moral and safety issues, very promising somatic gene therapy treatments would come to a halt. According to them, there are a number of reasons to be concerned about germline gene editing, including safety issues such as mosaicism, off-target risks, and the fact that side effects may only appear after several years, as well as the risk for a slippery slope towards human enhancement and the fact that, in some cases, some good alternatives are available. However, there is also this concern that premature clinical applications before safety and ethical issues have been properly addressed could backfire and, thus, jeopardize promising lifesaving somatic research and application.

A moratorium strategy, if modeled on the Asilomar example, seeks to achieve two things, according to Guttinger (2018): to limit risk of harm in the context of use while allowing for safe and contained research. The core of this strategy is a two-step process. The first step is to to limit risk of harm by separating the research context from the use context and to ensure that risks are limited

to the research. The second step is to use the safe space for research created
to further study the technology and expand knowledge. This means, Guttinger
argues, "that in order to be successful the Asilomar approach has to fulfil two
conditions, namely (1) that the containment strategy actually works and (2) that
the safe space that the containment creates allows researchers to do the right
kind of experiments, i.e. experiments that can assess the potential of modified
microbes/DNA to create harm." (Guttinger, 2018, p. 1088).

Guttinger (2018) argues that, although a moratorium on germline editing could
successfully contain risk from clinical applications, it cannot in the meanwhile
acquire the level of knowledge about risk to make a different decision without
allowing the transferal of edited embryos to a uterus. We could study off-target
risks in basic research (Guttinger, 2016; see also Guttinger 2020), but the same
cannot be said about the study of other risks. In particular, he argues that the safe
space does not suffice to study full range of effects on the organism since these
may be systemic and could "affect any stage of the life cycle of the organism." To
study systemic and long-term effects, "researchers would have to test all stages
of the ongoing life cycle, which ultimately means that modified embryos would
have to be transferred and allowed to fully develop into adult human beings"
(Guttinger, 2018, p. 1091). To do this would however violate the requirements of
the first step: to contain risks to the research context. As Guttinger points out:
"Such a course of action clearly violates the containment that forms the essence
of the two-step process" (Guttinger, 2018, p. 1091).

In other words, model organisms, research on human embryos limited to the
14-day rule, and animal testing can only provide limited knowledge about the
actual effects of germline gene editing. In the end, we will need to study these
effects on persons born with such edits to know their long-term effects and potential risks. Guttinger writes: "the final test will always be to assess the effects on
the actual organisms of interest" (2018, p. 1092).[5] Cwik (2020a) makes the same
point: "No matter how much progress is made on translation of GGE for clinical
use, the long-term effects of GGE on health and development will not be completely known until there is a sufficient sample of individuals born from edited
embryos walking around in the world." A similar concern was, in fact, raised by

---

[5] "The research that needs to be done to address the uncertainties cannot be done in a safe
space, as the two conditions (creating a contained space and doing research to assess the dangers of the technology) clash with each other. The release of the modified human embryos
will have to be part and parcel of the safety assessment, because the whole life cycle of the
organism will have to be assessed to get an insight into the potential dangers (and benefits)
each modification carries for the organism as a whole" (Guttinger, 2018, p. 1093).

Lappé (1991, p. 625) in an early paper on germline modifications (before the rise of CRISPR).

For this reason, according to Guttinger (2018), the Asilomar strategy will not work. Even if research can be conducted in a safe space without venturing into clinical applications, this research will not be enough to reliably conclude it is safe before being tested on actual individuals born with such edits. The "soothing promises of the Asilomar ban—'There is a safe and responsible way of doing more research on new molecular tools'—falls apart in the CRISPR-Cas9 case," he writes (p. 1093).[6]

Others have, by contrast, sought to provide ways to ensure this kind of knowledge by means of human modeling and multigenerational animal studies. Evitt et al. (2015), in their regulatory framework, address the same problem from a different angle. Should proposed germline research pass through the initial studies, it must also be "validated in multigenerational animal models of increasing complexity (e.g., rat, pig, dog, etc.) before consideration for human clinical trials" (Evitt et al., 2015, p. 27). However, this in itself is not sufficient, according to them. In order for the risk–benefit balance to allow for germline gene editing, reversal must be possible: "Any CGET [CRISPR germline editing therapy] should include a companion reversal mechanism ... Obviously, significant research is needed before such reversal mechanisms are made a reality" (Evitt et al., 2015, p. 26).

Hurlbut raises a different concern about the Asilomar strategy. Should a moratorium allow for germline research, this could preclude the moral decision. Thus, critical of Baltimore et al.'s piece in *Science*, and their "prudent path forward," he argues that "prudent restraint ought to extend to scientific search agendas and not merely to eventual applications" (Hurlbut, 2015, p. 13). He points to the differences in the two high-profile statements, in *Science* and *Nature*, respectively. While Baltimore et al. "supported increased research to evaluate the safety and efficiency of germ-line applications," the parallel statement by Lanphier et al. in *Nature* called for "prohibiting both clinical applications of these technologies and the forms of research that would make such applications possible" (Hurlbut, 2015, p. 13). What Hurlbut finds problematic in the Baltimore statement is that it is limiting the ethical issues only to applications and thus "profoundly

---

[6] Guttinger (2020, p. 62 ff.) expands upon the above ideas. Whereas off-target risks could be studied successfully without imposing risk, there are limits to what we can learn about unintended on-target risks, especially when considering polygenetic diseases and the extended knowledge about the contextual influences on genes. He argues that whereas a temporary ban may be justified for rare monogenetic diseases, a permanent ban may be warranted for polygenetic diseases (Guttinger, 2020, p. 69).

constrains the opportunities for collective ethical judgment." He reasons as follows: "Judgments that are confined to clinical applications alone are reduced to answering a yes or no question, a choice between prohibition and acquiescence to an already established technological trajectory" (Hurlbut, 2015, p. 13). This is to sell our ethical responsibility short, according to him: "Responsibility requires that our aspirations and values inform trajectories of innovation themselves, and not merely their eventual applications." (Hurlbut, 2015, p. 13).

The moratorium position is a temporary halt, and in a sense, it is also a temporary conclusion. It is not a final word on the ethics of germline editing but is meant to pave the way for such a conclusion eventually. Its immediate benefit would, of course, be that, while more information is gathered, there will be no clinical applications that could prematurely cause harm. Its other, more indirect, benefit is that it could provide time for reflection, debate, and collection of more knowledge to enable a more informed conclusion at a later stage. Thus, as Hurlbut points out, if such a moratorium is to provide space for a moral assessment, it cannot preclude the eventual conclusion. Hurlbut repeats a similar concern about the NASEM (2018) report (Angrist et al., 2020). Essentially, according to Hurlbut, this would be to put the science cart before the ethics horse. There is tension here: Should the temporary ban be limited to application and not research, it may make it more difficult later on to insist on a categorical ban on ethical grounds. Conversely, should the temporary ban include research, then it might not be possible to make a sufficiently informed decision on the grounds of risk, or to provide a safe translational pathway for the technology after such a decision was made.

3.3   Proceed with Caution

In addition to advocating a ban and moratorium respectively, there is also a more liberal and optimistic position. This position is largely in favor of proceeding with the new technology and applying germline gene editing in the clinic, on the condition of it being safe and the intended uses being justified, among other things. It is marked by distancing itself from more categorical positions rather than by advocating that we proceed with germline editing now. It still agrees with the general consensus that it is currently not sufficiently safe nor efficient. In practice, this position would still strongly advise against germline editing under the current circumstances, but the focus is on the expected benefits. The moral question here is less about the permissibility of germline editing as a unified category and more about under which conditions, moral and scientific, it would or would not be responsible to proceed. Rather than taking the ethical and safety concerns as reasons to oppose germline editing, they are regarded more as obstacles to be overcome. For instance, NASEM reasons as follows, in their 2017 report:

> Heritable germline genome-editing trials must be approached with caution, but caution does not mean they must be prohibited. If the technical challenges are overcome and potential benefits are reasonable in light of the risks, clinical trials could be initiated to only the most compelling circumstances and subject to a comprehensive oversight framework that would protect the research subjects and their descendants; and have sufficient safeguards in place to protect against inappropriate expansion of uses that are less compelling or less well understood. (NASEM, 2017, p. 189)

Here, the NASEM report moves away from a ban, without precluding any moral conclusions either way. The focus, though, is shifted towards ways that ensure a future path forward could be sufficiently safe and motivated. A second report published by the National Academy of Medicine and the National Academy of the Sciences in the U.S. together with the Royal Society in the UK (2020) had a more detailed translational pathway presenting various conditions to be met. However, the deeper moral questions were largely left unanswered and delegated to individual countries and public consensus (see Angrist et al., 2020 for reactions to this report). The Nuffield Council's second report (2018) was similarly noted for its move away from a categorical stance.

Similarly, Daley et al. (2019) argued that, even though He Jiankui's experiment was rightfully condemned, it would be "unwise" to call for a moratorium or ban on germline research (Daley et al., 2019, p. 1). Instead, they argue that there has been both scientific and ethical progress, including increased precision and efficacy, between 2015 and 2018. This somewhat surprising claim is substantiated by the slight shift in recommendations in "the 60-plus groups that have reported on the scientific and ethical landscape of genome editing." It is backed up in particular by the fact that some of these groups have alluded to the possibility of future permissibility of germline gene editing, subject to "achievement of greater scientific understanding and broader societal acceptance of specific clinical uses" (Daley et al., 2019, p. 2). However, some of these conditions are understood as surmountable obstacles, by developed standards for safe translational pathways on the one hand, and broad societal support and regulation on a national level on the other. They note, "The prospect of genome editing to prevent genetic disease, if determined to be safe, enjoys wide-spread public support, as shown by published opinion polls and engagement activities" (Daley et al., 2019, p. 3). In other words, the authors seem to take the various reports' calls for more safety and public engagement, together with public support for certain kinds of germline editing, as a somewhat sufficient answer to the moral issues raised.

Others echo the importance of letting research proceed. Sykora and Caplan (2017a) make the same observation as Daley et al. (2019) above—that there has been significant technical progress in terms of addressing earlier concerns about precision and off-target risks. They argue that the European Council's 20-year-old ban on heritable alterations to the human germline "no longer makes sense from an ethical point of view" on the grounds that the risks that originally warranted such a ban are likely to be resolved as research progresses: "With further improvements, gene-editing technology therefore has the potential for safely modifying the human germline for prophylactic and therapeutic purposes" (2019, p. 1871).

Brokowski and Adli (2018) are concerned that unnecessary bans may stand in the way of making informed decisions about the technology, given that we would need to pursue research to better understand the risks. Unless we can pursue the relevant research, we could neither know whether nor how it could be made sufficiently safe:

> The potential benefits of such revolutionary tools are endless. However, like any powerful tool, there are also associated risks raising moral concerns. To make truly informed decisions about areas of ethical controversy, well-controlled, reproducible experimentation and clinical trials are warranted. Currently, this is difficult because many international laws discourage or ban such research and/or inhibit its funding for certain types of investigation. Thus, widespread data about benefits and risks are unavailable. It is critical, however, for countries to examine their reasoning behind these prohibitions to ensure that they are not simply arising out of fear and without reasonable justification. (Brokowski & Adli, 2018, p. 8)

Thus, in light of the potential benefits, we need to revisit previous bans, so that we do not unnecessarily put obstacles in the way of developing important new technologies with many anticipated benefits.

Savulescu et al. (2015) want more explicitly to shift the burden of proof to those who want to ban research. Thus, rather than advocating further research in order to determine whether the benefits outweigh the risks, they assume as a default that the benefits of research are greater and that risks are manageable.

> To date, the weight of reasons favours continuing gene editing research, rather than banning it. Those who believe that gene editing research should be banned or discouraged need to explain why this technology needs to be treated differently to other technologies and other reproductive practices. Moreover, they need to explain how the expected risks outweigh the expected benefits, and why the risks cannot be appropriately managed with more specific legislation. (Savulescu et al., 2015, p. 478)

According to Savulescu et al., we ought to proceed with both research and clinical applications (Savulescu et al., 2015). It is generally assumed that the expected benefits are very likely to outweigh the risks and costs, once the technology is sufficiently safe (Sykora & Caplan, 2017a; Gyngell et al., 2017; Harris, 2015). Others suggest that there are strong moral arguments to proceed beyond the medical treatment of severe diseases. Harris (2009) argues that we have a moral obligation to enhance if it can be "demonstrated to be safe enough," and that a change to the germline as opposed to the somatic line is merely one of efficiency—it is better to perform the edit once than repeat it for every generation (Harris, 2009, p. 136).

In all of the above examples of this third optimistic position, the focus has been on ethics as a question of risks and benefits, where the risks of pursuing germline editing are presumed to be mangeable, while the benefits are presumed to be substantial. Furthermore, given that the risks can be managed and controlled with various kinds of restrictions and regulations, the only morally relevant aspects left to consider are the benefits and those risks that remain when the relevant restrictions are already in place. Other kinds of non-quantifiable moral concerns are largely ignored. There is thus a certain element of "techno-optimism" here with a greater focus on benefits compared to the other two positions (cf. Braun, 2005).[7] For instance, Sykora and Caplan (2017b, p. 2086) suggest that, given the possible medical benefits of germline gene editing, it would be wrong to let concerns about eugenics block promising research. They write, "general worries about the distant possibility of eugenics should not be permitted to hold hostage emerging research to develop cures for the sick and disabled."

The question is whether such optimism is warranted; in other words, to what degree the moral issues can be captured in terms of balancing risks and benefits in a narrow sense, and to what degree the risks can be sufficiently managed and controlled.

---

[7] We could compare the following description of "techno-optimists," which describes some of these voices fairly accurately in their overall optimism about technological solutions, the controllability of risks, the focus on technologically delivered benefits, and their contempt for more "categorical" objections as irrational or emotional. "Techno-optimists do not necessarily approve of any new technology, but they emphasize technology's potential benefits, welcome enhancement of choice, and believe that society is able, in principle, to calculate and to control potential risks. Since they regard rejecting potential benefits and limiting choice as irrational—as a stance that can be credited to religious or ideological emotions or beliefs—the conflict over biomedicine is often interpreted as a battle between rationality and knowledge on the one hand and ignorance, emotionality, and moral fundamentalism on the other—in short, as a battle between modernity and antimodernity" (Braun, 2005).

3.4   The Ethical Landscape: What is Broadly Agreed Upon?

It is worth stressing that none of the three positions discussed above suggests it is *currently* advisable to apply germline editing in the clinic. In fact, the broad consensus is that it is currently *not* safe to edit the human germline in the clinic (Thrasher et al., 2016; Birnbacher, 2018, p. 55; Braun et al., 2018, p. 8; Cwik, 2020a).[8]

The first position advocates a ban and categorical ethical arguments for not proceeding. Most arguments defending this position appeal to core moral concepts such as human dignity, human rights, or particular concerns such as fear of injustice, eugenics, and so on. The second position views germline editing as potentially greatly beneficial but currently too unsafe, and/or the moral question as not fully resolved. Many advocating a moratorium also see democratic dialogue or stakeholder involvement as crucial to proceed legitimately, and thus the decision to permit germline editing, even if safe, cannot preempt such a conversation. The third position tends to disregard any categorical objections, instead viewing the ethical questions in terms of potential progress and those currently suffering from genetic diseases.

The relevant moral issues informing the third position are largely limited to questions of safety and regulation By contrast, those advocating a ban have largely appealed to categorical moral arguments, while those defending a moratorium are a more varied group appealing to moral and democratic concerns as well as concerns about risk and safety. Between the hardline ban position and the moratorium position, there are a number of stances with a more complex understanding of the ethical issues beyond risk and safety, but falling short of categorical arguments.

In sum, it seems that in the recent debate on CRISPR there has been a slight shift from the categorical positions of the past towards more conditional positions based on precautionary concerns. However, when the Nuffield Council (2018)

---

[8] Cwik (2020a) expands the current point of agreement to four points, albeit with the admission that there are exceptions to this majority view. These four are: "(1) GGE is nowhere near ready for clinical use, and there should be a worldwide moratorium on creating pregnancies from edited embryos for the foreseeable future; (2) research on in vitro editing of human embryos and ex vivo editing of other germline cells (such as gametocytes) should continue, subject to existing ethical guidelines and best practices; (3) translational research should be confined to 'therapeutic' applications of GGE, and should eschew research into uses of GGE for 'enhancement'; and (4) GGE is a matter of serious societal concern, and moving forward with GGE should not happen without input from all of the relevant stakeholders and a transparent and inclusive public discussion." (Cwik, 2020a, p. 127).

released their report on human germline editing and suggested that there were no moral grounds for a categorical objection, but many ethical (and other) conditions that need to be met, this was largely seen in the media as opening the door to "designer babies." Thus, even if the categorical position has not been so prominent in the most recent publications on CRISPR and germline editing, it is still very much an actively held position.

Three Moral Perspectives on the Permissibility of Germline Editing

4

Across the whole spectrum of positions on human germline editing, there seems to be a wide agreement on two issues; (a) *it is currently too unsafe and there is currently too much epistemic uncertainty* for it to be acceptable to apply germline editing in the clinic and promote it on a large scale; and (b) *there are important ethical issues (among others) to address* before we could do so. Powell summarizes the first point very well:

> At the present time, human germline modification is neither safe nor effective, and it is widely legally prohibited. Significant technical and epistemic hurdles would have to be overcome before large-scale human genetic engineering could be realized. (Powell, 2015, p. 670)

This position is shared across the spectrum, from bioliberals to bioconservatives, medical scientists to bioethicists. According to Howard (2017), the most common policy position is "some version of no" to germline editing in the clinic. In a review of 11 expert groups, statements and policy recommendations, Ormond et al. (2017, Table 1) found the majority view is that we currently ought not to proceed with clinical use and that we ought to do so only when safety and efficacy, as well as societal agreement, has been achieved. In short, even though the ethical views on germline editing (in research, in the clinic, and for enhancement) varies greatly, all seem to agree that at the moment we ought not edit the germline and that it is urgent that the epistemic, scientific, democratic, regulatory, and ethical issues are addressed before we head down that road. It has also been noted that the pace of adoption and use of CRISPR has left little time for ethical reflection (Doudna, 2015; Baltimore et al., 2015).

© The Author(s) 2025
M. Hayenhjelm and C. Nordlund, *The Risks and Ethics of Human Gene Editing*,
Technikzukünfte, Wissenschaft und Gesellschaft / Futures of Technology, Science and Society, https://doi.org/10.1007/978-3-658-46979-5_4

Many, if not most, policy and opinion pieces also express the view that along-side technical and scientific issues, there are ethical issues to be solved. The view expressed by the European Academies' Science Advisory Council (EASAC) may, in this respect, be typical:

> It would be irresponsible to proceed unless and until the relevant scientific, ethical and safety and efficacy issues have been resolved and there is broad societal consensus. (EASAC, 2017, p. 28)

In other words, alongside the technical and scientific issues of safety and efficacy, there are also ethical issues that must be addressed, and we proceed with editing the human germline only once it is both safe and morally acceptable. Further-more, there ought to be broad consensus supporting such a move. But even if a majority view is that there are ethical issues to be addressed, agreement is far less forthcoming on what these ethical issues are, what makes them ethical, and what it would take to address them successfully. Moreover, for some, solving the ethical issues and achieving broad societal consensus seems to be more or less the same thing.

Therefore, even though most commenters agree it is currently too unsafe to proceed with germline editing, and that there are important ethical aspects to con-sider, views on what these ethical aspects consist in, what is required to address them, and what makes an issue "ethical" in the first place differ significantly between various writers and texts. This situation is not new. Braun (2005) writes the following about ethics and ethical experts entering the political arena: "in the context of biomedicine, people may mean different things when they argue that policies should be informed by ethical considerations. In such controversies, not only values and principles, but also the very meaning of 'ethics' and its proper role in politics are at stake." (Braun, 2005, p. 42).

The three positions on the germline—that of a categorical ban, a moratorium, or a call to proceed when safe—reflect very different perspectives on the ethical aspects. We could refer to these as the *Technical View,* the *Democratic View,* and the *Moral View.* All three views are, in a sense, moral perspectives: they are about values and priorities, and what constitutes doing the right thing. Thus, depending on the perspective, we get vastly different reasons about what ought to be done, what would be good if it were done, and what never ought to be done. In particular, the position that we ought not to edit the human germline (at present), takes on very different meanings depending on the perspective.

4.1   The Technical View

The Technical View is a reductionist perspective of sorts and appears to be the dominant perspective among scientists. This view sees ethical questions as primarily questions about risks of harm—we must not proceed with germline interventions until we know that they are safe, medically motivated, and sufficiently efficient. The main concerns, from this perspective, are off-target risks and unexpected side effects of the technology itself—problems that are best solved with more research, a sound and safe research practice, and appropriate regulation, as well as a possible temporary moratorium on premature clinical application before it is sufficiently safe. Strictly speaking, right and wrong are determined by technical success. Thus, it is wrong to introduce technology that does not work or could result in unexpected side effects, but it is also wrong to postpone technological development that could offer more efficient ways of doing things, or expand upon what can be done (with some good in mind). Sykora and Caplan (2017a, p. 1871), for instance, question the ban on inheritable human germline interventions of the Oviedo Convention, since it, according to them, "no longer makes sense from an ethical point of view." They argue:

> The main rationale was that classical genetic engineering technologies in humans were inefficient and imprecise. The risks were simply too great. But the risk assessment was based on recombinant DNA technology, which is much less precise than the new genome editing technologies—with the flagship CRISPR/Cas9 system—that are much more efficient and precise. (Sykora & Caplan, 2017a, 1871)

Others, of course, take a more cautious view of the risks. The point here is that from a technical perspective, the only ethical issues are those of safety, precision, and efficacy. If germline editing is sufficiently safe, there are no further moral issues to be addressed. Many are generally framing the moral issues on gene editing in this way. Consider the following statement by Qiu regarding the 2015 Napa and Hinxton meetings on CRISPR-Cas9:

> Although genome editing technology has the advantage of being simple, easy, fast and inexpensive, its problems include lower targeting efficiency and high off-targeting rate. It is neither possible nor permissible to apply this technology to humans as long as these two problems are not overcome. But the solution to these two problems can be obtained only by basic and preclinical research. (Qiu, 2016, p. 316)

In light of the above, Qiu mentions one of several conclusions from the Napa meeting (NAS, 2015): "Intensive basic and preclinical research is clearly needed and should proceed, subject to appropriate legal and ethical rules and oversight." Here, ethics is only used to provide the framework for how responsible research ought to be conducted, not as a means of asking the fundamental questions of what research we are morally obliged, permitted, or not permitted to carry out, and on the basis of what fundamental values. It is the degree of *safety* that does the moral work (presuming that research is conducted within the standard ethical framework of responsible research).

The Technical View, although influential, also has its critics, particularly among the proponents of the Democratic View. Although everyone would agree that the technology needs to be safe before use would be ethical, the Technical View holds that safety more or less exhausts the ethical issues. The gist of the criticism against the Technical View is thus that is reduces the ethical issues to something that can be technically addressed rather than hard issues about values and moral obligations. For example, while Jasanoff and Hurlbut (2018) admit that "[i]f the ethical stakes of human germline genome editing are limited to questions of physical safety, for example, then the technical evaluation of particular bio-logical endpoints (for instance, off-target effects) might offer sufficient answers" (Jasanoff & Hurlbut, 2018, p. 437). According to them, the ethical stakes are much larger than that and include "the central question of how to care for and value human life, individually, societally and in relation to other forms of life on Earth." (Jasanoff & Hurlbut, 2018, p. 437) In short, the Technical View does not seem to cover or probe deeply enough to fully address the moral issues. Further-more, it does not take into account the fact that implementing a technology such as gene editing might affect not only the life and health of individuals, but also society at large, in a fundamental and perhaps problematic way.

4.2   The Democratic View

The Democratic View stresses that ethical concerns are value considerations and thus fall outside the scope of science and technology. Instead, such concerns call for consultation, public dialogue, and stakeholder involvement that are broad and democratic (Jasanoff et al., 2015). The key idea is that we must not let research agendas and scientific and technological trajectories determine what kind of society we want to have (Hurlbut, 2015; Sarewitz, 2015). Instead, science and technology—especially the publicly funded kind—ought to be in the ser-vice of democracy and promote the sort of society we want. This view thus challenges the classic model of "responsible self-regulation" among scientists, which was propagated at the conference on recombinant DNA in Asilomar in

1975, and later on at similar meetings on CRISPR. Hurlbut is highly critical of the implicit idea of the Asilomar, "that those who are in a position to make the technological future are also the most competent to declare what possible futures warrant public attention." This, he argues, "gets democracy wrong" and "renders society and its institutions inevitably and perpetually reactive." (Hurlbut, 2015, p. 12). Instead, he argues, "[i]t is our technologies that should be subject to democratically articulated imaginations of the futures we want, not the opposite." According to him "Science and technology often claim to be servants of society; they should take that promise seriously. Imagining what is right and appropriate for our world—and what threatens its moral foundations—is a task for democracy, not for science." (Hurlbut, 2015, p. 12).

According to the Democratic View, ethical matters cannot be solved by science alone and are, in fact, value issues that we must address by way of striving for a broad consensus.

Science and technology have social impact and ought to be guided by the democratically decided ends. However, at the core of the Democratic View, there is also a stronger claim: that to address ethical issues of societal impact is primarily to have such conversations aiming for a broad consensus. In other words, the Democratic View, takes ethical issues from scientists, arguing that they are matters of value, and hands them to the demos. The calls for various forms of conversations as a means to resolve the ethical issues is ubiquitous in the CRISPR debate (Juengst, 2017; Dabrock, 2018). However, the nature of such conversations differ considerably across the various proposals: from merely relaying information to the public (about the technology and its risks and benefits) or from the public (about their values), to explicit attempts to place ethical decision-making in the hands of those directly affected, namely "all of us" as members of the human race (Baylis 2019). Here, the Democratic View encompasses such conversational practices as the preferred means to address moral issues and broadly regards ethical issues primarily as political and democratic issues.

There is no sharp boundary between the Technical and the Democratic views. Most writers seem to frame the ethical issues as a combination of risk issues to be scientifically addressed *and* value considerations to be discussed in democratic dialogue. The difference between the two views is thus largely one of weight and scope. However, from the vantage point of the former, it is ultimately about making sure the technology is safe and morally accepted. From that of the latter, scientific and medical progress cannot determine what kind of society we want technology to promote, as it is ultimately a democratic issue.

Sometimes the difference in weight and scope is significant. In certain cases, calls for stakeholder involvement and reflection are understood as something that can largely be addressed by means of quantitative and qualitative social science research and communication. Based on a critique of the Asilomar "self-regulation" model, as well as a wish to involve as many groups of people as possible in the debate, scholars in the UK created an online survey early on to capture the public response to the development of CRISPR-Cas9, including what images, ideas, and associations come to mind when people think about the technology. The organizers, Marks and Camporesi (2015), state, "Capturing this aspect of the public response is important as imagined futures can shape the boundaries of the ethical debate and the thinking of policy-makers". Such surveys might, indeed, capture a range of opinions regarding, for instance, ethical problems that differ from the scientists' own. However, although such opinions might be thought provoking for policy makers, they will hardly solve any ethical questions.

Ormond et al. (2017) have proposed another interesting model. Their point of departure is the following: "At this time, given the nature and number of unanswered scientific, ethical, and policy questions, it is inappropriate to perform germline gene editing that culminates in human pregnancy" (Ormond et al., 2017, p. 172). They then proceed to suggest what must be in place for such issues to be resolved. First, thresholds for off-target risks and unintended consequences must be established and agreed upon before any germline editing in the clinic can occur. Second, they claim, without much moral justification, that there is no reason to prohibit in vitro germline editing on embryos and gametes "with appropriate oversight and consent from donors, to facilitate research on the possible future clinical applications of gene editing". Third, they propose four minimum criteria that must be fulfilled before germline editing (once it is safe, etc.) could proceed in the clinic: There must be "(a) a compelling medical rationale, (b) an evidence base that supports its clinical use, (c) an ethical justification, and (d) a transparent public process to solicit and incorporate stakeholder input." Here, it is unclear on what grounds these recommendations rely: They exceed scientific concerns about safety, yet they are neither based on a moral framework nor on broad democratic conversations. If anything, they seem to offer a variety of recommendations based on what is generally understood (among scientists) as being relatively uncontroversial and already covered by moral consensus and/or regulation, and what is more controversial and thus needs to be studied empirically and discussed in stakeholder groups. Although, they clearly distinguish between "ethical justification" and the "transparent public process," both seem to largely describe empirical studies of public opinion. The first via social scientific methods and the latter via stakeholder dialogue. They write that "ethical and social values regarding germline genome editing need to be solicited and considered" and then go on to describe the means to achieve this in terms of "conducting primary research; conducting secondary analyses of published literature on the perceptions, acceptability, quality of life, attitudes, or values of stakeholders; and commissioning an expert review." (Ormond et al., 2017). Here, ethics seems to be interpreted as something akin of the express view of the larger population.

These two strategies, ethical justifications and stakeholder input, imply a largely empirical view on ethics. A similar view is expressed by Howard et al. (2018, p. 3), who argue that responsible development of gene editing technologies suggests that we prioritize "conducting careful scientific research to build an evidence base, conducting ethical, legal and social issues (ELSI [Ethical, Legal, and Societal issues]) research, and conducting meaningful stakeholder engagement, education, and dialogue (SEED [Stakeholder Engagement, Education and Dialogue])." They write:

> Research on the ELSI and impacts of human gene editing should be conducted in tandem with the basic scientific research, as well as with any implementations of gene editing in the clinic. Appropriate resources and priority should be granted to support and promote ELSI research; it should be performed unabated, in a meaningful way and by individuals from a diverse range of disciplines. (Howard et al., 2018, p. 5)

Here, although very crucial moral issues are listed, the fact that the research is intended to work *alongside* technological development, and ethical, legal, and social issues are grouped together, suggests that the limits for ethical investigations are already determined and that ethical issues are more or less reduced to matters of regulation and policy.

At the other end of the scale, some advocates are wary of moral issues being reduced to expert questions, as this will separate the questions from the fundamental social values at stake. Instead, according to this view, it is paramount that the ethical issues be recognized as fundamental questions about our own existence, our future society, and the limits of technology. Hurlbut writes:

> ... we need not and should not wait for a scientific declaration that the time for deliberation has come, nor should we leave it to scientific experts to determine when a moratorium is necessary or that society needs to play catch-up. Neither should we silently defer to expert judgments that the state of science in any field makes ethical deliberations premature. (Hurlbut, 2015, p. 13)

He continues, alluding to Baltimore et al. (2015):

A truly 'prudent path forward' requires recognizing that the technological possibilities that we find before us already reflect prior moral commitments about what choices are appropriate, what powers of control we command, and what moral imaginations should regulate and restrain our technological aspirations. Those commitments belong to all human societies; they demand unflagging democratic attention and the cultivation of capacities to sustain it. (Hurlbut, 2015, p. 13)

Overall, the CRISPR debate agrees that there are ethical issues to be resolved. The two most dominant positions on those ethical challenges are to either look at the safety and efficacy of the technology to ensure that it is safe, or to look to stakeholders and engagement with the public. What remains largely unanswered is what such broad consensus is expected to achieve and how far this would take us in terms of providing moral answers.

In fact, to many, the ethical challenges seem to be mere democratic challenges. Decisions about these challenges must not be determined by experts alone, from this perspective, but rightfully belong with those affected by those decisions. When science and technology are associated with serious risks that might affect individuals and society as a whole, it is not sufficient only to consult ethicists and social scientists:

Risk is more a political and cultural phenomenon than it is a technical one. Turning its framing over to scientists and other privileged experts, such as ethicists and social scientists, is to turn politics and culture over to them as well. Scientists are not elected. They cannot represent the cultural values, politics and interests of citizens—not least because their values may differ significantly from those of people in other walks of life. (Sarewitz, 2015, p. 414)

Although the claim that societal issues require democratic solutions and democratic decisions is uncontroversial, the Democratic View extends this logic of democratic justification to the domain of ethics, and thus equates "what we can democratically agree upon" and/or "what majority believe is right" with "what is morally right/wrong/obligatory/etc." This is a controversial view at least in moral theory since this would remove any possibility to argue on moral grounds against the majority position on any matter. The charge could thus be made against the Democratic View, that it conflates the political and the ethical, but also that it undermines the full force of ethics. That said, part of the challenges attached to a future with or without various gene editing applications may be political as much as it is ethical. Overall, it is unclear how broad consensus exercises are meant to resolve the ethical issues as ethical issues.

4.3   The Moral View

The Moral View, in contrast to the two other perspectives, is both present in and absent from the debate. It is present in the way that moral concepts, arguments and sometimes also theories, are named when presenting the ethical dimension of germline gene editing. It is largely absent in the large debate, when solutions to these ethical issues are discussed given that the Technical and Democratic Views dominate.

Thus, the broader debate is ripe with mention of key moral concepts, such as "human dignity," "human rights," "autonomy," "costs and benefits," "future generations," "informed consent," and so on. For instance, Sugarman (2015, p. 1) mentions three substantial arguments in a single sentence: "There are several arguments against manipulating the human germline. To name just a few, these include that it is unfeasible to provide intergenerational consent, that the consequences are impossible to predict, and that such manipulations pose a threat to human dignity." Presumably, all of these have been discussed at length in earlier bioethical literature, and perhaps they only need to be named here. Still, it is noteworthy that it seems to be more common to refer to than to investigate such arguments in the recent debate. The moral view is largely present in the descriptions of the moral issues and questions that need to be addressed. The ethical diagnosis is generally on point and moral concepts are used to describe these issues accurately.

What there is less of is in-depth ethical analysis. The Moral View is to a large degree absent from the proposed solutions to the moral issues described. As mentioned, part of this has to do with the dominance of the Technical View and Democratic View and their proposed solutions. Some scholars are also very skeptical about turning ethical matters over to some kind of moral experts as part of a broader concern about experts making decisions that ought to be made by us all via democratic deliberation. Key to the Moral View is that moral issues require moral analysis in order to investigate what we objectively have most reasons to believe, given all that bears on the matter, including facts, interests, and normative theories, what the stakes attached to those beliefs are, and what, in the light of the this, we have most reason to do.

Those who have engaged with the moral issues in some depth seem to either come from broad collaborative teams that include ethicists, such as the Nuffield Council, or from bioethicists and philosophers who publish papers somewhat outside of the bigger debate in the natural science venues. However, the debate in the more bioethical and philosophical literature is not as representative of the full breadth of moral philosophy as one might expect, but certain views dominate the recent publications. There seems to be an unexpectedly large proportion of ethical publications with strong utilitarian and bio-liberal leanings that is not quite representative of moral philosophy as a whole.

Thus, even though the Moral View is present in the recent debate, it does not seem to be fully exercised. How else could moral questions be addressed? The simple answer is *to seek to answer* them as best we can, given all that we know. This, then, would be the mark of what we call the Moral View: moral questions pose serious dilemmas that we need to answer as best we can. We need to seek the most informed and relevant *reasons* for possible answers to the questions at hand.

We can now specify that the Moral View entails two essential parts: (a) an understanding of moral questions as evaluative questions rather than descriptive questions and (b) an approach to address such questions by theoretical rather than empirical or social means. It asks the big questions, such as "What *is* the right thing to do, morally speaking, with regard to germline editing?," but it does not find the answer in statements such as "the majority support somatic therapy but not germline editing" or "once the benefits are known there will be little opposition." What then? If the answers cannot be found by agreement or consensus, how can they be found? From the Moral View, these are ultimately philosophical questions that can best be addressed by a combination of our best knowledge of morally relevant facts (about human nature, what is valued and what is not, and so on) and more principled reasoning about the kinds of things that ultimately matter and the kinds of principles that seem to best arbitrate what is right and wrong, given what we know.

The Moral View consists in a perspective and approach to moral questions that does not reduce moral issues to technical issues about safety and efficacy, nor to democratic issues to what can be agreed upon at a particular time among particular populations, but views morality as something that asks for moral foundations and moral answers to questions in a more impartial way: What ultimately matters? What do values consist in? What makes something right or wrong? In essence, from the Moral View, ethical questions must be addressed as ethical questions. That means that they cannot be addressed as descriptive facts to be collected through quantitative studies, stakeholder involvement, consensus conferences, focus groups, and so on. These are the methods of social studies. Nor can they be addressed through shared decision-making, compromise, and consensus, as with political decisions.

There is a difference between making the most optimal decision politically and the right decision morally. The former will need to balance our best conception of what is right and just with the actual political will of those concerned. Ideally, this may overlap, but when they do not, political legitimacy cannot be ignored. Such legitimacy is a core value in political decision-making. In fact, the more technical, scientific, and democratic moral views all come with implicit values that influence the conclusions that are drawn. The epistemic values of science are applied to germline editing when framed as a science project. The medical values of putting the patients' interest first are applied to germline editing when it is framed as a medical project. Democratic values of public decision-making are applied to germline editing as a policy issue. This is all reasonable, but from the Moral View, it does not address the heart of the moral matter and the questions of what the foundations are of moral goodness and moral duty, and what makes an act or a decision morally good or morally obligatory (permissible, impermissible, and so on).

From this perspective, there is a more fundamental moral question: Does germline editing ultimately promote what is genuinely good? And, is there something about editing the germline that violates a fundamental moral norm or principle? Such questions cannot be answered by any of the methods suggested above (more research, more stakeholder involvement, or more democratic decision-making). They pose a more abstract and difficult task requiring careful moral analysis, critical and scholarly reflection, and consideration. It does require something we could call moral expertise, but this does not mean that there is a moral expert who can provide the right answer.

4.4 Discussion

From a technical perspective, any conclusion that we ought not to edit the human germline will always be conditional and premised on the relative safety of the intervention in question. Thus, on this view, it makes sense to claim, "We must not, at this moment, edit the human germline, since it is not, at this moment, sufficiently safe to do so." It also makes sense to claim, "We must never edit the human germline since it will never be sufficiently safe to do so." This latter claim stands or falls on the premise being correct, and it is not subject to change with future research and development of the technology. In either case, any stance against germline editing will always be conditional on contingent facts concerning the safety of the clinical applications of the technology (for patients and their offspring) in a technical sense.

From a democratic perspective, any conclusion that we ought not to edit the human germline will always be conditional and premised on the democratic support for such applications. On this view, it makes sense to claim, "We must not, at this moment, edit the human germline, since we have not thoroughly involved the public and they have not had their say on the matter and have not fully reflected upon, discussed, and carefully considered the matter." It also makes sense to claim, "We ought not to edit the human germline, since there is not a broad consensus in support for this (yet)" or even that "We ought never to edit the human germline, since there will never be sufficient societal support for this." The last claim stands or falls on this claim being objectively true: public opinion would or could at no point support clinical applications of the technology. In either case, any stance against germline editing will always be conditional on contingent facts of societal decision-making, consensus, and broad public deliberation and support.

From a moral perspective, any conclusions that we ought not to edit the human germline must be founded on foundational moral premises about moral value and permissibility. On this view, it makes sense to claim, "We must not, at this moment, edit the human germline, since the requisite moral requirements are not yet fulfilled," but also, "We must never edit the human germline since the necessary moral requirements can never be fulfilled." Here, "never" is not based on any contingent facts, but on what could never even in principle be fulfilled. In other words, there is something about the essence of germline editing that makes it intrinsically problematic and immoral.

On the Moral View, rightness and wrongness do not stand or fall with particular facts or circumstances prone to change, but on assumptions regarding the nature of goodness and evil (in the form of final values), permissibility, and impermissibility (in the form of principles), permissible degrees of risk (when variables affecting value or permissibility variables are uncertain), and morally required degrees of certainty (when all is not known). These must be justified on moral grounds, not on contingent grounds such as safety or societal approval. However, from a moral perspective, it could be the case that the only morally relevant principle is one of safety and medical health, in which case the Moral View collapses into the Technical View, or the only morally relevant principle is one of democratic deliberation and societal approval, in which case the Moral View collapses into the Democratic View.

That said, from a moral perspective, such views seem highly unlikely to be true given how we think of other matters: We care about many things that are unrelated to health and safety and we are concerned about other kinds of wrongs that risk or disregard democratic input. In both of these perspectives, there is a tendency to conflate "acceptable risks" with "accepted risks." From the Moral View, these are two very distinct matters. Thus, we cannot answer any moral question in any serious way without asking what ultimately matters and is of value and what the foundational principles are for moral permissibility and moral obligation.

These three perspectives do not only suggest different ways of understanding the moral issues as such, but also different ways to legitimately respond to the moral challenges in question. What needs to be done, given that there are ethical challenges, thus differs.

From the Technical View, the main ethical challenges come from the risks involved in the technique and its premature release. Thus, what is primarily required is more control (while the technology is not known to be safe), and secondly, more knowledge and development in research. From this view, it makes sense to call for a moratorium (until it is known to be safe), more research, and various forms of transparent and predictable regulation and oversight. In terms of an ideal guideline, this would come in the form of the right kind of precautionary measure to ensure that the technology is not used prematurely (or before the public is ready).

From the Democratic View, the main ethical challenges come from the fact that moral issues are about values and that technology may have far-reaching social consequences for individuals, various groups, and society as a whole. From this perspective, it makes sense to call for more public engagement, debate, and democratic dialogues. The ideal approach would be a process that is sufficiently inclusive to ensure democratic legitimacy, such that technological development does not determine our shared future.

From the Moral View, the main ethical challenges come from the demands of morality and the fact that we risk doing what turns out to be morally wrong. From this perspective, what needs to be done is to seek the moral answers for where the lines of permissibility are and which moral reasons are ultimately weightier. What is needed is more analysis and careful reflection, and, in want of true moral answers, to find principles that help us to err on the safe side of morality.

In short, all three views are concerned with risks, but of different kinds. Thus, the relevant precautionary measures also differ. Indeed, we could conceive of a pluralism of meanings of precaution, depending on the kinds of risks sought to be prevented.

Thus, these three views ask different moral questions:

1. Is this sufficiently safe and efficient for it to be morally acceptable to apply it to the germline of future individuals?
2. Are the risks of a kind and level that we can accept and the benefits of a kind that we have reason to value? Is the technology instrumental to the kind of society we want to see?

3. Is this the morally right thing to promote and allow? Does it, overall, make the world a better place? Is it compatible with justice, fairness, dignity and autonomy, and other moral values?

The first views the moral questions as questions of acceptable risk and benefit. The second interprets them in terms of democratic preferences currently held in society. The third takes moral questions as having a bearing on core moral concepts and values in an objective sense. To answer the first, we must understand the technology and its risks and effects, and have some kind of measure for what is to count as morally acceptable levels of safety. To answer the second, we need to empirically collect the moral values and attitudes of the public in one way or another to make sure that public decisions reflect democratic views. To answer the third, we must analyze the core meaning of moral concepts and their nature, or draw on previous work where this has been done and see how the technology measures against those concepts and where the moral hurdles lie.

In sum, three positions have come to dominate much of the debate on editing the human germline. These could be divided into more categorical positions on the germline (as in the ban) or more conditional positions (as in the moratorium or cautious research moving forward). This book is interested in the kind of reasoning such positions appeal to, particularly the moral reasons. There could be technical grounds for a ban ("it will never be safe enough"), even though it would not appeal to categorical reasons, and there could be democratic grounds for a ban ("it would never be supported by the vast majority"). But there could also be moral reasons for such a ban ("it is morally wrong to do so, even if it is safe and even if a majority thought it acceptable"). The same is true for more conditional positions on germline editing. There could be technical, democratic, and moral grounds for not editing the germline now. Such reasoning could point to various factors that could change, and if they were to, germline editing would be perfectly acceptable. From the Technical View, the acceptability of germline editing would depend on it being sufficiently safe, efficient, scientifically motivated, and rational, given the options. From the Democratic View, one of the necessary conditions for the moral acceptability of germline editing would be whether it has been democratically discussed and has gained broad democratic support. From a moral theory perspective, the acceptability of germline editing would depend on whether it would violate any fundamental moral principles or not, and whether it would promote what is genuinely good.

In the following chapters, we will focus on ethics of germline editing from a moral perspective, starting with an introduction to moral theory and moral reasons. The matter of risk and its varieties and how this complicates the ethical picture will be addressed in Chap. 9.

Moral Theory and Moral Reasons

5

In the previous chapter, we argued that there are broadly three ethical outlooks in the debate on germline gene editing: the Technical View, the Democratic View, and the Moral View. These views also draw on partially overlapping and somewhat distinct moral arguments. The Technical View draws largely on consequence-based arguments limited to the technology itself and its more direct effects. The Democratic View draws on consequence-based arguments, but is more focused on indirect and societal effects, as well as on arguments based on political values such as democracy and justice. The Moral View draws on consequence arguments in a broad sense, as well as more principle-based arguments or deontological appeals to liberty, autonomy, and dignity. These arguments thus broadly overlap with the two dominant kinds of moral arguments in moral theory: consequentialism and non-consequentialism (or deontology).[1] In the next chapters, we will examine various categorical, that is one form of non-consequentialist arguments, and consequence-based arguments in more detail. Here, however, we will first take a closer look at the moral logic that underpins these arguments.

Consequentialism considers *the value of the consequences,* or states of affairs, to be the morally decisive aspect of moral actions.[2] Thus, a moral action is

---

[1] This distinction is well-established in moral philosophy, at least on textbook level. Yet the distinct categories come under various names and with slightly different meanings. An earlier version of the distinction was that between teleology and deontology. However, it is not without critics, see e.g., Vallentyne (1987) on why the teleology/deontology distinction should be replaced. Sometimes the distinction is drawn between the two dominant kinds of each, such as utilitarianism and Kantian ethics.

[2] The term "consequentialism" was originally coined by Anscombe (1958) but has largely become the preferred term to the slightly narrower term "utilitarianism" or the distinctly

© The Author(s) 2025
M. Hayenhjelm and C. Nordlund, *The Risks and Ethics of Human Gene Editing*, Technikzukünfte, Wissenschaft und Gesellschaft / Futures of Technology, Science and Society, https://doi.org/10.1007/978-3-658-46979-5_5

right only if its overall consequences are better than the alternative actions. Non-consequentialism considers *moral boundaries, principles, and norms* to be the morally decisive aspect of moral actions, in addition to, or irrespective of, consequences.[3] Thus, a moral action is permissible only if it does not violate any

---

broader notion "teleology." Consequentialism broadly covers all normative theories that take consequences to determine what is morally right and wrong. The paradigmatic cases being various forms of utilitarianism, such as those proposed by the classical utilitarians such as Mill (1998 [1861]), Bentham (2011 [1789]), Sidgwick (1907), and Moore (2005 [1912]). For overview and classical introductions see Sinnott-Armstrong (2021), Scheffler (1988), Smart and Williams (1973), and Sen and Williams (1982). In the applied area, Singer's book *Practical Ethics* (2011) deserves a special mention given its impact it has had over the thirty years since it was first published in 1979. See also Singer (2015) on effective altruism as a recent development of consequentialism. Beauchamp and Childress (2019) hugely influential attempt to combine consequentialist principles with non-consequentialist principles in the context of medical ethics has shaped large parts of the bioethical debate. Notably, at least partially consequentialist reasons can be found to be addressed in terms of their Principle of Beneficence (Beauchamp, 2019). The classical utilitarians preferred happiness, utility, or simply pleasure and pain (cf. Bentham, 2011 [1789]). The recent literature tends to speak about "wellbeing" in a broad sense (see e.g. Crisp, 2021; Fletcher, 2015; Griffin, 1988). In all the above the basic core to morality is the same: to bring about good outcomes and minimize bad outcomes and often in a way that can be aggregated across states and individuals. For this reason, cost–benefit analysis and similar ways of measuring costs, risks, and benefits in the policy area, can be understood as a kind of applied consequentialism (Hansson, 2007; Adler & Posner, 2001).

[3] Non-consequentialism is here defined as any normative theory where consequences do not suffice to determine what is morally right and wrong. It is most often applied to rights-based ethics, Kantian ethics and various related theories such as contractualism. For an overview of non-consequentialism, see Larry and Moore (2021). Rights-based moral theory often tends to go back to Locke (1988) [1689]) and similar accounts of natural rights theory. Nozick's *Anarchy, State, and Utopia* (2006 [1974]) has given a particularly clear expression of a moral account of rights and the idea of rights being moral constraints on actions. More recent literature on rights, include the works of Raz (e.g., 1986), Thomson (e.g., 1986, 1992), Dworkin (e.g., 1977) and others. Classical Kantian ethics has also been revived and developed in recent years by several contemporary writers, Korsgaard (e.g., 1996), Hill (e.g., 1992), Herman (e.g., 2007; 2021) and O'Neill (e.g., 2013) belong to some of the most influential ones. O'Neill has also addressed more applied issues including those related to bioethics (2002). Recently, Scanlon's every influential *What We Owe to Each Other* (1998) has given rise to a distinct form of contractualism where principles, to put it very briefly, need to be such that no-one could reasonably reject them. Principles of autonomy, justice, consent, and human rights are also well-researched in philosophy of law and elsewhere. Parts of Beauchamp and Childress (2019) theory that focus on principles of justice, autonomy, and consent also belong here. All of these approaches to ethics broadly falls under the category we might describe as non-consequentialism.

particular moral principle that prohibits it, and a moral action is obligatory only if there is some moral principle that makes it imperative.

The differences between these moral theories have real implications when it comes to what conduct is morally right and morally wrong. If what makes an action right is wholly determined by consequences, then there is no ground for moral objections that do not appeal to outcomes and their value. Violations of rights or autonomy, infringed liberties, and undermined dignity will not matter unless it will affect outcomes. Conversely, if moral rightness is determined by moral rules or principles independent of consequences, then the consequences can never determine the moral rightness of an action. For instance, if we are never permitted to violate human rights or dignity, then this would hold irrespective of how much opportunity for greater prosperity we thereby risk foregoing. Thus, Häyry (1994, p. 202) argues that deontological objections are "in a sense more fundamental" than the consequentialist ones. He explains:

> What I mean by this is that if deontological theorists are right, they can establish the moral status of human activities—such as genetic engineering—quite independently of the expected consequences of those activities. One valid deontological objection against gene technology would be enough to put all consequentialist moralists out of business in this field. (Häyry, 1994, p. 202)

This is not a controversial point; it follows from the different kinds of logic underpinning the two basic kinds of moral arguments. The main purpose of this chapter is to illuminate these differences and their influence on the arguments in the debate.

The underlying difference also has epistemic implications. In order to know whether human germline gene editing is morally right or wrong from a consequentialist perspective, we need to know whether the consequences are overall better or worse compared to the alternatives (see e.g. Hayenhjelm & Wolff 2012 for discussion). The less we know for sure about what the actual risks and benefits are, the less certain consequentialist conclusions will be. This also means that we may not know whether germline gene editing is morally permissible, impermissible, or obligatory until after we have acted: Should we, on good grounds, believe that germline gene editing will be largely beneficial, but overlook some grave risks that ultimately fully outweigh those benefits, then our initial conclusions would be wrong. To know whether germline gene editing is morally right from a deontological or non-consequentialist perspective, we must know what the relevant moral principles are and how they apply (see Hayenhjelm & Wolff, 2012; Hayenhjelm, 2018). As long as we know that the moral principles from which we depart are correct, and that we have applied them correctly, we will also know that we have acted rightly. There are significant epistemic challenges in both lines of argument, but of different kinds. The epistemic challenge for consequentialism is largely epistemic ignorance about future outcomes and how these compare to the relevant alternatives. These aspects are likely to change as new alternatives develop and knowledge grows—any more precise moral conclusion is likely to change as knowledge grows. The epistemic challenge for deontology is more limited to moral uncertainty and the difficulty in knowing what is actually morally decisive, beyond consequences.

Both kinds of moral arguments are abundant in the germline gene editing debate. There are consequentialist arguments for and against germline editing based on the anticipated benefits and risks. There are non-consequentialist arguments for and against germline editing on more principled grounds, based on concepts such as liberty, autonomy, rights, and dignity. Most arguments for germline gene editing tend to point to the value of its benefits, while most opposing arguments are more broadly divided into two categories: categorical objections and consequence-based objections based on slippery slopes.

These two categories are not always recognized as different kinds of arguments, and sometimes they are simply listed together without this difference being made explicit.[4] As an illustration, we can read Sugarman's brief indicative list of ethical arguments: "There are several arguments against manipulating the human germline. To name just a few, these include that it is unfeasible to provide intergenerational consent, that the consequences are impossible to predict, and that such manipulations are a threat to human dignity." (Sugarman, 2015, p. 879).

These arguments differ greatly from a moral perspective. First, Sugarman refers to the problems with achieving consent; that is, a deontological argument— here, faced with a practical hurdle in that it cannot be fulfilled. Second, there is a reference to consequences, framed in terms of a practical hurdle in the form of difficulties in predicting these consequences. Third, the categorical objection that it would threaten human dignity is mentioned. These kinds of lists risk lumping together very different kinds of concerns. If we knew that germline gene editing was a threat to human dignity and that this was a hard moral rule, then this would suffice to conclude the matter.[5] In that case, it would be impermissible to edit the

---

[4] However, see Sparrow (2011) for a particularly explicit discussion about the implicit moral assumptions in Harris and Savulescu's reasoning.

[5] Especially in a Kantian framework (2019), we owe respect to persons because of their inherent dignity as autonomous rational beings. See e.g. Dillon (2021, p. 2.2) and Hill (2014). For dignity in bioethics, see Sulmasy (2008).

human germline, no matter the consequences. If we knew that consent is necessary for germline editing to be morally permissible, and we know that it cannot
be obtained (and that parental consent would not suffice), then this would also
settle the moral matter. However, if consequences determine the matter, it could
be either right or wrong, but unless we know enough about the consequences, it
would be difficult to conclude one way or the other. Furthermore, the consequentialist conclusion would only hold for as long as the parameters that determine
the comparative value of outcomes hold. Thus, should a better solution appear,
then it might be wrong to apply germline editing in the older way and only right
to apply it in the newer one. Furthermore, difficulty in anticipating consequences
only matter to the extent that consequences matter. Should morality predominantly have to do with abiding by the right rules or acting from the right reasons,
we need not know what the consequences are, as long as we know that we have
abided by the right rules. Feasibility of consent is only of consequence should
consent be required, and this typically only applies to actions that would otherwise constitute rights violations. However, if being born with an edited germline
was not a rights violation in the first place, then consent would not matter.

The more difficult questions are, of course, the morally substantial ones. Are
there valid moral principles that apply to germline gene editing, and if so, would
they permit or prohibit germline gene editing? Do consequences fully determine
the morality of germline gene editing? These questions are general and not limited to germline gene editing. It cannot both be the case that consequences fully
determine the morality of outcomes, irrespective of categorical concerns, and that
categorical concerns determine right and wrong independent of consequences.
These moral theories are not random but take as their point of departure common
moral intuitions, and, jointly, the kinds of things that could affect the morality
of an action is not limitless. The kinds of things that could affect the rightness
of the agent's reasons or the act and its consequences could not arise from any-
place, but only from a very limited number of possible sources of normativity:
From the goodness of intentions, the rationality of reasons, the goodness in the
consequences, and the rightness of actions according to some moral principle.

We will take a closer look at the various arguments, both categorical and
consequentialist, in the next few chapters. In this chapter, we will explore the
underlying logic of the dominant arguments in the debate in order to make it
clear where the various arguments belong and on what moral premises they
depend. The short exposé in this chapter is thus not meant to be an introduction to moral theories. Instead, it is a map so that the underlying logic in the
various kinds of arguments in the debate can be identified and understood. In this

way, their underlying moral premises and their ultimate implications will become more obvious.

5.1   Three Kinds of Moral Logic

Thus far, we have distinguished between two kinds of moral arguments, consequence-based and principle-based, and two dominant moral theories, consequentialism and non-consequentialism (or deontology). These two theories are based on two different kinds of moral logic: value promotion and permissibility logic.

Consequentialism is based on *value promotion logic*. More often than not, it is based specifically on value *maximization*. This means that what ultimately makes an action right or wrong is whether it creates the most value compared to the alternative actions.[6] Deontology is based on *permissibility logic*.[7] This means that, unless there is some principle that makes an action impermissible, it is

---

[6] The paradigmatic example here is act utilitarianism and Bentham's (2011) "happiness calculus" aiming for the greatest happiness for all. Classical hedonistic act utilitarianism teach that an action is right if and only if it will bring about the greatest possible amount of happiness over all other options. Contemporary consequentialism and utilitarianism consist of various kinds of theories aiming to increase the good and assess moral rightness based on outcomes that depart from the classical view in various ways. For overview see Sinnott-Armstrong (2021).

[7] The paradigmatic example here is that of right-based ethics, or perhaps even more clearly Mill's (2008 [1859]) Harm Principle that permits any action if it does not harm another person. The basic idea is that the rights of others (to not be harmed for example) marks out the boundaries of what is impermissible. Nozick (2006) makes this very explicit in his take on Locke. It seems that modern contractualism also works this way: we are free to act in various ways unless we violate some principle that all affected persons could not reasonably reject. Similar thoughts can be found in Kant but only with regards to "perfect" or negative duties: there are certain things that we must not do because we thereby violate the moral law (see Johnson & Cureton 2022). However, the negative or restrictive take on morality neither exhausts the moral theories of Kant or Scanlon. There are also positive duties, things that we must do for others or value to promote. Herman (2007) has an interesting argument about obligatory ends in her attempt to develop a Kantian ethics in response to challenges from virtue ethics. In any case, there is not anything equivalent to the "maximizing" notion in non-consequentialism. There are things you are morally obliged to refrain from doing, there are things you are morally obliged to work towards, such as happiness, and there are things that morality does not oblige you to do, but that would be morally good to do. Kant (2019) refers to the first category as perfect duties (to oneself or to others) and imperfect duties (to oneself or to others). Wolf (1982) wrote a seminal paper on "moral saints" about moral goodness that goes beyond what is required.

permissible. If there is such a principle, it is impermissible. An action could also be mandatory, in which case it would be impermissible *not* to do it. Even if these two kinds of logic largely underscore the standard versions of consequentialism and deontology, respective logic is not limited to either theory and could be understood independently from them. Furthermore, newer versions of these moral theories tend to use more than one kind of logic.

We could add a third kind of logic to the two above, which, in want of a better name, could be referred to as *the logic of ideals*.[8] This logic is the protection, maintenance, and manifestation of ideals, which in this sense, is about promoting value as much as the first kind of logic. However, here, the value is not thought of as measure of a possible outcome of a single action. In fact, the values we are interested in are most often thought of as things in their own right, as ideals that we can manifest or seek to move towards. In contrast to the values in value promotion, the ideal may not be achievable but only approachable. Take something like world peace. It is an ideal in that it is considered to be good and something to promote and work towards, even if we could never fully achieve it. However, we can measure our actions in terms of whether it brings us closer or not to such an ideal. Such ideal states of the world would be unachievable but approachable ends. Other ideal states of the world could be thought to already exist, such as concepts of a world in natural harmony or ecological balance. Here, the right kind of action is that which seeks to protect and maintain that existing order or balance.[9] The ideal state of the world itself, in this sense is not the outcome of action at all, but one upheld by action. In both cases, actions are judged not by a quantitative measure of how much of a particular good they create, but whether, on the whole, the action is on the right track or does the right kind of job in the bigger picture of things when assessed against an ideal.

Let us contrast the three kinds of logic in terms of germline gene editing. Value maximization tells us that we ought to act in such a way that our action creates as much of the relevant outcome value, typically well-being, as possible

---

[8] In contrast to the other two theories, this is not an established theory. However, virtue ethics and perfectionism, could broadly fall under such a category. It would be largely teleological, in that the ends are morally decisive, but not necessarily as outcomes of singular actions and certainly not as aggregation of value, but rather a striving towards certain ideals. There is an element of this in Moore's ideal consequentialism. There is also an element of this in parts of Kant's philosophy such as his notion about regulative ideals or Kingdom of Ends. Ideals obviously also play a part in Plato's philosophy as in various other classical theories such as classical virtue theory found in Aristotle, but also in Stoics, Cynics, Epicureans, etc.

[9] Ideas in this direction can be found in some strands of Asian Philosophy, such as the Confucian notion of "harmony."

compared to other alternative actions. Hence, we ought to edit a human germline only if such an edit would increase overall well-being in the world compared to alternative actions. For instance, if germline gene editing would increase parental liberty and happiness, increase the overall health, prosperity and longevity of the population, and the total sum of this well-being increase significantly outweighed any expected harm from risk and was better than all alternatives, then we ought to promote such kinds of germline gene editing.

Impermissibility logic tells us that we ought to act in such a way that we do not violate any moral rules, typically restrictions derived from universalization and equal rights. Hence, we ought to edit a human germline only if this is allowed by the relevant moral rules. We must not edit the human germline of a person if it is morally impermissible to do so. For instance, if we all have a universal right to be born with unedited genes, then it would be impermissible to edit the germline of a future baby. Or, if certain germline edits would violate human dignity, then we must not perform those kinds of edits. Alternatively, if we have a moral right to be born with the best genes possible, then it might be obligatory to edit the germline of future children whenever that option becomes available. These kinds of arguments tend to focus on the individual and what they are entitled to, what we must not do to a person, and what would benefit humanity universally.

The logic of ideals tells us that we must act in ways that are compatible with the protection, maintenance, or manifestation of the greater ideals that we believe in. Such an ideal could pertain to human excellence, harmony between species, a just and fair society, or even a religious ideal about maintaining a cosmic order, and so on. Thus, we ought *not* to edit the germline when this is either incompatible with the protection, maintenance, promotion, or manifestation of the relevant ideal, or seems to lead us further away from such an ideal. Most often, these regulative ideals are implicit, and we ask moral questions with them already assumed. When considering whether to build a new hospital or university, we do not need to contemplate whether health-caHre or higher education are essential to the kind of civilization we believe in. or whether knowledge and learning has any social value. Rather, we look at the needs, costs, and benefits, and so forth. Most moral questions are similarly situated within already accepted ideals; however, some questions put things in a new light. The question about whether to abandon planet earth and instead colonize a different planet cannot be resolved by merely analyzing benefits and costs; instead, it forces us to rethink our place in the universe, our home and identity, and what ultimately matters most to us. The idea here is that the "ought we or ought we not to" question posed by germline gene editing cannot be fully answered by theories of permissibility or wellbeing given that what is at stake is not violating boundaries within our current conditions or adding costs and benefits to our current situation but applying tools that could radically change those background conditions. If so, what we need is a tool for comparing different worlds more than assessing pros and cons within a fixed world.

Some of our current values and ideals only make sense in a given world. The moral questions thus shift from being about improvements and permissibility to being about the kinds of values and ideals that matter and their necessary background conditions. For example, if justice and equality are perceived as fundamental ideals then, all else equal, we ought not to edit the germline if we believe that this could undermine such ideals. If, by contrast, we think that the most important ideal is one of human perfection and that human germline gene editing could bring us closer to this ideal, then we ought to edit the germline, all else equal. The "all else equal" qualifier is important here: An ideal does not specify means, and even though an ideal tells us where to go, all routes to that end may not be permissible.

5.2 Value Maximization

The first kind of logic, the value promotion logic, views the rightness and wrongness of actions wholly in terms of whether such actions result in more or less value. The most common logic of this kind of *maximization* can be found in, for instance, dominant strands of utilitarianism and cost–benefit analysis. Rightness and wrongness depend on the overall balance of positives and negatives, whether understood as cost and benefit, utility and disutility, harm and happiness, good and bad, preferences satisfied or frustrated, and so forth. On the maximization version, only that action, among the available options, that scores the highest in terms of net good is right, and all other actions are wrong. This is, however, not the only prominent version of this logic. There are also *satisficing* versions, which suggest that an action does not need to be the best action in terms of promoting value, but merely sufficiently good in creating net value (Byron, 2004).

From a value maximization perspective, it would be morally right to edit the human germline *only* if such actions would maximize net value more than all other available options. This means that for all cases where germline editing is the best option (provides, on average, the most utility minus disutility) over the alternatives is it the morally right option. In all cases where it would *not* be the optimal option, it would be morally wrong to pursue. Whether germline gene editing is the optimal or not, is likely to vary across cases, depending on how safe it is, how efficient it is, how many alternative treatments there are and the quality thereof, how great the expected benefits are, how great the costs are, how great the risks are, and so on. Value maximization not only means that "the good" (as in outcome values) has priority over "the right," (as in moral principles), as Rawls (1988) put it, but also that "the right" is determined by the good. We only know what is permissible, obligatory, impermissible, and so on, once we have defined what is good, or, to put it differently, what has value. This means, at least on the standard monist accounts of value, that there is no role for specific moral concepts such as "dignity," "autonomy," "consent," "democracy," and so on unless these are necessary or instrumental in maximizing the good. In short, if morality per definition is what maximizes the good, and the good is determined by a single concept (such as maximizing the overall well-being of all), then the fact that a specific act that would maximize such well-being over all other actions must be acted upon. This remains the case even if that act were to violate autonomy or dignity; that is, unless such violations would be so harmful to the overall well-being that the action would no longer be the action that maximizes well-being. In other words, goodness or value is what determines moral obligation.[10]

There is, on this view, no grounds for a *categorical objection* to human germline editing in the sense of there being something intrinsically wrong in editing the germline. The only kind of reason that could justify anything close to a categorical position on this view, are risks or costs such that expected benefits could never outweigh those risks. If germline editing were to cause more harm than its benefits can justify, then it must not be done. However, as soon as germline editing causes more overall net well-being than the comparable options, then it must be performed on the same logic.

There is a certain flexibility in this logic: If there are a certain number of steps that will cause overall more well-being than harm, and others where this is not the case, then we must act on the former. It is, in other words, hard to draw any firm

---

[10] There is plenty of room for relevant caveats here, and there are many versions of consequentialism. It is therefore hard to say something general enough without it being inaccurate for some specific versions. The classical version of utilitarianism is the hedonistic act-utilitarianism, where there is only *one* final value (utility understood as *well-being or happiness* aggregated over all affected individuals) and this value ought to be *maximized* (that is, the only right action is the action that brings about *the most* happiness and all other actions are wrong), assessed on *an act-by-act* basis (rather than generalized over many actions following the same rules), *compared* with other actions that were available at the time, and where such happiness is assessed as *actual* consequences (rather than as anticipated). All of these variables have alternatives; there are thus pluralistic accounts, sufficiency accounts, rule-based accounts, prospectivist accounts, etc. Here, the point is to make the general core idea clear and disentangle its distinct logic from those of more deontological conceptions of morality. See Broome (2002).

boundary at all on this logic, since what causes harm and what causes well-being will change with skills, circumstances, and so forth. Thus, if research that does not harm anyone would create value, then it must be done. Similarly, there are no grounds for objections appealing to "consent," "violations of rights or dignity," and so forth, *unless* these tip the overall balance of the good. This flexibility is both its strength and weakness; it means that we can assess the morality of things as we proceed and allow some steps but not others as our skills and knowledge progress. However, it also means that there is little ground for firm boundaries on moral grounds and prohibiting certain options and characterizing them as "off-limits." It also allows for the interests of individual subjects to be overruled in the name of overall happiness. "Informed consent" has little bearing on this logic. Only if such consent were to affect the overall wellbeing calculus would it be of moral relevance. The point here is to, in the starkest relief, illustrate the logic so that the inherent differences between the two kinds of logic become obvious. For actual moral work, there is plenty of sophisticated versions that deal with common objections and flaws in elegant ways.

The rightness and wrongness depend wholly on how the expected benefits outweigh the costs and risks *compared to alternatives*. It is thus not a simple matter of "the ends justify the means," but rather "the *comparably best* option assessed in terms of maximized final value compared to all other options." This logic highlights the alternatives; we cannot say whether germline editing is morally permissible or not until we can rightly assess how good the alternatives are. Thus, if newer technologies become safer, then this could make to use CRISPR impermissible, and if it were overall better to adopt a child than give birth to a genetically edited child, then this is what we ought to do.

Now consider what Ramsey (1970) referred to as the genetic eschatology: the concern that the gene pool (as a consequence of progress in medicine and science and the fact that health is no longer necessary for successful reproduction) is slowly deteriorating until it will, at some point in the future, threaten our species. If we pair these two concerns together: a concern about overall minimization of health and an imperative to maximize well-being, we can see how one can arrive at the position held by some liberal utilitarians or bioliberals that we have an imperative to edit our genes for reasons of overall well-being. It is also in this context that we must understand Savulescu's (2001) argument that parents have a moral obligation to select the child with the best chances of well-being, and if this means editing the genes of the child for the best possible prospects, including enhancement, then this is their duty.[11] (Of course, this is premised on this technology being sufficiently safe; but again, how safe it is can be viewed as a technical problem to be solved by further research.)

The same kind of logic can also be found in a cost–benefit analysis: We compare the various options, calculate the expected value of each option and select that which has the best overall outcome. Translated to the context of germline editing, we must for each considered kind (and token) of gene editing ask what the alternatives are and assess the expected overall increase of value, and then subtract the expected risk of harm from that value. Thus, we must ask whether it would be an overall good thing to develop the technology to treat and prevent various predispositions for disease for enhancement purposes, and so on. The morality cannot be determined conclusively, as it depends on how high and frequent the risks are and how valuable the particular outcomes are compared to the alternatives.

Two crucial aspects emerge here: the question about *alternatives* and *the assessment of risks*. What the alternatives are depends on how the decision is framed. We could frame gene editing as a case of parental choices and, in such a case, the alternatives could cover various gene editing methods, but also prenatal selection (in some cases), and the choice not to have a genetically related child (and instead adopt or not have a child, etc.) However, if the concern is for the genetic deterioration of the human gene pool over time, there may be no comparable option to germline editing (other than more classical eugenics programs, somatic engineering of each person born, etc.), at least not if the gene pool has been left to deteriorate over a long time.[12]

---

[11] Savulescu supports a principle he calls *the Principle of Procreative Beneficence*: "Couples (or single reproducers) should select the child, of possible children they could have, who is expected to have the best life, or at least as good a life as the others, based on the relevant, available information" (Savulescu, 2001, p. 415). The "best life" can be understood as "the life with the most well-being" (p. 419). This principle, however, is meant to direct *selections* of children as part of IVF and he is keen to point out that there is a different selection procedure (among a range of gametes, embryos, and fetuses) and genetic interventions of a single gamete, embryo or fetus. The point is that if we, on good grounds, select the embryos with the best chances of a good life and the person later develops cancer, we have done no harm to them by not selecting another one, but if we edit a particular embryo in such a way that that intervention later causes cancer, we have harmed that person. Likewise, Savulescu also points out that the principle of selecting the child with the best prospects for the future is not the same as the principle of acting in the best interest of the child, since that principle does not apply to selection, but only to how we must act towards a particular person (p. 419).

[12] Ramsey (1970) discusses the worry about a "genetic cul-de-sac," or even a "genetic apocalypse," as described in "writings of H. J. Muller" at some length (Chap. 1, esp. pp. 22–30).

Similarly, to be able to draw any conclusions about the overall balance of the expected net value, one would need to not only correctly assess the size and probability of benefit, but also the size, nature, and probability of harm that could arise as a consequence. Many cost–benefit calculations on emerging technologies may ultimately wholly miss entire ranges of harm that was not known and hence not factored in when assessing its value. Regardless of whether germline editing is thought to be something performed in the near or distant future, all arguments rest on some version of the "but only once it is sufficiently safe" clause. This is problematic for epistemic reasons and therefore also for moral ones. Since even "technical" risks cannot be fully excluded, deeming a particular procedure "sufficiently safe" will depend on epistemic and moral judgments (Holm, 2019).[13]

According to the value maximizing logic, we cannot say whether an action is right or wrong until we know of all its positive and negative consequences and how they compare to the alternatives. Germline editing could be morally wrong

---

Ramsey writes, "Within a period of a few million years, according to Muller, provided that during this period our medical men have been able to continue to work with the kind of perfection they desire, 'the then existing germ cells of what were once human beings would be a lot of hopeless, utterly diverse genetic monstrosities.' Long before that, 'the job of ministering to infirmities would come to consume all the energy that society could muster' leaving no surplus for general or higher cultural purposes." (Ramsey, 1970, p. 23 f.; Muller, 1959, p. 11; see also Muller 1950). For discussion on Muller, see Lappé (1972) and Paul (1987). According to Lappé the worry about a genetic apocalypse is a "red herring." This concern, although in a less dramatic form, is what underpins Powell's (2015) argument for enhancement and gene editing. Powell defends germline enhancement as a means to preserve our current baseline of genetic health. He argues as follows: "Even if we do not have moral reasons to genetically 'enhance' our children relative to the current status quo of normality, germline interventions still emerge as a *pro tanto* moral imperative so long as we have good reason to sustain the levels of genetic health that we presently enjoy for future generations— a goal that should appeal to bioliberals, biomoderates, and bioconservatives alike" (Powell, 2015, p. 670 f.). He continues, "Merely preserving important genetic and phenotypic aspects of the human species—and perhaps even human dignity—will require that we overcome the remaining technical obstacles and make germline genetic therapies legal and widely available to healthcare consumers" (p. 671).

[13] See Holm's (2019) careful analysis of the "only when safe" clause in the gene editing debate. Holm distinguishes between four meanings of harm in this context. Essentially, these are: (a) intentional harm; (b) technical inefficiency and mosaicism; (c) efficient but causing unwanted side effects "on its own, in combination with parts of the organism's (epi-)genome, or in combination with some infection or environmental exposure, either immediately or during the life-time of the organism"; and (d) off-target effects. However, as Holm points out (after disregarding the first kind of harm in the medical context): "The likelihood and magnitude of these harms can be estimated from research evidence, and may be reducible by future research and development. It is, however, as with all technologies, unlikely that the risks of these harms occurring can be removed completely" (Holm, 2019, p. 102).

in all instances if some outcomes is so great as to never outweigh the risks, or
the risks so great as to never be compensated for by the expected benefits, or the
alternatives so great that germline editing is never a better option. However, the
germline cannot be considered *a moral boundary*, based on the value promotion
logic, unless we know that all cases of germline editing will under all circumstances always lead to less well-being than all alternatives in all circumstances.
In all other cases, it can merely be defended as a heuristic, which is most often
the case, or as a temporary measure until it is safe and yields maximum overall
well-being.[14]

5.3   Permissibility and Impermissibility

The second kind of logic, the logic of *permissibility*, views the rightness and
wrongness of actions as a separate issue from the degree to which it promotes
value. To simplify greatly for the sake of clarity: The ends are not sufficient
to justify the means, as some means are simply impermissible, regardless of
the rewards. Instead, actions are assessed against general principles of moral
impermissibility. A central task for such theories is to find the right principle
or criterion to identify the correct subset of possible actions that constitute all
impermissible actions. Morality demands that we do not act in a morally impermissible way. However, in contrast to the value maximization logic, we are free
to do whatever is not impermissible even if sub-optimal.[15]

The focus, with this logic, will consequently be on principles that divide
actions into those that are permissible and those that are not, based on some
theory about what property in moral actions determines this difference. Classical
contenders for this role are actions that violate rights, undermine autonomy and
human dignity, and so on. For instance, an action that violates the rights of individuals, on a rights-based version of this logic is always wrong, but we are free

---

[14] However, it is not an exact science determining how valuable a certain outcome is; it is a
value judgment. What, in fact, maximizes well-being depends on *whose* well-being counts
(for instance, only humans or all sentient beings), what counts as *well-being* (preference,
satisfaction, happiness, flourishing, etc.), what counts as *disutility* to be subtracted from the
overall well-being, how far into the future and how widely *a consequence* reaches, and so
on. How to measure wellbeing is a literature onto itself, see e.g. Broome (2004) and Griffin
(1988).

[15] This difference can be observed in the classical challenge that consequentialist theories
are "too demanding"—an objection that has occasionally also been raised against contractualism, though less often (Sinnott-Armstrong, 2021, §6; Ashford, 2003).

to perform all actions that do not violate any rights. These particular concerns stem from a core notion of treating others as moral equals and rational moral agents. It is essentially a Kantian notion. Furthermore, if an act violates rights, this can be overridden if the person whose right it is consents to the act.

In sum, for our purposes, it is important to see that, on this logic, the focus will be on risks and moral wrongs in order to delineate a small subclass of impermissible actions. The moral goodness of an act may or may not factor into the moral assessment of the act, but fall within the freedom of the moral agent (from a rights-based perspective), or it may fall within duties to aid, help, assist, and so on (from a Kantian, neo-Kantian, or contractualist perspective). Kant famously divided moral duties into four categories: imperfect and perfect duties to oneself, and imperfect and perfect duties to others. Perfect duties include duties to not do harm, lie, and so on. Imperfect duties include duties to promote what is good, such as happiness. What makes the latter kind imperfect is that such duties cannot be satisfied in the same way as a duty not to kill, but requires a continuous endeavor to promote good without any end-point. Kantian theory thus has elements of both a permissibility logic and a logic of value promotion. Rights-based ethics is typically wholly a permissibility-based theory.

Applied to the question of human germline gene editing, if we adopt this kind of logic, the moral permissibility is not a question of weighing benefits and risks, but whether it belongs to the class of permissible action at all (irrespective of outcomes). We typically view genocide and biopolitical eugenics programs (at least of the Nazi and Fascist kind) as impermissible—no matter how beneficial its potential long-term consequences turn out to be (for instance, in terms of thriving states and populations generations later): that is simply irrelevant if the action is not permissible. The moral permissibility of the eugenics experiments of the past, on this logic, are determined by the fact that they were contrary to human rights and dignity and no long-term gain (in terms of the rise of UN, human rights frameworks, long-term peace in Europe, etc.) could alter the fact of its moral impermissibility. The mere fact that individuals were treated as means alone settles the moral matter. This is where a strictly consequentialist or value promotion logic differs: From this perspective, the morality of eugenics is wholly determined on whether, in the long run, it resulted in the most benefits over all alternative options. (An advocate of the value promotion logic would here most likely dispute any conclusion that would suggest that such actions were morally right by appealing to sub-optimality when comparing the actions taken to potential alternative courses of actions not taken.)O

What could render an action impermissible, on this logic, in the context of human germline editing? In the CRISPR debate, and the preceding bioethical debate, there are frequent appeals to autonomy, dignity, consent, rights, and the like—all of which have a distinct Kantian or deontological connotation. In particular, they are associated with Kantian ethics and its derivatives and (natural) rights theory, but also include Scanlonian contractualism (Ashford & Mulgan, 2018; Johnson & Cureton, 2022; Scanlon, 1998).

Classical Kantian ethics would render all actions whose "maxims" violate the categorical imperative as morally wrong. Essentially, this suggests that all action based on reasons and rationales that could not serve as a universal moral law to all are morally wrong, or simply put, not "universalizable." This rules out all actions that allow for moral exceptions for some (not to abide by the same moral duties as others, or not to be treated with the same respect as all others)—or as Kant put it, treats the humanity in others or oneself merely as a means and not also as an end. The crucial point is whether we treat the humanity in ourselves and others respectfully, where humanity here primarily points to rationality and autonomy.

What does this mean for the case of germline editing? It means that we are never permitted to use others as a means for our own ends: Thus, to edit embryos or gametes for the interests of the parents, where those are not also in the interest of the child, or to edit the embryos or gametes for political or economic interests (to serve the ruling class, etc.) is not permissible. However, to edit the DNA of a future person in such a way that they will have greater capacities and thus increase their autonomy would be permissible (but, in contrast to the value maximization logic, this does not make it obligatory to do so, since we only have a duty to avoid what is not permissible, not to always do the best out of all permissible actions.) The key to whether we may or may not edit the germline lies not so much in whether the intervention is inheritable or not, but whether it is in the interest of humanity (as a whole) and humans (individually)—does it promote autonomy and human dignity?

Whereas "autonomy" and "dignity" are frequently mentioned in the debate on gene editing, there has, thus far, been little straightforward Kantian analysis of the topic (*pace* Gunderson, 2007). More prominent in the debate is an appeal to rights frameworks, presumably because "rights" influence not only ethical theory, but also law and public documents and declarations. Thus, if there were a right not to be born with modified DNA, then it would be impermissible. However, rights must be rooted in morally relevant interests that would warrant such rights. Nevertheless, some (Gunderson, 2008) have argued that the rights framework will do more harm than good in the context of germline editing.

Contractualism appears even less in the actual debate, but it would be a possible candidate, given its prominence in much of moral theory (Ashford & Mulgan,

2018). In this case, only those actions that are compatible with principles that no one would have reasonable grounds to object are permissible (Scanlon, 1998). Thus, the important question is whether there are any potentially affected parties who, on good grounds, could object to a principle that made germline editing permissible and universally accessible across purposes (provided it was sufficiently safe). Currently, any representative of future generations could reasonably object to germline editing on the grounds that it was unsafe. Furthermore, current representatives and advocates for the disability and function-variation communities could reasonably object to germline gene editing if they have reason to suspect either that their particular genetic variation will largely be edited away or that genetic variations beyond the norm largely will be so, and thus reducing diversity and inclusivity in society.

Both Kantianism and contractualism are meant to assess principles or reasons rather than individual actions. We could thus refine the moral questions for various purposes and to various degrees of epistemic certainty and risk. We could ask: Provided germline editing was perfectly safe and we knew this with certainty, should such germline editing be generally available to prospective parents at their discretion? For medical purposes? For eugenics purposes? Furthermore, we could ask: Are there reasonable grounds to reject a principle that allows future children to be born such that they carry the burden of risks from germline editing research before we know whether it is safe? The answer at least to the last question, would most certainly be affirmative given that such a principle would allow for individuals to be treated as mere means, and hence go against Kantianism, and those affected would have good reasons to object to it, and hence go against contractualism.

The point is that once we have established whether any of the possible uses of germline editing are impermissible, the rough contours of the moral landscape are in place. We must *never* go beyond that line; no matter the alternatives or consequences—or we must never go there, unless there are preestablished rules or legitimate grounds for such exceptions (such as consent or no alternatives). This kind of logic is appealed to when it comes to murder, cannibalism, torture, genocide, and so on—there are certain acts to which we cannot respond "well how much can be gain by it?" to the question "when is *x* permissible?" Murder is wrong; it is not simply a question of adding "murder" to the "cons" of a pro and con list. However, almost all such seemingly categorical boundaries come with exceptions: *ceteris paribus*. Even if murder is generally strictly impermissible, there are limited contexts where it is permissible, notably self-defense and war. Even if torture is generally impermissible, there could be exceptions if that were the only way to prevent evil. Even if it will always be a rights violation to steal, break into a property, and so forth, rights can be infringed upon, violated, and restored.

5.4   The Pursuit and Protection of Ideals

The third logic, to which we have referred as *the logic of ideals*, may seem indistinguishable from the first logic, given that both determine morality in terms of ends (*telos*) and the value of such ends. However, whereas the first logic evaluates acts individually and assesses their moral worth by means of the aggregate value of their consequences compared to alternatives, this logic is not primarily about the value of consequences, but the value of ideals that determine the value of actions and a good life. To act rightly is to be guided and motivated by such an ideal, and to work towards such an ideal and not against it. This is wholly compatible with such ideals not being realizable by any single act, or even any set of acts. It may, for instance, be morally valuable, and even obligatory, to work towards a world of perfect peace and harmony, even if such a world could never be fully achieved. Such ideals could serve as motivation and point us in the direction of moral worth.

The idealistic logic is normally less about the evaluation of individual actions and more about the overall picture, and it often forms the basis. An individual act is seldom sufficient to promote or undo an ideal in any case. Certain kinds of acts, however, bring the matter of ideals into sharp focus. This applies particularly to actions that may completely change the course of events and lead to fundamental change, but also when certain ideals have been abandoned, outgrown, or challenged by others. In such circumstances, this could lead to a reassessment of ideals hitherto taken for granted. Examples would be prosperity based on colonialism and slavery, or obedience in child-rearing.

The question about what kinds of actions are permissible is not the same as the question about what ends are worth pursuing. Furthermore, the question of whether a particular action will, overall, yield more happiness than suffering is not the same as the question about what kind of ideal or non-ideal future state it brings us closer to. For instance, being colonialized and enslaved by an invading army but drugged to a state of bliss may maximize our happiness, but it would run counter to the ideals we believe in. Given that some actions are categorically impermissible, and some too costly in terms of suffering, ideals can never determine right and wrong on their own. It can, however, illustrate a bigger picture that would make some sense of wrong and right in terms of the kinds of futures they enable or prevent.

For instance, we may value a world of beauty and harmony over one of efficiency, even though both have the exact same aggregate happiness. We may value a world of justice over one of liberty, or vice versa. We may value one based on scientific truth over religious dogma, or vice versa. Such questions, whether to value the cultural riches of a more superstitious way of life, vulnerable to medical illness but rich in meaning and culture and closeness to nature, over one that is based on rationality and efficiency, successful in advanced medicine and prevention, but high in environmental pollutants and mental health problems. Usually, these kinds of questions do not arise, because we already depart from a particular worldview where these ideals are implicit. Nonetheless, they have been asked, especially in the context of colonialization, politics, and global collaboration. In the context of germline gene editing, the question is not limited to whether or not it is conducive to happiness and health, expands upon parental liberties, and so forth, but includes what kinds of futures germline gene editing could promote and enable, and whether those are closer to or further from our ideals of a good state of the world and society. The disagreement between the transhumanists at one end and the theological conservatives at the other seems rather to be a disagreement about the kind of future we would want to promote in this grander sense than a disagreement about what is and is not permissible or what would and would not increase human happiness.

We could value one possible world over another, because it was closer to an ideal that we had. We could prefer one possible future world to another, even if they provided exactly the same amount of happiness, because one world felt more like home to us and like a place we belong to or want to belong to. We could prefer one possible future world to another, because it would come closer to our political ideals than the other. We could prefer a possible future world to another, because it seems like a place that comes closer to a world full of beauty and harmony; we could prefer one possible future world to another, because it comes closer to a metaphysical or religious ideal; or we could prefer one possible future world to another, because it is based on science and rationality, and we consider this important. The liberal view is that such ideals should not be determined by the state and are up to the individual to pursue. An alternative view is that there is an objective truth to the matter, based either in culture or dogma, or in universal objective ends, and that it would be wrong not to pursue those ideals once known. Another possibility, is to see ideals as something we culturally and collectively construct. In either case, this perspective adds a dimension that is not fully covered by the former two kinds of logic; it is about the selection of ends or final values.

How can ends matter unless they describe possible outcomes of individual actions? First, they may primarily work as *motivations and reasons* for action and as states of the world too grand for any individual to achieve, but which could be worked towards as a shared vision.

Second, values relevant to actions, *could to some extent precede and be independent of* the values of outcomes, such that human obligations consist either in protecting or appreciating such values. An example of the former would be to protect, and not upset, sustainable ecological systems. An example of the latter would be to rejoice in life itself.

They could also serve *as a map*; a clear idea about where we want to guide actions in a different way, rather than a clear measure of individual acts in terms of, for instance, maximizing happiness. An individual act is not made permissible or impermissible on account of expressing, being compatible with, being motivated by, or promoting liberty. Rather, liberty is a property of a complex state of the world, which individual acts can support or undermine, some of which are permissible, while others are not. Such values need not be political and could, for instance, be religious.

Much of what Hurlbut and Jasanoff, among others (Jasanoff & Hurlbut, 2018; Hurlbut et al., 2018; Hurlbut, 2015; Hurlbut, 2020) claim concerning germline gene editing could be understood in this light. A key point is that germline gene editing could affect our future society in various ways and, as such, it ought to be subject to democratic decisions. It should not be science and technology that determine our future, but we should all be part of the decision. For instance, Hurlbut (2015) argues that "It is our technologies that should be subject to democratically articulated imaginations of the future we want." (2015, p. 12).

Here, the crux is not to determine what is permissible or not, or what would promote well-being the most, but to ask questions about what kind of future we want to promote, what kind of beings we want to see in the future, and what kind of societies we want to create. These questions are not strictly questions of morality—at least, they need not be. The reason for this is that, unlike permissibility and impermissibility or maximization, these questions need not have a single truth, and there could be many different kinds of answers to them. Most likely, there is more than one way a civilization could thrive and be prosperous and harmonious. Yet, changes that determine the kind of future that will be possible is significant, and some trajectories may make certain ways of life impossible or difficult for certain kinds of beings to prosper and thrive. Evans' (2019) call for a "thick debate" about human flourishing can be viewed in this light. Such a debate would be a debate "about the ends and goals that we should or should not pursue by means of a technology, with ends and means being considered together" (Evans, 2019, p. 48). He contrasts such a debate with a "thin debate" that would involve a discussion about ends in a more limited sense, such as autonomy, beneficence and justice (i.e., those that are part of Principlism) but take on human well-being or flourishing as composite moral concepts (Evans, 2019, p. 48). According to Evans (2020) this kind of logic was more at the forefront of the earlier debate on gene technology until the 1980s, but it seems to have fallen into the background since.

The major difference between value maximization and the pursuit of ideals pertains to the relation between the parts and the whole. The value maximization logic tends to view maximum happiness as something achieved by actions that seek to maximize happiness in the most efficient way. By contrast, the pursuit of ideals focuses on the end state as a complex whole that can be contributed to or promoted in various ways, the only common denominator being that these actions are guided by that ideal. On the former view, we focus on the individual action: What should person P do in situation S in order to achieve maximum happiness? On the latter view, we focus on the nature of the ideal: What, in the end, is it that we want to achieve? In the former case, the ideal is implied from the outcomes of individual actions; in the latter case, the individual actions are inspired by the ideal. This third logic thus focuses on the end state in a more direct way, forming a vision of an ideal state of affairs and finding ways to approach it, much as utopian thinkers and visionaries have a clear view of the desired state of affairs. This end state motivates and explains moral actions.

The maximization logic implies that we would be at a moral loss, unless we knew how to compare actions and outcomes and how to measure happiness and pain. The pursuit of ideals implies that we would morally be at a loss unless we have some vision of where we want to go and what kind of society we seek.

5.5 Ends, Means, and End Goals

The three kinds of logic discussed in this chapter are not necessarily incompatible, but could be viewed in many ways as complementary, since they address different questions. All three seek to answer the broad questions of morality: What should we do? How should we live?

The first two kinds of logic focus on and answer these questions in *the permissibility of actions*. According to value maximization logic, we ought to act in a way that promotes what is most valuable and is, hence, permissible (and obligatory). Permissibility, here, is wholly determined by the amount of value created, or the amount of value that it is expected to be created, as a consequence of a particular action. If the action in question is expected to—or will certainly—create more benefit than harm compared to all other alternatives, then it is permissible. If not, then it is not.

According to permissibility logic, permissibility is determined, at least in part, independently from consequences by what is "morally right" as distinct from morally good. Thus, even if an act consequently creates more happiness than other actions, but it does so by, say, killing a substantial number of individuals, this makes it impermissible, regardless of its benefits. The moral wrongness of the means makes the act impermissible: Killing people as a means to happiness is typically impermissible and morally wrong on most accounts. The exact theoretical explanation for the nature of this wrongness varies. It could be explained by appealing to concepts such as human rights, human dignity, respect for persons, autonomy and consent, justice, fairness, not treating others as mere means, and so on.

According the third kind of logic, *pursuit of ideals*, we ought to act in a way that maintains, sustains, and protects morally crucial orders of society, the world, or the universe—or we must seek to bring our own character, actions, society, civilization, world, or universe closer to some ideal. Here, an individual act is measured not by the amount of value it produces, but by whether it agrees or disagrees with a bigger picture, order, or trajectory, and whether it protects some existing order or brings us closer to some desired end state of the world.

Returning to the topic of germline editing, these three kinds of logic with their three different moral foci give rise to three different moral questions:

1. The moral question about *expected benefits and risks* compared to the alternatives: What are the expected benefits and risks and how do these compare to the alternatives? Are there risks or potential harms that germline editing could cause that could not, even in principle, be outweighed by the benefits? Do the potential benefits suffice to make it preferable to the alternatives?
2. The moral question about *permissibility*: Is germline editing morally permissible or does it (categorically) violate some fundamental moral value or rule, such as justice, fairness, human rights, or human dignity?
3. The moral question about *ideals for the future*: What kind of future is germline editing, if adopted on a large scale, likely to give rise to, and would such a future, overall, be worth promoting and striving for? To what extent would such a future be objectively good or widely desirable, and in the interest of all? When considering the ideals we envision for our future, to what degree

would germline editing promote or obstruct the pursuit of such ideals? To what degree would they be compatible or incompatible with such ideals?

The three kinds of questions are very different, but all three have been discussed in the literature on germline editing. Representatives of the "proceed with caution" position, as well as the Technical View, tend to focus on costs and benefits, and often dismiss the other two kinds of questions as irrelevant. Appeals to human dignity, human rights, or even precaution are either reinterpreted in terms of costs and benefits, and the question about the ideals for the future are either replaced with deterministic positions on scientific progress that cannot be stopped or techno-optimistic futures (such as the transhumanist vision) where deliberately and genetically perfected humans are part of that vision.

Representatives of the more cautious or even categorical oppositions tend to focus more on the permissibility aspect and potential harm to individuals, as well as its long-term implications about who we are and the kind of society that will evolve, and concerns about genetically amplified injustice and discrimination. Less focus is typically placed on the potential benefits and comparative strengths and weaknesses.

When it comes to the question about ideal futures, this is probably where the most profound moral disagreement lies. For some, such as the transhumanists, the very prospect of perfected humans constitutes a necessary part of the idealized future. For others, the mere prospects of playing around with our own nature risks jeopardizing all that is of ultimate value. For others, the worth of the project is wholly determined by its actual costs and benefits, and some potential uses, if they are sufficiently safe, may be very valuable in combating challenges we want to eliminate in an ideal future, but other uses may be too risky or unsafe to consider.

The pursuit of ideals has perhaps been the most pronounced in the Democratic View: Given that technology can completely determine and alter the society and the kinds of lives possible, the worth of any technology must be assessed in terms of a vision of a future that we democratically elect to pursue. The value of a particular ideal stands or falls on the kind of consensus or majority we can form to support it. This takes a subjective but collective view on what the ideal future is: it must be democratically agreed upon. Others take a liberal view: the choice must be there, but ideals are a private matter of belief and preference.

Some view the ideal future, or the ideal state of the world, as an objective matter: certain end states are good, while others are not. Some theologians promote a different kind of ideal future that is largely a religious one where perfection lies with God, and the virtue of mankind lies in loving one's neighbor or seeking a Thomistic or "beatific" vision (Deane-Drummond, 2019). Others argue against germline editing on the grounds that it may lead to a dystopia of some kind, a topic imaginatively exploited in Hunter and Hasselbring's "genomic thriller" *CRISPR: Apocalypse* (2018). The debate between bioliberals, transhumanists, bioconservatives, and some theologians, draws much of its force from clashing visions of ideals. The transhumanists envision a future of perfected humans, or even posthumans, with longer lives, greater beauty, greater strength, greater moral and mental capacities, and so forth, as the ideal. Yet, from a different perspective, a society that glorifies perfection also risks being a society that discriminates, lacks humility, suffers inequality, risks making people obsolete, and has no appreciation for the natural—which no amount of "perfection" can outweigh.

All three kinds of logic point to important moral aspects in answering the question and all three have internal weaknesses when applied as the only logic.

The maximization logic is helpful in that it can take into account both benefits and losses and can deal with nuances and the prospect that seemingly comparable actions can be better or worse. What it cannot do is draw definitive lines against particular kinds of actions that are always off-limits: such as using individuals for the benefit of the collective, or violating rights. There is nothing in the logic that prohibits exploitation, suppression, and other kinds of injustice, as long as it is the best option for maximizing the good.

The permissibility logic is helpful in that it can protect individuals from exploitation, suppression, and other kinds of injustice, now and in the future. There is, however, nothing inherent in the logic to allow for balancing losses with benefits or allow for degrees of badness—something either violates a boundary or it does not. Furthermore, the permissibility logic, as found in rights-based ethics, does not determine what is morally good, required, or mandatory, but leaves it open. There is what we are free to do (i.e., that which is not impermissible) and what we are not free to do, but no higher aim or ideal to realize or pursue as a given.

Therefore, even if the permissibility logic is in one sense Kantian, it is in classical Kantian notions such as autonomy, dignity, and respect for a person that serves as the foundation for moral boundaries; permissibility logic does not recommend what we ought to do, only what we ought not to do. In order to address the latter, we need to address what has final value. From a Kantian perspective, the same moral notions that serve as foundations for rights and impermissibility also serve as basis for what we ought to promote; namely, the autonomy of rational beings, happiness, dignity, and so on. This means that from a Kantian perspective, the morality of germline editing might depend on to what extent such edits would *promote* values such as autonomy, happiness and dignity of the persons as much as it could be ruled out by violating rights and boundaries based on them. This is also what Gunderson (2007) argues.

The question about desirable end goals contextualizes the moral issues. We cannot make informed moral decisions by merely viewing each next step in isolation—at some point, we need to ask whether the overall direction is worth pursuing or not. The more serious concerns about germline editing seem to articulate this larger moral question: Would a widespread use of germline editing for all sorts of purposes generally be an improvement and part of a thriving society where humans flourish, or would it put obstacles in the way of an ideal society? Part of the answer to that grand question lies in what one ultimately considers to be of value: liberty and personal perfection, the equal worth of all and a shared humanity, a democratic society that only moves in directions that are both to the benefit and agreed upon by all, medical improvements and scientific progress above all else, maximizing human autonomy, profit and progress, or minimizing all causes for suffering? The weakness is that (a) everyone will not sign up for the same kind of ideal and such deep disagreements may never be resolvable; (b) a particular ideal, even if agreed upon, or even if objectively good, may never be achievable or may come at great cost (or may only be reached through impermissible routes); (c) a particular ideal, even if agreed upon or objectively good, does not necessarily tell us anything about what we ought to do or what is permissible—it can thus at best serve as merely a partial moral guide when supplemented with some idea about what makes certain acts impermissible.

Thus, valuable ends do not tell us anything about what is permissible, and ideals may never be realized or even realizable, and they may not unite all, but instead give rise to conflicts. However, we are convinced that moral analysis based solely upon permissibility logic and value promotion logic would be incomplete and shortsighted without addressing also long-term visions or ideals.

Categorical Objections to Germline Editing

6

In this chapter, we will take a closer look at the categorical objections to germline editing that state that it is categorically wrong to edit the human germline. We could refer to this basic idea as *the Categorically Wrong Claim.*

> Categorically Wrong Claim (CW): Every act of human germline editing is categorically morally wrong.

These arguments have in common that they support the claim that even if germline editing were to be sufficiently safe and efficient (in a technical sense), and even if there was broad public support in favor of such edits, it would still be wrong to edit the human germline.[1]

Now, the term "categorically morally wrong" is vague. On the one hand, it is a general claim that applies to germline editing categorically rather than differentiating between various kinds of germline editing, or various moral aspects that suggest different kinds of moral conclusions for different cases. On the other hand, "wrong" is merely an evaluative term that does not strictly translate into a precise deontic claim, such that it is categorically *impermissible.* A moral act can

---

[1] This position also overlaps with how Primc (2020, p. 41, n4) defines bioconservatism: "In this context, the characterization as bioconservative refers to positions that for some reason believe that germline manipulation represents an ethical limit that should not be transgressed, even though it could eventually be regarded as sufficiently safe." This definition is, however, both too narrow and too broad, since one can be bioconservative and draw the line elsewhere, or apply a principle that does not operate on a line at the germline, or not specifically take a stand on germline editing, but only as a part of a broader stance, or one could support such a line for non-conservative reasons; for instance, on grounds of fairness or resource allocation.

© The Author(s) 2025
M. Hayenhjelm and C. Nordlund, *The Risks and Ethics of Human Gene Editing*,
Technikzukünfte, Wissenschaft und Gesellschaft / Futures of Technology, Science and Society, https://doi.org/10.1007/978-3-658-46979-5_6

be morally wrong but still permissible in certain circumstances; say, if the alternatives are worse, unavoidable, or similar. For instance, it may be categorically wrong to kill but permissible for reasons of self-defense. In general, however, it is reasonable to presume that whatever is morally wrong is *ipso facto* also morally impermissible.

There are at least three kinds of arguments for these general claims against germline editing. The first argument is an argument based on intrinsic properties: It is morally wrong because germline editing is *intrinsically wrong*. Here, this would mean that because of the kind of act that germline editing is, it is wrong. However, since germline editing does not refer to precise moral properties that make it wrong, this line of argument requires further explanation. Some of these arguments draw on theological aspects, such as germline editing constituting a case of human hubris, it being a case of "playing God," or it commodifying humans and transgressing some boundary of naturalness.

The second argument is an argument based on *violated moral principles*. It is morally wrong, because it violates a categorical principle, such as moral rights. Thus, should we in every case of editing the human germline also cross some moral line, such as the categorical imperative, or violate human rights, then this would imply that it is categorically wrong. In the recent debate, more moral work is done with key deontic concepts, particularly "dignity," "autonomy," and "rights." The idea is that germline gene editing is incompatible with human dignity and/or violates human rights and/or human autonomy and is therefore morally wrong. These arguments often draw on more than one of these concepts and there is a significant overlap between arguments based on rights, on dignity, and on autonomy.

The third kind of argument agrees with the overall conclusion that every act of germline editing is morally wrong, but not because it is necessarily intrinsically wrong, nor because it violates some moral principle, but because it would *open the door to a slippery slope* to truly worst-case scenarios, such as eugenics, genocide, designer babies, or a future dystopia divided between genetically enhanced and unenhanced humans. These arguments are not, strictly speaking, categorical arguments, since it is not germline editing that is morally wrong per se, but they lead to a similar categorical conclusion on germline editing based on the perceived risk for such outcomes. It is morally wrong, because it *would necessarily open the door* to even worse moral actions or a worse state of affairs, such as eugenics or deep injustice.[2]

---

[2] Engelhard (1998, cited in Primc 2020, p. 41) similarly points to three kinds of arguments raised in support of a categorical position against "germline genetic engineering": "(1) such

All three kinds of arguments defend some categorical and general stance on germline editing that always applies to all cases. This could be contrasted with the view that we must assess the morality of germline editing on a case-by-case basis or along a more precise moral classification of various kinds of germline gene editing interventions that lead to different moral conclusions.

All of these arguments could be taken as support for the notion of the germline as a moral "red line." If this notion could be supported, then it would certainly settle the moral issue: If it is the case that every act of germline editing is morally wrong, then it would not matter how beneficial or safe it is, given that it would always be wrong. For this reason, we will address these kinds of arguments before we turn to the consequence-based arguments in the two chapters that follow.

6.1 Germline Editing as Intrinsically Wrong

The most straightforward argument in support of the claim that germline editing is categorically wrong would be an argument that germline editing is intrinsically wrong. In other words, if we could argue that there is something about germline editing that makes each such act morally wrong, then, of course, such an argument needs to highlight some such property that would make the claim plausible. In the literature, three core moral concepts have been called upon to perform this job: (a) dignity when attached to human life right from the start, or more abstractly to humanity as a whole attached to the human genome; (b) appeals to "naturalness" as a basis for moral limits; and (c) appeals to theological boundaries, such as the charge of "playing God" or hubris. Here, we will address the first in the next section and the other two jointly in the following section.

---

alterations are intrinsically wrong because of the status of the human genome, (2) there are obligations to others or rights possessed by others that would be violated by such undertakings, or (3) such undertakings would on balance cause more harms than benefits." The first two overlap with two of the kinds of arguments listed above. The third kind does not: that germline editing would on balance be more harmful than beneficial is a consequentialist argument and could not support a categorical position, since this would preempt the actual outcomes. However, appealing to worst-case scenarios, if realistically possible and relevant, could warrant such a categorical stance if realistically possible. Similarly, certain kinds of slippery slopes that assume that a certain outcome is either unavoidable (because it necessarily and deterministically follows) or the possibility that it will occur cannot be ruled out, could also warrant a principled stance. In short, a categorical position needs categorical reasons as justification; it cannot be justified by relative reasons that apply in some cases or on some estimates but not others.

6.1.1   Dignity and Human Genome as the Heritage of Humanity

Should germline editing be intrinsically wrong, then there must be some reason for this to be the case. A common notion is that of dignity: If dignity is fundamentally attached to human worth and human life, then harming or taking such a life would be wrong for this reason alone. This is the classical conservative pro-life argument. Here, however, the question is not one about life and death, but about edits to human DNA. Thus, we would need some additional premise to explain why such edits would be a violation of dignity.[3] One such premise that has been discussed relates to the notion of the right to be born with an untampered or unaltered genome. Thus, according to this argument, should we have the right to be born with a "natural" or "unaltered genome," then any editing of the germline would be categorically wrong. Another version of this argument is more abstract: We, as the human collective, have a shared interest in our unaltered human nature and the human genome deserves protection as a kind of shared human heritage and basis of our common human nature. We could therefore, along with Braun, Shickl, and Dabrock (2018), divide dignity arguments into two categories: those that argue that germline editing would violate the dignity of a particular future child and those that argue that germline editing would undermine the dignity of humanity as a whole.

The first argument looks somewhat indistinguishable from rights-based arguments, which will be discussed in the next Sect. (6.2). Here, the dignity of the human embryo provides the basis for a right against instrumentalization (being used as a mere means) for some end that is not their own. This idea is closely connected to ideas about a right to be born with an unaltered genome, and we will therefore discuss these kinds of arguments in Sect. 6.2.2 below together with other arguments for the rights of the individual (here, the developing child or embryo).

The second argument is, according to Braun, Shickl, and Dabrock (2018, p. 6), "based on an abstract image of humanity, or the human species, and its identity as an intrinsic value" and involves an obligation by the state to protect human dignity. This kind of notion can be found in the much-discussed Universal Declaration on the Human Genome and Human Rights issued by UNESCO (1997), which states:

---

[3] Indeed, Bostrom (2008a) argues that dignity could speak in favor of human enhancement in various ways.

> The human genome underlies the fundamental unity of all members of the human family, as well as the recognition of their inherent dignity and diversity. In a symbolic sense, it is the heritage of humanity. (UNESCO, 1997)

The notion, here, is that the human genome constitutes the heritage of humanity and therefore deserves protection. However, assigning moral status to the human genome does not provide a very compelling case. Braun, Shickl, and Dabrock (2018, p. 7) point out, "However, due to genomic variation there is no such thing as a 'human genome' shared by all of humanity (The National Academies, 2017). And if there were, it is unclear why it should not be altered to prevent diseases (BBAW 2015)." It seems hard to find a convincing case for the sacredness of the human genome without some kind of essentialist assumption about human nature (see Juengst 2013 for discussion). Harris argues in *the Guardian* (2 December 2015) that the position is absurd. De Miguel Beriain (2019a) argues that the idea that the human genome somehow is intrinsically value rests on problematic essentialist assumptions. In short, the fact that we tamper with the human genome is not a moral reason in itself, and it is unclear why this would have any moral significance. We alter the human genome in various other ways (epigenetic effects); it is not a constant, and, in any case, we do not object to altering genes in somatic gene therapy to cure disease.

6.1.2 Theological Objections: "Playing God," Going Against "Nature," and "Hubris"

Another set of categorical objections is the so-called theological ones or charges of "playing God," tampering with nature, or acting on hubris (e.g., Peters, 2017, 2018). Häyry (1994) sums up the core notion as follows:

> Many theorists and a number of laypersons seem to think that gene technology is somehow inherently and irrevocably "immoral", either because it is against the higher laws of God or nature. The objections based on these ideas are genuinely categorical, since the immorality of the practice under evaluation is supposed to be intrinsic (or conceptual) and therefore beyond empirical testing. (Häyry, 1994, p. 204)

Thus far, these kinds of objections seem to converge with the notion that there is something inherently wrong with genetic engineering of the human germline: the act itself crosses a moral boundary. According to Ramsey's (1970) classical book on the ethical issues raised "by the new biology," nothing less than the "humanity of man is at stake" (p. 122). Ramsey contrasts "the man of serious conscience" to "the man of frivolous conscience." (p. 122) According to him, the man of frivolous conscience "announces that there are ethical quandaries ahead that we must urgently consider before the future catches up with us." Ramsey elaborates: "By this he often means that we need to devise a new ethics that will provide the rationalization for doing in the future what men are bound to do because of new actions and interventions science will have made possible" (p. 122). The man of a serious conscience, by contrast, "means to say in raising urgent ethical questions that there may be some things that men should never do. The good things that men do can be made complete only be the things they refuse to do." (p. 122).

Here we are examining the arguments that human germline gene editing could be something that we ought never to do. Weckert writes, "the wrongness might derive from harms caused but it is not always seen in this light. It might rather come from the fact that something is being done that humans have no business doing" (Weckert, 2016, p. 87).

Ramsey himself discusses four arguments in relation to humanity being its own "self-creator": overstretching our wisdom (i.e., a kind of hubris); threats to the "nature and meaning of parenthood"[4]; aspirations for godhood; and "species-suicide" (Ramsey, 1970, p. 123). These arguments are more directly concerned with what falls into the category of enhancement, or even transhumanist projects, than germline editing, and will be discussed in later Chaps. 8 and 9. Furthermore, the arguments about species suicide are based on losses and worst-case scenarios and will be addressed as such (see Chap. 9).

Thus far, two different routes to a categorical line against germline editing have been presented: it might constitute a case of hubris and "playing God" and thus be at least theologically objectionable, or it might constitute a case of violating the laws of nature in some sense. To complicate matters further, there is no sharp distinction between these two objections: Sometimes the "playing God" objection is interpreted as tampering with nature, and sometimes tampering with nature is discussed as part of "playing God." Peters writes the following: "By 'playing God,' we mean manipulating the intricacies of nature so that human nature becomes something other than what it is. We mean changing nature" (2017, p. 173). Here, we will however treat "unnaturalness" and "playing God"

---

[4] It is worth noting here that Ramsey's concern about parenthood is about replacing sexual reproduction and parenthood as an essential part of being human with "hatcheries" and, as such, something of an objection to nature. This contrasts later concerns about values of parenthood being lost when the meaning of parenthood changes from appreciation of a child as "given" to one of designer and product (see Sect. 8.6).

as two separate but related charges. It is noteworthy that neither of these arguments has been convincing in the literature, and they are mostly found at the enhancement end of the spectrum.

Weckert approaches the notion of playing God as a case of going "beyond our rightful place" to a place "rightfully beyond human interference" (2016, p. 87). On religious grounds, this kind of objection, at least initially, seems to make sense; there is a rightful domain for humans and a rightful domain for the divine. However, it has been suggested that this is primarily a Greek, not a Christian, notion. It goes back to the ancient myth of Prometheus, who, in hubris, stole fire from the gods. According to Peters (2007), there is no Christian ground for arguments of playing God; what matters is not whether or not we infringe on God's territory, but whether new technologies promote goodness and love (Peters, 2007, p. 182). Coady (2009) points to three different traditions within Christianity that determine this relationship: dominance, stewardship, and co-creation, and "to the degree that we are co-workers with God, as much Christian tradition teaches, and I dare say other traditions as well, then playing God is no accusation" (Coady, 2009, p. 156). German Roman Catholic Theologian Rahner (1968, discussed in Ramsey, 1970) argues that "there is nothing *possible* for man that he ought not do," and that creative freedom is part of what it means to be human (Ramsey, 1970, p. 140).

The hubris charge can, however, be interpreted in another way. On this version of the charge, we must not do what would truly require capacities well beyond us. Certain things are such that they require omnipotence, omniscience, and possibly even supreme benevolence to be done successfully (see Hamilton, 2013, p. 180, cited in Weckert, 2016, p. 87; Coady, 2009, p. 161 ff., esp. p. 163). As Coady puts it, "The great achievements of science and the prospects they open up for us can lead us to an exaggerated sense of what we know, to misplaced confidence in our own moral deficiencies" (Coady, 2009, p. 164). This version of the hubris argument could be applied to germline editing: To edit the human germline in a responsible way would require skills, capacities, and judgment of a kind that are simply beyond our intellectual and technical capacities, and doing so could lead to dire consequences that we are unable to fully comprehend, foresee, or take responsibility for. History also demonstrates that some advanced medical treatments in the past, such as early hormone therapy, have had unexpected and undesirable effects, sometimes more serious than the problems they were initially meant to alleviate (Nordlund, 2007).

Ramsey discusses both of these ideas, the theological concern about playing God and the wisdom required for man to self-create, and writes, "Men ought not to play God before they learn to be men, and after they have learned to be men they will not play God" (Ramsey, 1970, p. 138). The hubris objection is largely directed at enhancement and taking control of human evolution. By contrast, Powell and Buchanan (2011) have argued that an evolution that is deliberate is to be preferred to one that is left to chance. The question is, Ramsey writes, "whether man is or will ever be wise enough to make himself a successful system or wise enough to being doctoring the species" (Ramsey, 1970, p. 123 f.). One particular concern is the kinds of mistakes we might make and the fact that things may go irreversibly wrong: "will we not be launched on a sea of uncertainty where lack of wisdom may introduce mistakes that are uncontrollable and irreversible?" (Ramsey, 1970, p. 124). The point is that, should we decide to design humanity according to our own ideas, we will no longer have any measure or map against which to navigate such changes, since what we usually take as our measure, our own nature, is what is being altered. Ramsey writes:

> The point now being made, however, may be cinched by saying that, from man's rape of the earth and his folly in exercising stewardship over his environment by divine commission, there can be derived no reason to believe that he ought now to reach for dominion over the modifications of his own species as well. It is almost a complete answer to these revolutionary proposals simply to say that 'to navigate by a landmark tied to your own ship's head is ultimately impossible.' (Ramsey, 1970, p. 124)

Part of the concern stems from the fact that we have no map to navigate by, and the consequences are unknown and will affect people in the remote future "whose values and milieu we have no means of controlling" (Ramsey, 1970, p. 125). It is thus not merely a case of hubris in the sense that we do not have the right knowledge to predict outcomes, we also lack the knowledge about the values according to which to assess potential outcomes, and those affected by such outcomes will be future individuals whose lives we take upon us to deliberately control. There are two parts to the concern: one is about being able to foresee and control the outcomes and the other is about having the moral judgment to be able to discern what the right action is when it comes to altering human nature. Thus, should germline editing be such that we do not know what we are doing, and should our moral nature not be so robust as to exclude the possibility of it being used to evil ends, then this could support a categorical stance against germline editing, since not opening up the possibility would be the only sufficiently safe option.

6.1.3 Against "Nature"

In addition to the charge of hubris and playing God, there is also the charge that germline editing constitutes an illicit tampering with nature. Again, there is more than one argument here, but they probably share more of a family resemblance than they respresent distinct arguments of the same kind. The simplest argument is, however, a version of the argument of hubris or playing God, where the role of God has been replaced by nature. Thus, certain kinds of activities would be either impermissible or such that the success of them "would require mortals to possess a degree of omniscience and omnipotence that has always been preserved for God or the great processes of Nature that are rightfully beyond human interference" (Hamilton, 2013, p. 180, cited in Weckert, 2016, p. 87). Such a statement makes sense of the categorical element of the objection, and similar ideas have been expressed about "the wisdom of nature," and so on. The problem is, of course, that nature is not all good, all-knowing, or omnipotent. The realm of the natural is also the realm of natural catastrophes, various kinds of human suffering, and human shortcoming. For this reason, it has long been argued that nature is a poor source of moral guidance (see e.g. Bostrom & Sandberg, 2009; Daniels, 2009). Consequently, Powell and Buchanan (2011) have argued that we have good moral reasons to deliberately take charge of evolution rather than leave it to chance.

Häyry has argued that "the unnaturalness objection" comes down to "a warning against making people whose human worth and dignity will be questioned either by themselves or by others." (1995, p. 213) That is, the concern is not about whether a future human being is "natural" but whether their human worth or dignity has been undermined in some sense. If this is right, then this would not constitute a separate argument but merely one version of the deontological objections.

In order to make sense of arguments based on the assumption that germline editing would go against nature, one would need to address what counts as "nature." According to Weckert (2016, p. 89 ff.), one could define "nature" in two ways: in contrast to what is "human" and thus including everything in the natural world except for humans, or in contrast to what is manufactured or artificial and thus including everything in the natural world, also humans. However, neither interpretation provides a convincing case that tampering with nature would in itself be wrong. Most things we do is to intervene with, control, and change nature. Just consider gardening. At the same time, many horrendous diseases are perfectly natural. It does not seem that what is morally good or morally bad necessarily coincides with what is natural or unnatural. In other words, it seems hard to defend "nature" as the mark of a categorical moral boundary (see Weckert, 2016 for discussion).

However, there is a third element to naturalness that is not about what is natural or manufactured as much as it is about the *human nature* by which we morally navigate. If so, the concern is perhaps less about individual violations of a presumed naturalness boundary and more about gradually undoing something that has come to serve as our only moral constant, as it were. These concerns seem to apply more to projects of enhancement rather than crossing the germline per se. Sagoff similarly states: "According to this widely held view, even if the human genome plays a more contingent, variable, and limited role in directing the human traits than analogies to blueprints suggest, it nevertheless connects human beings as individuals and a species to a natural evolutionary and ecological order" (Sagoff, 2005, p. 72). Thus, he argues, one need not "favor nature over nurture to believe, with Ramsey and other critics, that the concepts of nature and the natural play a critical role in guiding our moral intuitions." (Sagoff, 2005, p. 72) Nor need one be a "genetic determinist or essentialist" to worry "that genetic techniques, if used extensively to alter germ lines, would remove a crucially important link that ties human beings to a common evolutionary heritage and other species in the natural world" (Sagoff, 2005, p. 72). Here, it is not the intrinsic value of what is natural that marks the boundary, nor some law of morality that forbids us to change what is natural. Rather, perhaps in a moral sense, the contingent role that nature has for our own identity and way of being and existing in the world is premised on our biological nature and history as biological beings, and it is our shared nature that gives us a place to navigate from.

In summary, how convincing are these arguments of playing God, hubris, and nature as normative notions? In short, appeals to nature do not seem to mark out a morally significant category: We do all kinds of things that could be considered "tampering with nature" and may seem morally unproblematic. Thus, this does not seem to be the moral problem, but rather something else, such as the risks involved in very pervasive technologies that we do not fully master. The objection of playing God does not seem to have any obvious theological foundation, but again marks concern about doing something that may simply be too risky.

6.2   Deontological Objections: Rights, Autonomy, and Dignity

Many of the categorical arguments against germline editing appeal to deonto-logical concepts, such as human dignity, individual rights, autonomy, or some overlapping combination of these.[5] It is in appeal to these moral concepts that the ban against germline editing is often motivated in legislation, as well as in the Oviedo Convention and the UNESCO Declaration of 1997 (see also Sect. 3.1). There are two key notions here: the notion of the human genome as a shared human heritage that deserves protection (UNESCO, 1997) and the notion of a child's right to an open future that would be violated if they were deliberately designed.

Each of the moral concepts of dignity, rights, and autonomy has a solid moral foundation in moral theory. The question with regard to germline gene editing is thus not whether these concepts do any moral work, but rather whether they apply in this case, and, if so, in what way, and whether they would support the idea that it is categorically wrong to edit the human germline.

6.2.1   Rights and Autonomy

What kinds of individual rights of future persons could potentially be violated by germline editing? Two kinds of individual rights have been discussed in the literature: the rights of parents, particularly in terms of reproductive choices, and the rights of their future offspring or future generations more generally. Given that the focus of this chapter is on categorical objections, we will only focus on the rights of the future child, given that only those rights would provide any grounds for categorical objections to germline editing. Parental rights are often cited as a reason for germline editing, especially if this would enable them to have a genetically related child if they would not otherwise be able to (see also Sect. 7.2), which would be a benefit of germline editing. The rights of the future

---

[5] The arguments in the debate draw from rather different theoretical frameworks. There is the Kantian tradition where dignity, human worth and respect for persons are rooted in the fact that we are autonomous, rational and moral agents who are able to act from reason (see, e.g., Dillon 2021 for overview). Here, dignity and autonomy are tied to our reason and rationality. Then there is the human rights framework that bases human rights on dignity (see UNESCO, 1997), as well as the strong focus on autonomy and our right to informed consent in the med-ical ethics context. It seems that these concepts carry different weight in terms of policy and in different countries.

child or the developing rights would thus need to be assessed against the rights of parents. The potential rights of a future child could be divided into two separate categories: rights protecting the welfare interests of the child and rights protecting the autonomy rights of the child. The former would protect from harm and the latter from decisions made without consent.

Welfare rights would be rights based on the welfare interest of the future person. An act of germline editing would violate such a right if it went against the interests of that person, or in other words, would be expected to harm that person. Here, one would need to spell out what kind of harm this would include. One example would be one of the two principles that Nuffield Council suggests must be fulfilled for germline editing to be morally legitimate: it must be such that the intervention is intended to secure, and is consistent with, the welfare of a person who may be born as a consequence of intervention using genome-edited cells (Nuffield Council, 2018, p. 75).[6] In a more negative sense, such a right would prevent actions that would harm them and thus undermine their chances for well-being. Such rights could, however, equally support germline editing, especially, if one presumes the technology to be safe and enable opportunities for a good life.

Autonomy rights, by contrast, would be rights based on the future person having a right to have a say in fundamental matters that affect them. Typically, in liberal thought, the idea is that individual rights demarcate the limits of what others may do. My liberty to do what I want ends where your rights begin. I may not do as I please with what is rightfully yours: your body, your property, your life. At least not without your consent.[7] The general idea of a right to give to or withhold consent stems from individual autonomy rights: I have a say in what is done to me. This can be justified from a Kantian perspective on respect for persons and a right to autonomy (lit. "self-rule") and a natural law perspective on self-ownership. In medical ethics, informed consent is often understood as an important part of what respect for patient autonomy requires (see, e.g., Beauchamps & Childress, 2019). Thus, in a medical context, invasive

---

[6] The full principle reads, "Principle 1: The 'welfare of the future person. Gametes or embryos that have been subject to genome editing procedures (or that are derived from cells that have been subject to such procedures) should be used only where the procedure is carried out in a manner and for a purpose that is intended to secure the welfare of and is consistent with the welfare of a person who may be born as a consequence of treatment using those cells" (Nuffield Council on Bioethics, 2018, p. 75).

[7] For instance, Nozick's (2006) Lockean account of rights paints rights as moral boundaries that should not be crossed and Mill's ([1859] 2011) harm principle limits moral freedom to that which does not harm others.

medical procedures are only thought to be morally permissible with the express consent of the patient, if possible (and by means of proxy consent, if not).

Consequently, one argument against germline editing concerns the impossibility of consent. When parents elect to edit the germline of a future child, they cannot do so with the child's consent. Yet, the consequences of such interventions could potentially be profound; they could affect the very kinds of lives their children could live. The fact that we can alter the germline of future persons without their consent can therefore be considered to be deeply problematic (Collins, 2015, p. 1). The argument about consent to germline editing is based on the following premises. First, any medical intervention is only morally legitimate with consent. Second, consent is impossible to obtain from a person who does not yet exist. Third, germline edits done to embryos or germ cells to be transferred to a uterus are performed on a future person who is not yet able to consent. Thus, since germline editing cannot obtain the consent of those affected, it is morally wrong to edit the germline.

However, objections against germline editing based on consent have been largely rebutted or dismissed, as we do not consent to our own genome, even without germline editing. In fact, it is equally impossible to consent *not* to being genetically edited as it is to being genetically edited. For this reason, Gunderson states that consent arguments are largely a "red herring" (2007, p. 94). Thus, although it is true that no one can consent to having one's germline edited before birth, "it does not follow from this that germ-line engineering restricts autonomy even though consent is not possible" (2007, p. 94). In essence, since it is not possible to either ask or give such consent, it cannot be a moral requirement. He writes, "[c]onsent functions to make permissible what would otherwise be impermissible. It is a normative tool for controlling the obligations of others." In other words, consent has no function or meaning when applied to those unable to even in principle to give it. This does not imply that they cannot be wronged or harmed, but it does mean that consent does not play into it. Gunderson writes: "The person who has been genetically engineered can forgive those who did the engineering or accept the engineering, but cannot consent to the engineering." (2007, p. 94) Gunderson's point is theoretical. The notion of consent only makes sense as a kind of exception within a framework of rights. Thus, although I do not have the right to make free use of your money, your consent for me to do so makes all the moral difference. Thus, there must first be a right not to have one's genome altered for consent to play a role. However, if there is a such right and consent is not possible, then we would be bound by that right.

Mintz et al. (2019) have, again drawing on Kant's moral theory, suggested that although a developing embryo does not have full autonomy rights, it has "anticipatory autonomy rights," which are rights in trust by which their prospective parents are bound. Their concern is that, should germline editing be used as a tool for parents to pursue what they consider to be better traits, or traits conductive to a better future for their child, they make decisions that are not theirs to make. Here, autonomy does not play a key role in consent, but as a future right of the child who must not be circumscribed by parental choices before birth. "In germline engineering," they write, "these anticipatory autonomy rights of the embryo are not preserved but are taken over by the parents' paternalism" (Mintz et al., 2019, p. 1419). Their argument draws in part on Feinberg's (1980) notion of a child's "right to an open future." The concern is that, should parents begin to "design" their future offspring and tailor their genes for excellence in a specific way, this may heavily circumscribe what the child can do and be in the future, and, hence, violate their right to an open future.[8] However, they argue, this does not support a categorical right not to have one's genome edited or a categorical ban on germline editing. For instance, it would be permissible to edit the genome in order to save a child's life (Mintz et al., 2019, p. 1419).

Furthermore, it does not necessarily justify all therapeutic interventions on the assumption that better genetic health automatically, and for all cases, would imply a more open future. This need not be the case. What is left is the child's autonomy right as a future right in trust. This obligates the parents to respect such a right and make assessments based on how such decisions might affect their child's autonomy in the future. Making such predictions is difficult, they argue, even in the case of disease prevention. A person with disease and disability may still have an open future, and "[p]redicting the openness of a child's future is especially difficult for late-onset and nonfatal diseases" (Mintz et al., 2019, p. 1421). As much as autonomy interests provide morally weighty reasons, they do not seem to provide much of a case for categorical objection to germline editing. Instead, they flag a serious risk that we could, but need not, violate such future autonomy interests of the child if editing their genome.

The appeal to the scope of future opportunities and options could also be in favor of germline editing and enhancement. Not being limited by a genetic disease or, as some bioliberals hope, securing a longer lifespan, greater cognitive capacities, and so on, could significantly expand someone's opportunities in life. If we take the right to an open future to imply that more choices are always better than fewer, this could imply that parents have *an obligation* to enable as many futures as possible, and thereby enhance their children if that would provide more

---

[8] Sandel (2009) makes a similar argument that once parents seek to perfect their future children, we stand to lose a sense of "openness to the unbidden" (see Sect. 8.6).

options for them.[9] This follows if one combines the idea that enhancement could expand upon the number of options available to one with a moral obligation to do what creates the most value; that is, applying the value maximization logic. Sparrow (2012) argues against the idea that parents would be obliged to provide a maximum number of choices, since the numbers themselves are not what is important, but rather that there is a range of options sufficient to ensure liberty and autonomy and that those options allow for a good life. For this reason, Sparrow has suggested that we replace the right to an open future with a right to a decent future, "understood as a future which promises a reasonable range of opportunities to lead a life of human flourishing." (Sparrow, 2012, p. 356) Thus, parents must not edit the germline of a child such that it would violate their right to a decent future.

Here, again, the appeal to rights seems to prohibit some cases of germline editing, but it does not make a case that it would be categorically wrong to edit the germline, only that it would be morally wrong to violate a child's right to a decent future. In most cases, such a right need neither rule out germline editing for therapeutic nor enhancement reasons.[10] Furthermore, it might not rule out giving birth to a child with genetic disease if the prospects for a good life are still decent. Sparrow writes, "Indeed, a concern for the child's right to a decent future might only rule out 'enhancements' that radically constrain the options available

---

[9] Sparrow sums up this line of argument in the following way: "A number of authors, including Nicholas Agar (1998; 2004), Jonathan Glover (2006), Dena Davis (2001), and Allen Buchanan, Dan W. Brock, Normal Daniels, and Daniel Wikler (2000), have therefore argued that 'openness of future' is, instead, the appropriate metric for evaluating the extent to which enhancement improve future individuals' life-prospects (see also Robertson [2003; 1994] and Baily [2005]). That is, what we should attempt to do is to preserve for our children the most options, so that they can make the decisions themselves about how they want to their lives to go. This in turn would require ensuring that they are born healthier, happier, and more intelligent, and with longer life expectancies, etc., on the assumption that these are all goods that increase the availability of options for those who possess them (Agar 1998). A concern for the openness of futures resonates strongly with the liberal intuitions and institutions of the societies in which most of the debate about regulation of PGD is taking place" (Sparrow, 2012, p. 361).

[10] Something that complicates the rights argument is that there are members of the disability community who defend a "'right to disability' as a version of a right to difference or a right not to be discriminated against" (Rixen, 2018, p. 19). The concern is that germline edits for the sake of a healthy, genetically related offspring, where genetic variations are eliminated, could diminish diversity and thus undermine equality and increase discrimination against people with those genetic variations. Essentially, this would entail a form of eugenics with very real costs, not for the specific child, but for those with disabilities. For a similar concern, see Sufian and Garland-Thomson (2021).

to the future child by shaping their genetics so that they could only succeed in a very limited number of life projects" (2012, p. 366 f.). Thus, if a right to an open future could be used to promote enhancement as well as medically motivated germline editing, and if a right to a decent future only rules out a limited case of enhancement, it seems that neither idea can provide any support for the Categorically Wrong Claim. We are left with two notions, one leaning towards maximizing options, which would entail an obligation to enhance, should that increase life options, and another leaning more to a sufficiency of valuable options, which is compatible with any action or inaction regarding the germline, as long as there is a sufficiently large amount of decent life options available, combined with a more Aristotelean notion of a good life as one of flourishing.

6.2.2 Dignity and the Right to an Unaltered Genome

Particularly in the German legal context, the concept of dignity plays a prominent role and is strongly connected to human life from the very beginning (Rixen, 2018, p. 24). A related and recurring argument that has been discussed in the literature is the notion of a right "to a pristine genetic inheritance" (discussed in Munson & Davis, 1992), to have genetic material whose integrity has not been tampered with (Resnik, 1994) or simply a right to "an unmanipulated genome" (Primc, 2018). Both of these notions imply that we wrong a developing child or embryo if we alter their genome; first, if it is the case that alteration of the genome would violate the dignity of the developing child, and second, if it is the case that we have a right to be born without any deliberate edits made to our DNA.

Dignity seems to play several moral roles in the debate. First, dignity could be understood in a Kantian sense, referring to the inviolable human worth and our unique value as ends in ourselves. In this tradition of thought, dignity is tied to our capacity for reason and autonomy. Secondly, dignity could also be understood in an Aristotelean sense, as being allowed to live and prosper according to our human nature (and pursue and perfect our nature, thrive, and develop our virtues). According to the first notion, we must never edit the human germline if this entails using another merely as a means and not also as an end in themselves. This seems morally viable, but it is hard to see how this could rule out all cases of germline editing. According to the second notion, we must never edit human nature in such a way that it undermines the dignity of that person or is humiliating, based on certain assumptions about human nature. These are not distinct notions, and the difference is mostly one of nuance and emphasis.

Dignity arguments could be used in this way to prevent one person being used as a mere means for someone else's interests or being mocked or humiliated. Of course, it may be hard to edit someone in humiliating ways without also using them. Although, one could imagine cases where someone was exploited or edited for someone else's agenda without being humiliated. Being bred to have fluorescent rabbit ears would be humiliating, since it would go against the dignity of being born human, whereas being bred to make an elite sports team would not be humiliating. Furthermore, dignity could be applied to someone who is not yet a full moral agent.

Braun, Shickl, and Dabrock distinguish between dignity arguments that appeal to instrumentalization and those that appeal to humiliation but find that both kinds fails in the case of germline gene editing. They reason as follows:

> … it can be argued, on the one hand, that the genetic modification neither instrumentalizes the embryo (for other purposes), nor violates its human dignity, since it is a medical intervention for the sake of the embryo's health and life (and therefore for his own sake). On the other hand, there is no sense in which the procedure humiliates the embryo, and it is doubtful that the born child or adult will complain about having been born healthy instead of diseased, or never having been born at all. Therefore, the assumed violation of human dignity can only lie in the alteration of the human genome itself. (Braun et al., 2018, p. 7)

Their argument, then, is that there are no convincing grounds for a categorical argument against germline gene editing based on dignity. Every case of germline editing is not a case of instrumentalization of the embryo and every case of germline editing is not a case of humiliation of the person born with such edits. Some cases will violate dignity in one or both of those ways and others will not. For instrumentalization to go against dignity, it is not sufficient to serve someone else's purposes; this purpose must also go against the interests of the person. Birnbacher (2018) argues that for instrumentalization to be a violation of someone's dignity, three additional criteria need to be met: they must suffer harm due to the instrumentalization, they must be deprived of their rights, and it must involve some kind of crippling of their human capacities (Birnbacher, 2018, p. 58). In any case, it would seem that appeals to dignity cannot make a good case for germline editing being categorically wrong. A categorical conclusion against the moral permissibility of human germline editing based on dignity, would require either an argument to the effect that every act of human germline gene editing violates the dignity of a person or that it violates the dignity of mankind and "the human genome." The first line of argument does not look very convincing across all cases. Why would it be a violation of a person's dignity to be edited such that one would not carry the genes for severe genetic disease, for instance? The latter line of argument looks even weaker, especially since "the human genome" is not a fixed entity but an evolving and changing one. Birnbacher (2018) argues that dignity "fails to be relevant in this case." Similarly, Braun, Shickl, and Dabrock (2018) dismiss this on the grounds that "due to genomic variation there is no such things as a 'human genome' shared by all of humanity" and, they add, even "if there were, it is unclear why it should not be altered in order to prevent diseases" (Braun et al., 2018, p. 7).

By contrast, Kass (2008) argues that only dignity can properly capture the full scope and depth of the moral issues at stake when it comes to biotechnology and enhancement. He writes:

> Neither the familiar principles of contemporary bioethics—respect for persons, benef-icence (or "non-maleficence"), and justice—nor our habitual concerns for safety, efficacy, autonomy, and equal access will enable us to assess the true promise and peril of the biotechnology revolution. Our hopes for self-improvement and our dis-quiet about a "posthuman" future are much more profound. At stake are the kind of human being and the sort of society we will be creating in the coming age of biotech-nology. At stake are the dignity of the human being—including the dignity or worth of human activity, human relationships, and human society—and the nature of human flourishing. (Kass, 2008, p. 302)

That there is something that needs to be explained and made sense of is not the same as persuading that dignity is the right concept for that explanation. Furthermore, high stakes do not equate to a categorical argument.

A different kind of argument points not to the direct harm of individuals, but to the undermining of our key moral concepts and ideas. Thus, it is not the dignity and rights of individuals or mankind that is at stake, but notions such as "dignity" and "rights"—and by extension, all that such concepts could protect from harm. Notions such as "rights" and "dignity" already presume that there is a shared and recognized human nature deserving of equal rights and a certain kind of respect. The threat is thus indirect rather than direct. Thus, should humans become too distinct from one another, we may no longer recognize each other as "one of us," deserving of the same kind of respect and treatment.

There are limits to how far we can go in changing our human nature with-out changing our humanity and basic human values. Because it is the meaning of humanness (our distinctness from other animals) that has given birth to our concepts of both human dignity and human rights, altering our nature necessarily threatens to undermine both human dignity and human rights. With their loss, the fundamental belief in human equality would also be lost. Thus, Annas (2000) raised the following concern about the threat to humanity lurking behind germline engineering: "If history is a guide, either the normal humans will view the 'better' humans as 'the other' and seek to control or destroy them, or vice-versa. The better human will become, at least in the absence of a universal concept of human dignity, either the oppressor or the oppressed." (Annas, 2000, p. 73, cited in Juengst, 2009).

Here, again, dignity is considered helpful in considering the farthest and morally most troubling aspect of germline editing and enhancement. However, there is no clear dignity-based argument for the categorical wrongness of human germline editing. Annas' argument is more of a worst-case scenario based on a concern about a potential threat to humanity and is, as such, more a probabilistic argument than a categorical one.

6.3   Worst-Case Scenarios and Slippery Slopes

The third kind of argument against germline gene editing is the slippery slope argument or, more broadly, categorical objections to germline gene editing based on what it might lead to further down the line. More than one kind of slippery slope is described (see, e.g., McNamee & Edwards, 2006, p. 516 ff.; Evans, 2020, p. 9 ff.; Baylis, 2019, p. 175 ff.) and more than one kind of worst-case scenario at the end of such a slope. However, the basic notion is the same; should we begin to edit human genes, we will eventually end up with some kind of dystopia as a result.

In this chapter, the focus is on arguments that could justify a categorical objection to germline gene editing. For this to be the case, the argument must persuade that there is a slippery slope in the first place that could not easily be avoided with regulation, and that the potential bottom of the slope is severe enough to warrant a categorical opposition to germline gene editing. Not all slippery slopes could justify such a conclusion.

There is a general case for the slipperiness of the slope: Given that the distinction between therapy and enhancement is too vague to draw a clear boundary, and given that there will be financial incentives for private IVF clinics to offer more reproductive choices to parents, and given that parents will have a strong motivation to give their children the best possible chances in life, it seems very unlikely that germline editing, if legal and acceptable, would come to a full halt at avoiding severe genetic disease and not venture any further. Furthermore, it seems equally unlikely that once very modest germline improvement was successfully offered and delivered, this would not give rise to new "genetic products." Once germline gene editing is offered, there seems to be grounds for a certain slipperiness at the top of the slope. The concern is that once we move past what would fit squarely into "therapy" or prevention of severe genetic disease, the slide will continue; first, to modest forms of enhancements that boost chances for health, then to more controversial kinds of human enhancements, and from there, potentially, all the way to some kind of dystopia.

The exact nature of this dystopia is not always articulated in the debate, but merely alluded to by using terms like "eugenics." Powell (2015) writes, in a paper that otherwise advocates extensive germline edits for the purposes of maintaining current levels of genetic health, that "Even if the present theoretical and ethical motivations are sound, there is still a worry that the coordinated, mass-scale manipulation of the human germline could encourage or otherwise facilitate a return to human rights-violating eugenics programs" (Powell, 2015, p. 683). This, he argues, is "one of the most serious moral objections to the development of germline modification technologies" (p. 683).

However, the dystopian arguments generally appeal to at least one of the following: a concern that enhancement may spell *the end of humankind* and human nature; a concern that some idea about enhancement will lead to *dehumanization*; a concern about *the return of eugenics* and human breeding; and a concern about *deep social injustice* along permanent genetically determined classes with no social mobility. These are not entirely distinct objections, as there is plenty of overlap here.

Evans (2020) also divides these objections into two main categories: a conservative and a liberal line of objection, each with their own take on what constitutes the final dystopian outcome. The conservative dystopian argument is largely one about dehumanization of humanity and the kinds of concerns that *Brave New World* illustrates (Kass, 1972; Fukuyama, 2003). Here, Evans cites Kass' claim that we are "witnessing the erosion, perhaps the final erosion, of the idea of man as something splendid or divine, and its replacement with a view that sees man, no less than nature, as simply more raw material for manipulation and homogenization" (Kass, 1970, p. 785, cited in Evans, 2020, p. 14). Fukuyama (2003) is similarly concerned about dehumanization and, again, finds the relevant illustration in *Brave New World*. According to Fukuyama, the more obvious problem with the kind of society that *Brave New World* illustrates is that, even though the people of the book are "happy and healthy," they have "ceased to be human beings" (Fukuyama, 2003, p. 6). He elaborates: "They no longer struggle, aspire, love, feel pain, make difficult moral choices, have families, or do any of the things that we traditionally associate with being human" (p. 6). In fact, he writes, they "no longer have the characteristics that give us human dignity" (p. 6). He continues this line of argument and claims:

> Indeed, there is no such thing as the human race any longer, since they have been bred by the controllers into separate castes of Alphas, Betas, Epsilons, and Gammas who are as distant from each other as humans are from animals. Their world has become unnatural in the most profound sense imaginable, because human nature has been altered." (Fukuyama, 2003, p. 6)

However, according to Fukuyama, this only constitutes part of the concern. The most important thing is the close relationship between our values and our nature. "So our final judgement on 'what's wrong' with Huxley's brave new world stands or falls with our view on how important human nature is as a source of values." It is here that we can find the most serious threat posed by "contemporary biotechnology," according to Fukuyama. The point is that the concept of human nature is crucial to our self-understanding and key to our human values.

> This is important, I will argue, because human nature exists, is a meaningful concept, and has provided a stable continuity to our experiences as a species. It is, conjointly with religion, what defines our most basic values. Human nature shapes and constrains the possible kinds of political regimes, so a technology powerful enough to reshape what we are will have possibly malign consequences for liberal democracy and the nature of politics itself. (Fukuyama, 2003, p. 7)

We will return to this particular concern in a later section that specifically addresses this in relation to enhancement (see Chap. 8, esp. Sect. 8.7). Here, it suffices to say that this kind of concern about dehumanization was raised by several writers in the earlier debate (well before germline gene editing), directed at earlier versions of biotechnology. Habermas reasons along similar lines:

> How we deal with human life before birth touches on our self-understanding as members of the species. And this self-understanding as members of the species is closely interwoven with our self-understanding as moral persons. Our conceptions of—and attitude toward—prepersonal human life embed the rational morality of subjects of human rights in the stabilizing context of an ethics of the species. This context must endure if morality itself is not to start slipping. (Habermas, 2003, p. 67)

The key concern is that all of morality and our self-understanding is based on the assumption that there is a firm line between the subjective and the objective, between the natural and the manufactured, or differently put, between "us" as moral agents and "things" we use for our own ends. Or, in Habermas' words, "obliterating the boundary between persons and things" (Habermas, 2003, p. 13). Once biotechnology turns its focus from external nature to our own nature, this line is blurred, and with it, the firm boundary between what we may not do to other persons but could do to things. Things, whether parts of nature or artifacts, can and may be owned. This does not apply to other humans; to treat them as mere objects for our own ends is to violate their dignity and human rights. With regard to the event of persons being born, not as accidents of nature, but as predesigned individuals, one has to consider whether our self-conception changes if we are born as manufactured objects. Additionally, the grounds for treating all other humans equally on the basis of being of "equal birth" would no longer exist.

However, according to Evans (2020, p. 14), the conservatives have largely left the debate to the liberals. The liberal dystopian argument is about deep inequality, increased discrimination, and permanent class divides along genetic lines, as illustrated by the film *Gattaca* (1997). Interestingly, Baylis lists the release of *Gattaca* among the defining events in human genetics (Baylis, 2019, p. 85; see also p. 81). According to Evans, *Gattaca* represents a different kind of dystopia than that of *Brave New World*. In this new illustration of dystopia, "children's genetic qualities are selected by their parents in line with a very rigid genetic hierarchy with no mobility between classes, resulting in durable social and economic inequality" (Evans, 2020, p. 14 f.). The main worry has thus shifted from a worry about the end to humanity to one of dramatically deep social injustice and the formation of new social classes along genetic lines.

According to Baylis (2019), this is the main argument against human germline gene editing. This eugenics concern is, of course, not new: it is a concern about sorting humanity into groups with distinct degrees of desirability. In the old eugenics, this decision was a top-down program, determining who should and should not procreate. Baylis describes the concern raised by "the opponents of heritable human genome editing" in the following way:

> They anticipate instead a new kind of eugenics and a widening of the gap between the "haves" and the "have nots." If so, the dramatic societal and cultural consequences will probably include increased discrimination, stigmatization, and marginalization––at first only of those with so-called undesirable genes, but eventually also of those with unmodified genomes. (Baylis, 2019, p. 92)

This concern about injustice and discrimination as a result of germline gene editing has been widely echoed; for instance, by the disability community (Sufian &

Garland-Thomson, 2021). The Nuffield Council (2018) made it a key requirement that germline gene editing must be compatible with a just society and "not increase disadvantage, discrimination, and division in society" for it to be morally acceptable. Annas (2010), in an early criticism, raised the possibility of genocide as a potential outcome in a future society divided between those with modified genomes and those without.

The appeal to worst-case scenarios will also need to rely on some kind of slippery slope premise if they are to support a categorical objection to germline edits. Slippery slope arguments have been classified predominantly as either conceptual or empirical. We could also view these kinds of arguments as worst-case scenarios, as found in ethics of risk. The aim is not to point to a specific series of steps that inevitably follow on one another. Rather, the question is whether the worst outcome is sufficiently likely to occur further down the line, whether norms and attitudes are likely to shift to enable such outcomes, whether technology develops in a way that would enable it, and whether there are firm boundaries that could prevent such outcomes. In order to warrant serious concern, these scenarios must be sufficiently likely and difficult to prevent if gene editing is promoted for some limited ends, such as to prevent severe genetic disease.

Annas writes, "What really seems to be in dispute then, …, is the probability of the worst-case scenario actually occurring, and how high that probability must be to justify actions today to try to avoid it" (2010, p. 260). Annas suggests that what starts as medically motivated interventions will inevitably lead to enhancements and attempts to create superhumans or posthumans:

> The project to make a better baby by genetic engineering begins with attempts to cure or prevent genetic diseases, but inevitably leads to the eugenic agenda of improving or "enhancing" genetic characteristics to create the superhuman or posthuman. (Annas, 2010, p. 257)

Similarly, Baylis and Robert (2004) argue that there is an inevitability about enhancement technologies in a society driven by consumer demand, profit-driven markets, free research, and free competition. Furthermore, we could add to this picture the social pressure on parents to use new technologies to enhance their children, once it becomes the norm. Future women who elected not to edit their child when they could have done so could be labeled "bad mothers" (Baylis, 2019, p. 90). In other words, it is not unlikely, once germline editing is offered as a consumer choice to prospective parents through private IVF clinics, that the available kinds of edits on offer will not be limited to preventing severe genetic disease.

In short, the rationale of a categorical position against germline editing based on worst-case scenarios depends on the probability of such scenarios materializing and to what extent they can be avoided. Thus, if it is possible to edit the human germline for medical purposes without it leading to such outcomes, then these arguments fail. More plausibly, worst-case arguments can provide grounds for pragmatic rather than categorical reasons to object to germline edits as a means to avoid possible, but not inevitable, worst-case outcomes.

6.4   Discussion

What shall we make of so-called categorical objections? The different objections reviewed above highlight several distinct concerns. Although they point to various potential reasons to be concerned about germline gene editing, the case for the claim that germline gene editing is categorically morally impermissible is weak.

The case for there being something *intrinsically wrong* about editing the human germline, or that doing so violates a fundamental moral right by tampering with what is natural, is probably the weakest of the three. The theological objections predate the germline-editing breakthrough and the event of CRISPR. It is therefore worth considering whether these kinds of objections hold the same kind of force against germline editing as they might have held against recombinant DNA and human cloning. More specifically, the moral concern about undermining human nature deserves more consideration than it is given—should an act or policy gradually undermine the humanity in us or the unity between us, it would be deeply problematic. However, it seems clear that this applies to cloning, which adds a whole new paradigm for reproduction, both in methodology and outcome, that would upset a fundamental aspect of our self-understanding and social relations in a way that certainly does not apply to germline edits to prevent disease, and possibly not to many kinds of enhancements either. The objection of playing God is not persuasive as a theological argument and, even if it was, it would be of limited force in a largely secular context. Some have interpreted this concern as one about "naturalness"; however, there is little to suggest that natural risks are in any way more benign than artificial ones, or can in any other sense serve as a moral boundary. The same argument understood as an epistemic concern about "epistemic hubris" will be explored in a later chapter (see Sect. 9.4).

The deontological objections fail to convince us that they would draw the line between what is permissible and what is not exactly at the point of germline editing. This holds for all three versions of the argument: dignity, autonomy, and rights. Certainly, it is not permissible to violate human rights. But, rather than object to germline editing as such, this would suggest that consent is required for the affected parties (in this case, from parents), and that edits to future persons are such that both parents would have to agree to them and they would have to be in the best interest of the child in a way that is not dubious (such as imposing an increased risk not warranted by the intervention or imposing changes that are controversial, such as non-medical ones). In short, it would seem that some cases of germline editing would be impermissible on a rights-based account and some not. Rights of future individuals are complex, and it is not clear to what extent non-existent persons can have rights. We can, however, assume that they have interests that warrant rights, and thus, should any interventions go against such interests that is, not be in the best interest of the future person, or risk not being so, then they would be impermissible. However, medical prevention of heritable diseases would clearly be in the person's interest, provided that it was sufficiently safe and known to work as intended and not risk unforeseen harm. The same goes for appeals to dignity and autonomy. Regardless of how one understands affronts to human dignity and autonomy, it is difficult to see how medical prevention of debilitating diseases could not support, rather than undermine, both dignity and autonomy.

The worst-case and slippery slope arguments depend on the plausibility of the dreaded outcomes. There are a number of slippery slope arguments in the debate. Some talk about slippery slopes from somatic to germline therapy, others from therapy to enhancement, and so on. However, even if the slope of medically intervening to prevent and treat disease to enhancing normality might be slippery, it is a stretch from parents paying for various genetic advantages to the kinds of dystopias imagined and borrowed from fiction, such as *Brave New World* or *Gattaca*. In any case, these worst-case scenarios might provide a stronger case for careful deliberation, precaution, regulation, and control, rather than the moral conclusion that germline gene editing is therefore categorically morally wrong.

Consequence Arguments for and Against Germline Editing

In the previous chapter, we looked at arguments supporting the claim that germline editing is categorically wrong. In this chapter, we will look at arguments that highlight the various positive and negative consequences of germline editing. First, let us contrast the Categorically Wrong Claim along with a general Conditional Claim on the permissibility of germline editing. It might look something like this:

> The Conditional Claim: The moral permissibility of any particular kind of germline editing depends wholly on the reasons for and against it. Whenever the reasons that speak for it are weightier than those that speak against it, it is, all else equal, permissible. Whenever those that speak against it are weightier than those for it, it is, all else equal, impermissible. There is no overall categorical degree of permissibility or impermissibility of germline editing independent of such reasons.

Stated in this way, nearly any kind of moral position would be compatible with it. In fact, it would be compatible even with categorical positions, since such positions would simply take "categorical reasons" to be weightier than all other kinds of reasons. In this chapter, we will more closely examine two versions of the Conditional Claim above: one weaker and one stronger. Generally, we will look at arguments for and against germline editing based on the possible consequences. We could make the underlying assumptions more explicit by substituting the broader category of "reasons" for "consequences" and then arrive at the following claim:

© The Author(s) 2025
M. Hayenhjelm and C. Nordlund, *The Risks and Ethics of Human Gene Editing*,
Technikzukünfte, Wissenschaft und Gesellschaft / Futures of Technology, Science and Society, https://doi.org/10.1007/978-3-658-46979-5_7

> The Weak Consequence Claim: The moral permissibility of any particular kind of germline editing depends on the consequences. Whenever the consequences in support of the action are weightier than those against it, we have stronger reasons to view it as permissible, and whenever the consequences against it are weightier than those in support of it, we have stronger reasons to view it as impermissible. There is no overall degree of permissibility or impermissibility of germline editing that is not, in part, determined by the consequences thereof.

The above claim merely states that in a moral assessment of germline editing, we must take consequences into account, which are likely to play a significant part. Such a broad claim is probably something that most of us would agree with. Note, however, that the claim is compatible with some kinds of germline editing being permissible, while others are not, and that it might be permissible when conducted under certain circumstances but not others. In any case, it would not support a strong position on the germline as a moral boundary for reasons other than precaution, or similar concerns. Now, contrast the weaker claim above with the following much stronger consequence claim:

> The Strong Consequence Claim: The moral permissibility of any particular kind of germline editing depends entirely on the consequences. Whenever the consequences in support of it are weightier than those against it, it is permissible, and whenever those against it are weightier than those in support of it, it is impermissible. There is no overall degree of permissibility or impermissibility of germline editing that is not determined by the consequences and how they compare to the consequences of available alternatives.

Here, there is nothing beyond consequences that could, even in principle, affect the morality of germline editing, other than whether the consequences would be overall for better or worse (compared to alternative actions). How these consequences are to be calculated is not specified in the above claim. If we specify this in terms of maximization, we will arrive at something like the following:

> The Maximization Claim: The moral permissibility of any particular kind of germline editing depends wholly on the consequences in support or against it. The only permissible course of action is that which is likely to produce the most valuable outcomes compared to the alternatives.

The most valuable outcomes could be understood in many ways. Typically, each outcome is assessed on the scale of some measure of what is considered good (such as happiness or utility). However, we need not view "most valuable" in this quantitative sense; instead, we could take "the most valuable outcome" to mean something like "most desired," "most favored by the majority in a democracy," or that which "embodies the highest values and ideals," and so forth.

In this chapter, we will explore various arguments based on consequences for and against germline editing. This comprises a very broad category of arguments that could support the germline as a moral boundary, but only in a weak conditional sense. Any "boundary" would effectively only be a conditional line as long as the benefits are outweighed by the risks, and it disappears as soon as that balance is not upheld. In other words, such a "boundary" could disappear when the expected benefits are thought to be greater than previously thought, or if the risks turn out to be less likely, less impactful, or could be mitigated to a greater extent than previously thought.

These consequence arguments could roughly be divided into two categories. We could refer to those that predominantly *describe* some morally relevant outcome in support of or against germline editing as Descriptive Consequence Arguments, and those that predominantly engage in the overall *normative* discussion about germline editing based on consequences as Normative Consequence Arguments.

Descriptive Consequence Arguments highlight reasons for and against germline editing based on the potential consequences of doing so. Such arguments could support any one of the three claims above: They could add to an overall deontological analysis (compatible with the Conditional Claim without subscribing to any of the Consequence Claims) or provide the sole moral input for consequentialist analysis (compatible with the Strong Consequence Claim and the Maximization Claim).

Furthermore, Descriptive Consequence Arguments highlight *particular kinds of beneficial or risky consequences* of germline editing. As such, they need not preempt any particular conclusion based on those reasons. Rather, there is nothing general we can say about permissibility and impermissibility of germline editing until we have assessed the overall balance of consequences.

The dominant consequence reasons *in favor* of germline editing tend to list one or more of the following prospective benefits: scientific epistemic benefits (acquiring more knowledge about the human genome, embryonic development, etc.); genetic health benefits for the individual patients born without a genetic condition; genetic health benefits on a population level; benefits of providing an option for parents not otherwise able to have a genetically related child; and hopes of enhancement for developing new capacities that exceed our current ones, or for leveling the playing field for those genetically less fortunate or to maintain current levels of genetic health. To this, we could add the financial prospects of those involved in the biotech and fertility industry.

The dominant consequence reasons *against* germline editing all point to some kind of safety concern or risk. There are two prominent categories of unintended effects. First, unintended effects in case it does not work as intended, such as off-target effects (at other sites of the genome than intended), unwanted on-target effects (inefficacy), and mosaicism—and by implication—unwanted risks for any child born with such edits. And second, unintended effects in case it does work as intended: psychological costs in the form of lost values in the parent–child relationship or for the child (loss of giftedness, imposed expectations on children, risk for obsoleteness and similar); social costs in the form of loss of diversity, increased intolerance of genetic difference and increased discrimination and/or general change in how we view others and humanity; social costs in the form of increased injustice due to the divide between those with access to genetic enhancement and those without, and the undermining of equality and fairness.

Normative Consequence Arguments typically engage with the value maximization logic (described in Chap. 5) and the views expressed in the Maximization Claim and the Strong Consequence Claim. From the Strong Consequence Claim and the Maximization Claim, it follows: (a) there are no principal objections to germline editing—given that morality is determined by consequences alone; (b) there is nothing intrinsically wrong with editing the germline—again, given that morality is determined by consequences alone; (c) an absolute ban could only be justified by appeal to the consequences (for instance, such that the potential harm could not possibly be outweighed by the benefits or that we could never achieve sufficient certainty to rule out such a prospect; and (d) as a general conclusion, the moral permissibility of germline editing depends on whether the positive consequences outweigh the negative consequences to a higher degree than the available alternatives.

Most arguments that discuss the normative implications of consequences attempt to do one or more of the following:

1. Highlight that *safety arguments* (or consequence arguments more broadly) are *the only relevant moral arguments against* germline editing (Gyngell et al., 2015).
2. Argue for the *irrelevance of categorical moral objections* and the irrelevance of appeals to non-consequential aspects such as human nature, reasons, values, and so on. (This follows from number 1 above, but is mentioned separately here due to the prevalence of arguments aimed either at categorical objections generally or specific versions of categorical objections.)
3. *Weigh the risks against the benefits* and reach some kind of conclusion based on the assessed balance; that it is currently not safe enough, that it will never be safe enough, that the expected benefits will outweigh the costs once it is safe enough, or that the prospective consequences make it imperative to proceed, and so on.

4. *Compare germline editing with the available alternatives,* in particular with PGD (preimplantation genetic diagnosis) (Ranisch, 2020).

The first two arguments follow from the Strong Consequentialist Claim and value maximization logic. In short, if the moral permissibility and the moral rightness or wrongness of germline editing are always only determined by its consequences, then it follows that nothing that does not fit into the category of consequences could be morally relevant. In particular, nothing could be taken as a relevant moral objection that is not based on consequences, including concerns about human dignity, human rights, autonomy, and so on. Furthermore, the only consequences that could speak against germline editing are those that point to some kind of ethically relevant drawback, such as direct harm, suffering, and costs. The first argument is a version of this focusing specifically on safety. The other two arguments make sense both as defenses for strong consequentialist positions and as part of broader ethical assessments that could include also non-consequentialist considerations.

On a consequentialist framework, there are no straightforward or categorically permissible or impermissible actions. Instead, the permissibility of a particular act depends on the comparative net benefits after risks and harms have been subtracted when the act is compared to alternative options. This means that in order to be able to say anything at all, we need to know what the options are, what their prospective outcomes, good and bad, are and how probable each one of those outcomes are, as well as exactly how negative any prospective harm will be and exactly how positive any prospective benefit will be. What does *not* matter on this view, is that which does not affect outcomes: ideals, principles, virtues, and motives. From this perspective, there are no special rights to acknowledge unless these bring about better consequences, and there is nothing intrinsically valuable about human nature and nothing special about remaining as we are. Furthermore, should the benefits be significant enough, they might very well outbalance the risks.

It is no surprise that most scientists and most bioliberals (including posthumanists) tend to argue from some kind of consequentialist framework (in this case, the value promotion logic). Should germline editing be safe and have clear medical benefits, then there is no reason not to proceed. We could then contrast the claim that germline editing is categorically wrong with a conditional and consequentialist claim that germline editing is morally wrong only when the negative consequences outweigh the positive ones, and morally right only when the positive consequences outweigh the negative ones. Such a view is likely to divide germline editing into a number of smaller categories, some of which are permissible and some of which are not, depending on how likely they are to promote overall well-being. Implicit in such a claim is the notion that the moral status of any prospective act of germline editing can only be determined by assessing the sum total of all the prospective negative effects and the sum total of all the prospective positive effects, and that everything else—appeals to precaution, rights, justice, dignity, and so on—is morally irrelevant, unless we can understand such concerns in a consequentialist way.

In addition to the above four arguments, there is also an argument that there is a moral imperative to pursue germline research and germline editing beyond treatment and prevention to improve the genetic starting points of future individuals. It has, for instance, been argued that there is a moral imperative for parents to create the best possible child (Savulescu & Kahane, 2009; see also Savulescu, 2001, 2014). Similarly, it has also been argued that it is imperative for us to enhance humanity, at least, to maintain our current levels of genetic health (Powell, 2015). Such conclusions also follow if one accepts that (a) enhancement is per definition improvement; (b) morality obliges us, in each decision, to maximally improve the world; and (c) there is nothing other than the totality of benefits that could affect what is morally required (including constraints of consent, justice, human nature as an ideal, and so on); and (d) the overall benefits are considerable enough to outweigh the risks (or the right level of safety can be achieved to make this the case). Consequently, we can add a fifth kind of argument based on consequences for enhancement:

5. Argue for *moral obligations to improve future generations* genetically or conduct research to this end.

The validity of any kind of consequentialist conclusion depends on the assumptions about the particular harms and benefits on which it rests. What counts as harm and what counts as beneficial are not definitive. There is great scope for disagreement; not only about what value to assign to various outcomes, whether a particular outcome would be on the positive or negative end of the value spectrum, or how much positive or negative value lies on that spectrum. Additionally, there is also great scope for disagreement in the assessment of how likely and impactful a particular outcome needs to be in order to be worth considering in the moral context. Should the cost–benefit calculus only consider the expected harm of off-target effects and the like, or should it also include the potential risk of genetic injustice and loss of human nature or negative impacts on culture? Should we only consider benefits in terms of medical benefits and health, or should we also consider benefits from potential superpowers in genetically enhanced individuals? It is worth noting, regardless, that all the dominant arguments *for* germline editing and enhancement are largely consequentialist in nature. Furthermore, such arguments are often strengthened by an expressed doubt about more categorical and deontological concerns. That said, some of the objections to germline editing and advocates for moratoria and bans are also largely based on consequentialist concerns.

7.1   Safety Arguments

The most dominant arguments *against* germline editing concern risk and safety. Regardless of the overall moral positions towards germline editing, safety inevitably factors into the assessment. On a descriptive note, there are three kinds of risks in particular that are repeatedly mentioned in the literature and that form part of the overall picture of germline editing: risks of *off-target effects*, risks of *unintended on-target effects*, and risks of *mosaicism* (see, e.g., Nuffield Council on Bioethics, 2016). There is consensus (as we saw in Sect. 3.4) that all of these raise serious questions about the overall safety of germline editing. Beyond that point, opinions differ. Let us refer to these three main risks as *the basic risks.*[1] What unifies these basic risks is that they do not describe harmful outcomes for persons in the form of physical, psychological, or social effects, but changes at the cellular level. This makes perfect sense from a scientific perspective; it is sufficient to know that there are serious risks and that we ought not to bring germline editing into the clinic until it has become much safer. However, for a moral context, we would need to know more about what kinds of *experienced outcomes* they could contribute to. There is consensus that the basic risks are serious enough to make it currently unwise to edit the germline. As stated, opinions differ beyond that point. In particular, there is broad variation across the following four points:

---

[1] For instance, as Baylis describes: "Children born of embryos whose genomes have been modified may experience serious health problems as a direct result of harmful off-target effects (edits in the wrong places), on-target effects (edits in the right places but with harmful consequences), and genome-wide effects (on different chromosomes and in different tissues). These are the same risks as with somatic cell genome editing for patients. But with germline editing, there is the added risk of mosaicism (incomplete editing). This is when some, but not all, of the developing embryo's cells are successfully modified and as a result the embryo has both non-edited and edited cells (as reportedly happened with one of the twins created by Jiankui He)" (Baylis, 2019, p. 90 f.).

1. How "safe"/"risky" germline gene editing is, especially when compared to alternatives (such as PGD).
2. The scope of relevant "safety"/"risk" considerations.
3. The moral exhaustiveness of "safety"/"risk" as the only relevant kind of objection.
4. The overall level of "safety"/"risk" as a preliminary assessment, especially in terms of whether it is "safe enough" to proceed or "too risky" to be permissible.

Let us take a closer look at the differences in these matters next. We could now ask the following questions: How safe is germline editing? What counts as safe? Are safety objections the only morally relevant objections? Overall, is it safe to proceed once the basic risks have been overcome?

7.1.1 How Safe?

How safe is germline editing? There is little disagreement that there are risks and that it is not currently sufficiently safe. Thus, it should come as no surprise that one of the main objections to germline editing is that it is too risky. We could refer to this as a *basic risk argument*: There are non-trivial risks involved and it is currently too unsafe to proceed with germline editing in the clinic. Ranisch (2020, p. 61) writes:

> Because of its inefficiency in introducing genetic changes, GGE [germline genome editing] is still seen as too risky for human reproduction. Gene editing tools sometimes cut non-targeted genes, leading to off-target effects, or do not reach all cells, causing mosaicism in embryos. Off-target effects or mosaicism have been detected in most experiments on human embryos.

Thus far, there is, as we have seen in earlier chapters (especially Sect. 3.5), broad agreement on this point across all ethical perspectives on the germline. The level of basic risk is, however, not static. In fact, some argue that the overall level of risk has changed over the last few years (see, e.g., Sykora & Caplan, 2017; Daley et al., 2019).

There appears to be a consensus that we ought not to edit the germline *until it is sufficiently safe* to do so (Birnbacher, 2018, p. 55; see Holm, 2019 for discussion). For instance, Savulescu et al. (2015, p. 477), who generally promote very liberal positions on germline editing, including enhancement, readily concede that "it would be highly unethical to bring modified human embryos to term unless we were very confident that the technique could be used safely. The risk would simply not be justified by any potential benefits." Where opinions and assessment differ is to what extent such basic risks are likely to be overcome any time soon (or at all!), how far the relevant safety concerns extend beyond basic risks, whether any objections other than safety ought to be considered, and how safe or unsafe germline editing on the whole can be considered to be.

A key aspect that underpins the safety concerns is the fact that any edit of the germline will be *heritable*. This heritability leads to at least two safety concerns: (a) *the multigenerational aspect* that will multiply each risk; and (b) *epistemic risks* of unknown and unpredictable outcomes. The first aspect is simply the fact that whatever we do to the germline will be heritable, such that we will not only affect one future person, but also all future persons who may come from that person. There are three things we could say about this. First, all risks (known and unknown) that would result from the edit would be heritable. Second, all benefits from the edits would also be heritable. Third—which we have not seen discussed in the literature—should the risks ultimately be more severe than anticipated, it could pose difficult procreative choices for those people in the future.[2]

The second aspect comes from the fact that we do not know how significant the gap in our knowledge is; thus, even if we were to know what the direct results were on a cellular level, we would not know what the direct and indirect effects were until this had been studied on live subjects. Furthermore, some effects might only appear after some generations. In other words, we will not know exactly what we are doing until after we have done it.

In addition to the above risks of the heritable aspect of germline editing, there are two other aspects that add to the overall picture of risk: the *pervasiveness* of the intervention, such that one edit affects all cells of the future person, and the likely *irreversibility* of such edits. Birnbacher (2018) writes about the first aspect that "correction of anomalies has to be attempted in the very early stages

---

[2] Thus, if the rationale for germline editing rests on the premise of having a genetically related child when that would otherwise not have been an option, we ought to, in all fairness, ensure that it does not come at the cost of removing that option for the next generation. That said, they might, in their turn, be able to edit the germ cells of their future child, or they might not—to speculate about what would be available technologically and to whom would require speculation about societies, economies, accessibility, political priorities, geopolitical speculation and such—even if the technological expertise is there, it is very difficult to comment on this. Here, the point is simply that, ethically, it makes little sense to provide an opportunity for couple *x* if it were at the same time to remove that possibility for couple *y*. Especially from a more consequence-dominated perspective (unless we assume some kind of priority for the interests of our current generation, etc.).

of a human individual's existence, at the stage of gametes, their precursors, the pronucleus, or the embryo in its very first stages of development. This implies that every single one of the individual's somatic cells will be altered by the intervention. A potential failure of the operation would leave traces in, and have potential impact on, the functioning of every single one of the individual's cells" (Birnbacher, 2018, p. 63). The second aspect is, of course, more speculative. However, as Birnbacher points out, "the alterations produced by genome editing are, as far as we can tell, irreversible" (p. 63).

Two comments are presented here: Given its pervasiveness, it seems highly unlikely that one should be able to reverse the edits for the person born with them. However, on an even more speculative note, it does not seem impossible that one could possibly seek to re-edit the germline of their offspring such that the original edits did not continue to future generations. Also, recall the insistence of Evitt et al. (2015) on making reversibility a requirement for germline gene editing (see Sect. 3.2).

Currently, it seems safe to assume that any resulting harm could be both serious, irreversible, and heritable. Thus, it is hardly surprising that most arguments for a moratorium on germline editing appeal to safety in some regard. The risks involved are regarded as justification for a moratorium. Should the risks associated with the technology be sufficiently severe, they may warrant the conclusion that we ought not to edit the human germline (Braun et al., 2018, p. 8). It could even be argued that, on grounds of safety, we ought not to even engage in research aimed at some future germline editing in the clinic. This is largely the view that Birnbacher has:

> There is, however, one consequentialist argument, that, in my view, calls into question the legitimacy of research directed at a potential clinical use of human germline genome editing: Namely, the improbability of meeting the challenge of making the method safe enough for clinical application…. Nevertheless, it seems to me that the safety issue confronts human germline genome editing with a substantial, and not only temporary, problem. My impression is that it is grave enough to make research directed at clinical application of germline genome editing in humans seem problematic from the start. (Birnbacher, 2018, p. 63)

Birnbacher notes that he is much more pessimistic than Doudna and Sternberg (2017), as well as the view represented by the National Academies of Sciences, Engineering, and Medicine (NASEM, 2017). He gives two reasons for this: the risks mentioned above (its pervasiveness, irreversibility, and heritability) and the fact that there is already a comparably safer alternative available in PGD and embryo selection.

Another concern is how we could get from here to there. It seems that in order to achieve sufficient safety, some embryos will need to be carried to term before it is known whether it is sufficiently safe. As Primc points out, we could not achieve sufficient safety without exposing certain people to unknown risks first. She writes, "An important question to be asked with regard to the possibility of therapeutic human germline editing is how the transition from a theoretical concept to a relatively safe medical option can be achieved in clinical practice" (Primc, 2018, p. 102). She adds, "Determining the point at which results in live animals and human embryos can be deemed good enough to risk the first live birth of an edited human being is a very challenging ethical decision" (p. 103). There are several challenges here. First, there is limited transferability from animal studies, thus studies on embryos will also be required. Second, embryos, or embryo models, studied in the lab differ from actual person's born in two important respects: life-span and environmental exposure. Conclusions about safety will therefore be limited. For this reason, Primc argues that the "first use in humans must be regarded as a risky experimentation" (p. 103). Thus, even if germline editing in theory could become sufficiently safe, it is not clear that we could bring it to clinical practice as a safe and tested method without exposing some initial persons to an unproven method (rather than as a clinical trial). Primc believes that the first persons exposed to germline editing will not be cases of closely monitored clinical trials (in contrast to NASEM, 2017, pp. 45–47, see Primc, 2018, p. 104, n8), but rather constitute a case an unproven method. It will not benefit an existing patient already suffering some condition (see Sect. 7.2.2 for discussion of this point) and there are alternatives already considered safe. Ultimately, "The transition to a safe clinical option involves the challenging ethical situation of a prospective newborn having to undergo all the risks of an unproven intervention, just to alleviate the distress caused to its parents by their intense wish to have a genetically related child." (Primc, 2018, p. 104).

7.1.2 What Counts as Safe?

Hauskeller (2019, p. 66) points out that "'safety' can and should be interpreted to mean different things." It could be understood in a narrow sense to refer only to such aspects that relate to the efficiency and precision of the technology itself or to include how those risks could play out (diseases, weaknesses) and affect individuals' future prospects in a broader sense. Do we limit our concept of the relevant risks to foreseeable technical risks of harm, such as off-target mutations, mosaicism, and unwanted on-target effects, or do we also include psychological and social costs that could occur if germline editing was brought to the clinic and proved successful in a technical sense? Do we count only risks of incurred losses and harms, or do we also count the costs of lost opportunity from not pursuing expected benefits?

Baumann (2016, p. 140) discusses the comment made by scientist George Church—"What is the scenario that we're actually worried about?" That it won't work well enough? Or that it will work too well?" (Vogel, 2015, p. 1301)—and subsequently reasons as follows:

> On the one hand, there are concerns about the safety of the therapy that alters the plan of each body cell in a human being. Such a therapy might prove irreversible and, in the event of unforeseen and harmful side effects, could pose a threat even to future generations.

> On the other hand, if CRISPR/Cas9 could be applied safely in the future, issues of injustice and accessibility might arise due to the likely high price of germline therapy, increasing the relevance of general ethical objections about enhancement and fear of eugenics. (Bauman, 2016, p. 140)

Presumably, most advocates for a more cautious approach to germline editing take both concerns as highly relevant in assessing its safety. It cannot be regarded as safe as long as there are real risks for irreversible harm to those born edited, and it cannot be regarded as safe as long as there are real risks for societal breakdowns of one kind of another.

What makes the question more difficult is that while we can, without actually imposing the risks on anyone, study what happens when we edit a germ cell in the laboratory, however, without actually seeing germline editing embryos born, the actual consequences as lived experiences will remain speculative. Furthermore, any social or otherwise interactive consequences could not be drawn from the examples of single individuals. This means that even if some worst-case scenarios seem both improbable and do not materialize, there might be other equally bad scenarios that we could not have predicted.

7.1.3   Is Safety the Only Relevant Objection?

Is safety the only relevant grounds for objection? Many of the more vocal techno-optimists of various stripes, tend to argue or imply that concerns about safety are the only grounds for objections to germline editing that merits consideration. This includes also bio-liberals. For instance, Gyngell et al. (2015) seem to be of the view that objections relating to safety are the only valid objections. The rationale behind this is based on the value maximization logic, according to which the consequences are the only thing that matters morally—the suffering we can avoid or alleviate and the happiness we can increase assessed against the suffering we risk imposing or increasing, and the happiness we risk diminishing. Principle-based considerations do not (typically) enter the calculation. (Many bioliberals do take principled-based considerations into account, but mostly in terms of liberty as a positive value, such that even if no objections were to remain, germline editing would fall within parental choice.) Depending on how broad a concept of safety we assume, almost all consequence-based objections could sort into the rubric of safety.

This position contrasts with those that view the safety aspect as merely one among several important conditions that need to be in place to make it morally permissible.[3] Specifically, this position means that any other kinds of objections, such as non-consequentialist objections, are deemed irrelevant. This applies particularly to more categorical arguments, such as that germline editing amounts to playing God or it goes against nature, human rights and dignity.

7.1.4 How (Un)Safe Overall?

How safe is germline editing overall? This is where opinions diverge considerably, as any conclusion about the overall degree of risk and safety will depend not only on what kinds of risk and probability for harm we take into account as well as the magnitude we assign it, but also how we measure the benefits and what our degree of optimism is for limiting and controlling risks.

The third kind of safety arguments are normative claims that preempt some conclusion about how likely germline editing is to be sufficiently safe in the near future and how severe the safety concerns are—something of a *permissible as soon as safe enough* argument (see Holm, 2019). There are arguments to the

---

[3] In their 2015 paper, which advocates continued research, Savulescu et al. do not argue that safety arguments are the only valid moral argument. However, they do write that concerns about unpredictability are insufficient, and that the assumed slippery slope is too weak, unless there is reason to believe that there is a direct causal link from one to the other. They also write that safety arguments are "the clearest ethical concerns" and they call upon those arguing for a ban "to explain how the expected risks outweigh the expected benefits, and why the risks cannot be appropriately managed with more specific legislation." (p. 477) They go on to argue that there is an imperative to continue with research, largely based on its expected benefits (once safer), such as "reducing the global burden of genetic disease," but also the hope that "gene editing could be used to delay or turn off aging in humans."

effect that any properly precautionary approach needs to weigh potential losses from missed benefits as much as the risks of potential harm (see Koplin et al., 2019). By contrast, others view the safety concerns as the only relevant objection, but also either likely exaggerated or outbalanced by the costs of maintaining the status quo and loss of opportunity.

From the consequentialist perspective, all moral considerations other than those of expected benefits or costs (in a broad sense) are groundless (A perspective that often coincides with the Technical View and therefore often seems to find scientific support). Consequently, some argue that once safety issues have been sufficiently addressed, and sufficient benefits have been demonstrated, then there are no remaining moral issues with the particular pursuit of germline editing (Harris, 2015; Gyngell et al., 2017; Sykora & Caplan, 2017a; Gyngell et al., 2015; see Holm, 2019 for discussion). In other words, if we accept the argument that only safety-based considerations are relevant, t, then there is no basis for objection to germline editing on other grounds. Should prospective technology not only be sufficiently safe and thus without any reasons to object to it, but also promise great benefits, then the matter is more or less morally settled: We must proceed and pursue germline editing. (Unless, we also assign independent moral value to liberty and choice in which case society ought to offer us such choices). As Harris puts it:

> Once a new and beneficial technology has been demonstrated to be "safe enough" for use in or by humans, any decent society will wish to ensure that citizens are not denied the opportunity to choose for themselves whether they wish to avail themselves of these benefits. (Harris, 2015, p. 33)

A similar position on research is defended by Gyngell, Douglas and Savulescu (2017, p. 510). After claiming to have shown that such research "can be conducted safely in ways that carry manageable and reasonable risk" and "that there is a significant medical case for pursuing GGE," that is, germline genome editing, and "a research case for pursuing this technology," they conclude that "the moral case in favour of pursuing is stronger than the case against. This suggests that pursuing GGE is both morally permissible and morally desirable." (Gyngell et al., 2017, p. 510).

To what extent we can now presume that germline editing will eventually prove to be sufficiently safe remains unclear (Holm, 2019). Some express confident optimism, others much greater pessimism. This is about two separate but interdependent aspects: safety and what we can know beforehand. Of course, the overall conclusion about whether the benefits outweigh the risks maximally compared to the alternatives may not depend so much on how severe and likely the expected risks are, but on how great the expected benefits are presumed to be, and how great the risks are compared to alternatives and the status quo. Should the benefits be so great that any realistic risk estimate will be more or less outweighed, then this seems to settle the moral question.

It has been argued, as we shall see in the next section, that not pursuing germline editing might allow for the human gene pool to slowly deteriorate (Harris, 2009) and that aging itself is a form of harm and disease to be overcome (Savulescu et al., 2015). Others have stressed that when we balance the benefits and risks, we must not prefer the status quo simply because it is the status quo, and that when we assess future prospects, we must weigh up the loss of opportunity to treat and prevent as a genuine risk (Bostrom & Ord, 2006; Koplin et al., 2019; see Hayenhjelm 2024 for discussion). It is thus not necessarily more daring to move ahead with germline editing than it is to maintain the status quo of not doing so (Koplin et al., 2019). Savulescu et al., notes Hauskeller, "have a very expansive understanding of what should count as a genetic birth defect, which includes fundamental aspects of our common human nature" (Hauskeller, 2019, p. 63). This follows if all negative aspects of humanity count as harms or losses in some sense and all positive aspects (speculative or real) as benefits or gains. Then, we should in any way we can improve on humanity by adding more positive aspects on the presumption that they would increase our capacity for general well-being, and in any way we can reduce any harm or suffering, whether considered "natural" or not. Recall the consequentialist logic that well-being is the only thing of moral relevance and, in a quantitative sense, whether something is natural or technologically manufactured is of no moral relevance. Thus, Savulescu et al. (2015) describe aging as something that "kills 30 million every year and disables many more" and is thus something that we ought to address, provided we have the right tools to do so without imposing greater harm in some other way.

Koplin, Savulescu and others have argued that those opposed pursuing the prospective benefits may suffer from an irrational status quo bias (Koplin et al., 2019; Bostrom & Ord 2006). Their argument is that we must not value current harms less than the loss of expected benefits. Savulescu has, in fact, argued that not enhancing a child would be to harm that child (Savulescu, 2019). In light of this, we can see how an objection like Comfort's (2015) could be raised, that there is a tendency among bioliberals to view all social problems as genetic problems that could be solved by means of genetic interventions rather than social ones.

7.2   Benefit Arguments

By far the most important argument for germline editing is one that appeals to its prospective benefits, particularly in terms of medical treatment and prevention. Furthermore, most of these arguments are comparative, claiming that germline gene editing is better than the existing alternatives. But what are these benefits exactly?

We could roughly divide the dominant pro arguments based on benefits into three categories:

1. *Arguments of medical benefits.* Germline gene editing could provide the benefit of being able to give birth to a genetically related child without genetic disease and erasing the genetic risk for such disease from a lineage.
2. *Arguments of population health.* Germline gene editing could provide genetic health benefits that improve genetic health on a population level.
3. *Arguments of enhancement.* Germline gene editing could provide benefits beyond what is considered normal capacities.

The first kind of benefit, that of treatment and prevention, is the least controversial in that its aims fall within what medical science is expected to do. It is, however, complicated by two troubling objections: Given that we only treat germ cells and embryos of not-yet existing persons or patients, and genetic disease could have been avoided by not giving birth to a genetically related child, it is unclear to what extent germline editing can actually qualify as a treatment or even prevention. Furthermore, its value seems to depend, in no small way, on the value we attach to having a genetically related child. We will return to all of these points in the next section.

The second kind of benefit also primarily focuses on medical or health benefits. Here, however, the focus is not on the medical interests of particular parents and children, but on those of the population as a whole. The notion that we must improve upon our gene pool to counteract a general decline in genetic health and ensure longer and better lives for those carrying genetic disease is old. As an end, it is also indistinguishable from the eugenics of the past. The question is whether the fact that, in this case, genetic improvements are merely allowed as an individual choice, and not state-imposed biopolitics, is sufficient to avoid the moral objections associated with past eugenics, or if it will undermine the notion of equal worth. We will expand on this later.

The third kind of benefit relates directly to possibilities of enhancement: The greatest benefit germline gene editing could have is improving upon humans and accelerating evolution. If germline gene editing, *ex hypothesi*, could improve upon all the qualities that we value most as humans, such as intelligence, memory, and altruism, then this is an opportunity to increase well-being. On consequentialist grounds, this last kind of benefit is, in a sense, the most morally compelling in that it clearly offers the greatest quantitative increase in well-being (if safe and successful). Yet, it is by far the most controversial; not in the least because any presumption of safety and success is mostly speculative and the risks remain largely unknown. Furthermore, any radical changes could turn out to have very different outcomes than expected in the grand scheme of things, and given that they are pervasive (nature-changing), largely irreversible and heritable, there are many reasons to be concerned, even when just assessing the consequences.

The main point here is to highlight that all arguments for germline gene editing based on its prospective benefits largely fit into the logic of value maximization. In turn, it is argued that, provided the gene technology can be made sufficiently safe, if it were the most efficient way to prevent genetic disease, enable parents to have a healthy and genetically related child, improve overall genetic health, and maximize human capacities for well-being, then there are compelling reasons to proceed.

7.2.1 Benefiting Prospective Parents and Future Persons

Most papers restrict the scope of benefits discussed *to treatment and prevention of genetic disease*. Rubeis (2018), for instance, writes, "It is usually agreed upon that the main clinical perspective of editing the human germline is disease." Some genetic diseases depend on a number of interacting genes and are thus less suitable for germline editing. However, when it comes to severe monogenetic diseases, there is a lot of promise in germline editing, which is often considered the main benefit. If we look at the nature of monogenetic diseases such as Huntington's disease or sickle cell anemia and the associated suffering, and consider the parents whose genetic predispositions prevent them from having a child, then the benefits of germline editing do seem compelling. The number of individuals that would benefit from such intervention could also be considerable. NASEM, for instance, suggests the following in their 2017 report:

> Thousands of genetically inherited diseases are caused by mutations in single genes. While individually, many of these genetically inherited diseases are rare, collectively they affect a sizable fraction of the population (about 5–7%). The emotional, finan-cial, and other burdens on individual families that result from transmission of such

serious genetic disease can be considerable, and for some families could potentially be alleviated by heritable editing. (NASEM, 2017, p. 111)

This suggests that there are substantial benefits to be gained here, and unnecessary suffering could be avoided. The suffering with each of these diseases is corroborated by what the Nuffield Council writes in their 2018 report:

> Inherited genetic conditions can represent significant burdens to many of those who are affected by them, whether directly or as family members. These burdens include physical, psychological and social impacts and privations as well as financial costs. These factors may be compounded, increasing the risk of co-morbidities, and the economic impact and socio-economic disadvantage of families with certain genetic conditions can be compounded through successive generations. (Nuffield, 2018, p. 17)

Furthermore, in many cases the only treatment of monogenetic disorders are relief of symptoms and palliative care (NASEM, 2018, p. 18). Sugarman (2015) writes, "germline editing might be the only means of treating genetic diseases, which are otherwise fatal in utero." For cancers and genetic disruptions of biological systems, other treatments may be available, including somatic gene therapy in some cases. Thus, considering both the suffering caused by genetic disease and the prospective benefits of germline editing, and setting risk and safety concerns aside, there seem to be good grounds for the claim that germline editing would overall be a highly beneficial choice.[4]

Thus far, these points taken together do seem to provide a compelling case for the benefits of germline editing. How compelling it is, however, depends on how beneficial and risky *the alternatives* are. If they could achieve the same ends with lower risk, they would be morally preferable to germline editing (Nuffield, 2018, p. 20 ff.). What counts as the relevant alternatives to consider depends on how the question is framed. If we only consider options that can provide a genetically related and healthy child, this will narrow the number of options down to two: germline gene editing and IVF with PGD and embryo selection. In comparison, Baylis mentions, in addition to PGD and embryo selection, the following alternatives: adoption; foster parenting; "other parenting arrangements"; and IVF using donor egg, sperm or embryos (Baylis, 2019, p. 29).

However, if we restrict the options to PGD and germline editing, which one is morally preferable? According to Ranisch, all positions on whether germline

---

[4] "Overall" most beneficial here implies that it is most beneficial when taking all affected parties into account, either as an average or a total; it does not refer to overall as the all-things-considered net balance when taking safety, risks and benefits into account.

editing is morally preferable to PGD and selective abortion can be found in the literature: that it is morally preferable, morally equal, and morally inferior (Ranisch, 2020, p. 62).

The notion that germline gene editing is the most efficient way to treat and prevent genetic disease, however, meets two fundamental challenges. First, it is far from clear that germline gene editing constitutes a case of treatment, or even a case of preventing disease, in the individual case. Second, it is far from clear what moral significance to afford the preference of having a genetically related child. Both of these points have been raised in the literature, and we will review them both briefly in the next two sections. Here, we must also add that, at least, the first generation of germline edited children will undergo, to some extent, an "unproven method" rather than a clinical trial, in that safe options exist for therapeutic ends (Primc, 2018, p. 104).

7.2.2   Neither Treatment nor Prevention

It is not clear that germline editing is *a case of treatment* in the ordinary sense of a person suffering from a disease being offered treatment of that same disease. The Nuffield Council has argued that, in fact, germline gene editing is neither a case of treatment nor prevention (Nuffield, 2018, p. 22 f., p. 25). They wrote the following in their 2016 report on genome editing (also quoted in Nuffield, 2018, p. 22 f.):

> Genome editing is not straightforwardly therapeutic in the way that gene therapy is therapeutic, treating an existing patient who is affected by an unwelcome condition; nor is it preventative in the way that some public health measures are preventative by addressing an imminent risk, since the risk itself can be avoided by not conceiving children. On the other hand, it is therapeutic, in the sense that it potentially overcomes infertility (albeit that the infertility is voluntary, a hard choice among an undesirable set of options) and it is preventative in that, taking the decision to reproduce as given (or, at least, one that a couple it entitled to make and should not be prevented from making), it may prevent any child they have being born with a serious or life-limiting disability.

Normally, when we talk about "treatment," it usually refers to some existing patient with an existing medical condition being cured or relieved from this condition by intervention. However, in the case of germline gene editing, there is neither a patient suffering from a disease nor a disease. It thus does not seem to be a case of medical treatment in the usual sense.[5] Furthermore, when we talk about "prevention," it usually refers to some medical condition that would have occurred had we not prevented it. But, again, there is no existing patient who is bound to suffer any disease without the editing. The risk for the medical conditions could equally have been "prevented" by not having a genetically related child, among other options. Thus, it seems that what germline editing provides is less of a treatment for disease than a remedy for having a genetically related child for parents who are at risk of passing on serious genetic disease.

7.2.3 A Genetically Related Child

The possible benefits of germline editing are largely premised on the significance of having *a genetically related and healthy child*.[6] There are undoubtedly numerous couples who have a strong preference and desire for a genetically related

---

[5] Gyngell and Savulescu (2016, p. 501), by contrast, reason that germline editing, as opposed to genetic selection, could actually cure a person from disease who would otherwise be born with it. They write, "Finally, genetic selection replaces one individual with a disease with a healthy individual. It does not benefit those with disease. Its benefits are impersonal. GGE on the other hand could provide benefits to individuals who would otherwise be born with genetic disorders—it could cure their disorders." In the case of somatic editing of an embryo or child this seems to be the case, but germline editing will occur before there is a person in any real sense. Thus, although there is not a choice of a healthy embryo over an unhealthy embryo, but a "correction" or "treatment" of one embryo, it is not clear that there is any person who benefits here. The reason for this pertains to when such editing must occur, namely prior to implantation and there being a pregnancy or a person. This means that there is no alternative scenario when the same embryo would have been carried to term but remained unedited. It is either the case that the parents know that they risk giving birth to a child with serious genetic disease and decide that the risk is too high to procreate naturally, or they do not know or decide this. Should they decide that the risk is too high, they would only have a genetically related child with that risk removed: i.e., through PGD and embryo selection, in which case an unhealthy embryo would not be selected, or through germline editing, in which case an unhealthy embryo could be edited. Should they not know or decide that the risk was too great to procreate naturally, they would presumably procreate naturally (if at all), but then the chances that any embryo would be exactly the same as the one that was edited in the other scenario are extremely low, given the number of sperms. This means that it is highly unlikely that the embryo to be edited would have existed without the decision to edit it. It thus seems that, just as in the case of selection, the future child benefits in being given the gift of life and being born, but not such that they were cured of something they would otherwise have suffered.

[6] The terminology in the debate is about "genetic relatedness." This is a bit simplified. More accurate would be to define this as the desire for a child that is both ii) genetically related AND ii) without the inheritable genetic condition that one or both parents are carriers of.

child. The question is how morally weighty such a preference is. It could gain moral weight in one of two ways; it could be the case that couples *have a right to a genetically related child* (as part of their reproductive rights and right to reproductive autonomy), or it could be the case that fulfilling such a preference *increases overall well-being* in the world more than any alternative course of action. The first would be an argument based on permissibility logic, while the latter is based on value maximization logic.

Most writers either simply take this preference as a given or appeal to the autonomy/liberty-based rights of parents. However, as the Nuffield Council (2018) has pointed out, there is a difference between *negative rights* (that no one has a right to interfere in procreative choices) and *positive or entitlement rights* (that one has an entitlement to aid and assistance, having a particular kind of technology available to one).[7] Negative rights are rights where others must refrain from doing something to the rights holder. Positive rights are entitlements that rights holders have that others are obliged to fulfill. For instance, a child has a negative right not to be harmed or exploited, but a positive right to food, shelter, emotional support, and education. The point, here, is that even if parents have a negative right to make their own autonomous procreative decisions and pursue a genetically related child if the legal options available enable this, there is no government obligation to provide such options if they do not exist. Had it been a positive right to be able to have a genetically related child, genetic relatedness would have outweighed the alternatives that would not allow for this, and the very fact that some couples cannot use PGD as an alternative would make germline gene editing morally right.

It could be worth asking to what extent being genetically related to one's child or one's parents is likely to increase well-being and on what grounds. Are there any good reasons to believe that *having a genetically related* child (in cases where this would involve germline editing) would promote happiness to a greater degree than having a genetically unrelated child (through adoption or other means)? Of

---

To describe this merely as a desire for "genetic relatedness" ignores the tension between that desire and the genetic diseases that such relations would risk to pass on to the child. To describe it as a desire as for both genetic relatedness and healthy, is too broad: since health in this context relates to the particular genetic conditions that would be strong enough reasons not to have a genetically related child. The following, "genetic relatedness" is a short-hand for the desire to have a genetically related child for prospective parents who would not want to pass on some genetic disease they are carriers of.

[7] On a rights-based framework, some interests are significant enough to oblige others to either not interfere with their pursuit of those interests (i.e., negative rights or liberties) or to provide them (i.e., positive/claim rights or entitlements).

course, given the strength of such a parental preference, at least the parents' well-being could viably be expected increase.

That said, it is not uncommon that we misjudge how we will, in fact, react to some future scenario when we try to predict it. The fact that parents *now* believe that they would be much happier with a genetically related child need not preclude that they would also be very happy with a genetically unrelated child. There is no lack of examples, at least not anecdotally, of parents who are happy to parent adopted children, foster children, or children from extended family arrangements, so it certainly seems possible to be a happy parent to non-biological child (Westerlund, 2004). It could, of course, be that some parents have such a strong preference for a genetically related child that they could not possibly be happy in any other way. That does not necessarily afford this preference significant moral weight if the preferences of others are to be considered as well, given that even on value maximization logic, it is always the total amount of well-being that matters and not just well-being for those most directly affected. In this case, it means that there must not be any loss in well-being that is greater than the gain.

Does it benefit a child to be genetically related in any significant way? Perhaps so, given the opinions of some donor-conceived persons. Some of these have been very critical towards egg and sperm donations, arguing, among other things, that it might have a negative impact on "the child's psychological development and its everyday sense of identity" (Primc, 2018, p. 105). In a culture where genetic relatedness is greatly valued, this could suggest that future edited persons might also benefit from being genetically related to their parents.

Another interesting aspect is *how stable* such preferences are. The Nuffield Council (2018, p. 61) writes, "What we can conclude is that the significance of genetic relatedness varies among people, between cultures and perhaps also over time and in response to personal experience." This might suggest that many couples who now think that their well-being is dependent on having a genetically related child might be equally happy having a genetically unrelated child when taking into account the IVF processes and concerns about risks to their child, and so forth. We could also imagine a future scenario when the worth attached to genetic relatedness was not considered as important as it is now, and, consequently, that the value of the future offspring being genetically related did not outweigh the risks at all.

Let us imagine a future scenario where genetic relatedness has lost its value. In such a scenario, should a person be born with significant risks as a result of germline gene editing and the only rationale for such editing was the parental desire for a genetically related child, then the parental desire would not justify the risks. We could further complicate this scenario to make the point even starker. Imagine that in the morality of the future, it was considered a grave wrong that there were children not cared for by anyone as their parents. In such a scenario, having been born as a result of a risky technology only so that one's parents could have genetically related children instead of caring for those already in need of a parent, could, if we allow a bit of speculation, perhaps become something of a stigma, like being born the heir of riches built on slave trade.

In any case, in order to apply the value maximization logic fully, we cannot look at the increased well-being of the parents or their children only; what matters is whether *the world as a whole*, or the sum total of those it affects, directly or indirectly, in terms of well-being, is made worse or better.[8] Value maximization logic as part of a consequentialist moral theory would require something more than merely maximizing the well-being of parents (and their prospective children): it is what creates *the most benefit in total (or on average).*[9] In other words, it is the totality of well-being achieved, not the optimal treatment of a particular patient that is often the focus of the medical ethical context, that determines what one ought and ought not to do. From this perspective, it is irrelevant *who* benefits.

This means that if one person who now suffers is relieved from that suffering and another person who previously did not suffer now comes to suffer to the same extent as the first one did, nothing is lost or gained. This also holds if one person who suffered at some unit of say -10 is relieved from that suffering,

---

[8] Here, let us point to an interesting contradiction. It cannot both be argued that germline editing ought to be promoted on the grounds of the value of similarity between parents and children and at the same time that we ought to promote human enhancement in order to speed up human evolution and the arrival of the trans- and posthuman. If anything would jeopardize the likeness value, it would be if the offspring belonged to a different species or had non-human properties. It seems that either the case for germline editing is weak (because the interest in a genetically related child is not morally significant)—if so, we could still argue that human enhancement is important—or, we could argue that likeness between parents is very important, but then it seems that we would have strong reasons to not slip into enhancement. And should germline editing risk sliding down the slope to enhancement, then this might be reason enough not to allow germline editing even for medical reasons in order to protect the likeness between parents and their offspring in the future.

[9] In fact, this is one of the important differences between standard versions of deontological and consequentialist theories and their respective inherent logic: doing what will contribute to the most happiness or the least suffering, or reach above some kind of threshold for moral duty or remain on the right side of what is permissible. Although, there are deviations to this general trend; for instance, some consequentialist theories point to sufficiency instead of maximization. Maximization has been the dominant idea in the consequentialist framework, and for this reason, an objection raised against consequentialism is that it is too demanding. A counter-argument has also been raised that deontology is too demanding (see Ashford, 2003).

and instead ten other people begin to suffer at the unit of −1. Again, nothing is gained or lost. Since the total amount of suffering is exactly the same, they are, on this logic, morally on a par.[10] Should it be the case that the excess happiness that prospective parents would experience by having a genetically related child (as opposed to adopting one) is not greater than the weight of a longer wait for adoption of children in need of new caretakers, then it would not be morally right, even from a well-being perspective.

Perhaps, genetic relatedness is of moral relevance simply because it seems to be vital to people; therefore, at least all else equal, it is something we should try to respect. This seems to be the position the Nuffield Council (2018). After having noted that "While it is clear that many people desire to have genetically related children, it is hard to demonstrate that having genetically related children, or even having children at all, is a good in itself" (Nuffield, 2018, p. 63). They continue to argue that "[t]his may be beside the point" for following reasons:

> In spite of attempts to demonstrate both that people should and should not have children—or have/not have them in certain circumstances—the complex motivations that people express seem rarely to be governed (or governable) by theoretical rationality. We may nevertheless have good reasons to respect them, and those reasons may not be that they are good desires, but that they are the desires of people for whom we should, a priori, have respect. (Nuffield, 2018, p. 63)

In summary, even if the value attached to genetic relatedness is undoubtedly vital for many prospective parents, at least in our time and culture, this desire does not directly translate into a moral value or something of such moral significance that it outweighs the risks. Nevertheless, the fact that it is considered important to many may still count for something.

7.2.4 Benefiting the Population

If the previous benefit argument focused on the benefits for the small family unit—for prospective parents, and possibly their prospective child, in terms of ensuring a healthy and genetically related offspring—the next argument focuses on the medical gains from a wider perspective. Given that germline editing can remove the heritable genetic risks for certain diseases, we are not just "curing"

---

[10] This is in sharp contrast to other moral theories, such as Scanlonian contractualism, that define morality in terms of what we may and may not do to individuals, and obligations that we owe each person affected (Scanlon, 1998).

a single patient but a whole lineage, and by extension, we would improve the overall genetic health in the whole population this way. "Using GGE to remove all disease-causing genes from an embryo will lower the total frequency of disease-causing genes in the gene pool, and therefore the incidence of such diseases in the future generations" (Gyngell et al., 2017, p. 501; see also Powell, 2015).

In 1992 already, Munson and Davis wrote, "If germ-line therapy were possible, practical, and widely employed, hundreds of genetic diseases might be eliminated from families." They continued, "Horrible diseases like Lesch-Nyhan, PKU, and Tay-Sachs would simply disappear as a nightmarish heritage in certain family lines." Munson and Davis also suggested that some "genes may cause more severe forms of a disease in succeeding generations" (Munson & Davis, 1992, p. 139). More recently, Powell (2015) has argued for the position that there is a *pro tanto* moral imperative to employ germline gene therapy in order to sustain current levels of genetic health (p. 670 f.). According to him, germline editing could be used as a means to combat a decline in genetic health and the cost of continuous medical somatic intervention (p. 681). He writes:

> Conventional medical intervention is often touted as less risky than germline modification because (inter alia) any harmful consequences of the intervention will be limited to the intervenee and not transmitted to the next generation. The flip side, however, is that if an undesirable trait is genetically heritable, then ameliorate modifications will be required on behalf of all descendants who express the trait, in perpetuity. In contrast, once the germline has been repaired, the remarkably accurate machinery of DNA replication, repair, and expression will do all of the intergenerational work for us, free of charge! The point is that we should not take our genes and the medical services they provide for granted. (Powell, 2015, p. 679)

The risks to consider are thus not only or even primarily those that follow from germline intervention, but rather those that follow from *not* intervening: the decline in genetic health and the cost of continuous medical somatic intervention (Powell, 2015, p. 681; see also Koplin et al., 2019). There is thus a *prima facie* duty (but not an all-things-considered duty) to work towards germline engineering, according to Powell. However, Koplin et al. argue that this makes it an "open question" as to whether it would be more precautionary to proceed with GGE or to refrain from doing so, since the risks on both sides seem largely symmetrical, with worst-case scenarios on either side (Koplin et al., 2019, p. 58).

Powell (2015) presents his argument for enhancement to maintain current levels of genetic health as a kind of middle ground position between enhancement for improved human capacities (beyond the species' typical functioning) and medical treatment, given that there is still enhancement, but only to the point of current normal functioning (at least in the first instance). There are strong arguments for this position, Powell claims, given that the human gene pool will otherwise decline due to the success of medicine in affording long reproductive lives, even with genetic weakness. Koplin et al. (2019) add two indirect consequences to this: increased medical costs and vulnerability due to increased dependence on medical technology.

This concern is, of course, not new. For instance, in the classic *Fabricated Man* (1970), Ramsey described the problem as conceived by his contemporary geneticists as follows:

> It is incumbent upon me, however, to describe in summary fashion mankind's problematic genetic situation as this is understood by certain contemporary geneticists. This would not be so bad if from generation to generation a more or less stable pool of genes were in passage, with its particular balance of physical, mental and emotional strengths or defects. The fact is, however, that in addition to the load of genetic deficiency from the previous generation, one out of every five persons now living (twenty percent) bears a deleterious mutation that has arisen with him and which he will pass on to or through any offspring he may have. The quality of human beings to be born could be maintained at its present levels if, and only if, twenty percent of us, become genetically extinct, either by failing to reach reproductive age or by not having children. The fact is that, because of our technical and medical competence and our proper concern for persons now alive, we are enabling people to reach the age of reproduction, and to reproduce when they do, in greater numbers than would have been the case in former ages. (Ramsey, 1970, p. 2 f.)

Gyngell et al. (2019, p. 521) add a *justice* twist to the above argument. They argue that "there is a strong moral imperative to develop HGE [heritable genome editing] as a matter of intergenerational justice." This argument draws on two premises. The first is a version of the deterioration of the genetic baseline argument above. "Modern medicine is removing selection pressures that humans have historically been subjected to. This is increasing the rate of random mutations accumulating in the genome and poses a risk to future generations" (Gyngell et al., 2019, p. 521). Thus, in a few generations, one can expect a "genetic deterioration in the baseline human condition" (Lynch, 2016, cited in Gyngell et al., 2019, p. 521). After listing examples such as shortsightedness, deafness, blood pressure problems and assisted reproduction, they argue that "In future generations, nearly all people may be reliant on technologies" for "basic functions" and that "society will become burdened by spiraling health costs" (Gyngell et al., 2019, p. 521). The second premise is an intergenerational justice argument: It would be *unjust* to let future generations suffer from poor genetic circumstances that could be avoided. We owe it to future generations to ensure that they can enjoy the same genetic starting positions as us. "Fortunately, there is a straightforward compensatory action—developing HGE [heritable genome editing]" (p. 522).[11]

Some argue that there are, in fact, significant risks to consider by *not* pursuing germline editing (Powell, 2015; Koplin et al., 2019). Koplin et al. argues that we could expect significant increase in both medical costs and increased reliance on medical technology in the future should we not opt for germline gene editing. The former would redirect resources from where they are better spent, the latter would increase vulnerability in cases of various kinds of catastrophes, they argue (Koplin et al., 2019, p. 58). They therefore conclude that there are risks on both sides of the matter; that is, editing the germline and not editing the germline, and these risks are "largely symmetrical." Thus, it is unclear which course of action is, in fact, the safer one and which course of action the precautionary principle would support (Koplin et al., 2019, p. 58). This uncertainty is related to what we know and do not know, and is thus something that may be overcome with time as we learn more.

However, the goal of increasing overall genetic health may not go according to plan. Baylis (2019, p. 92 f.) argues that widespread germline editing could prove harmful to the gene pool either by adding harmful genes, replacing certain bad genes with others, or reducing genetic diversity. Such decreased diversity could increase the risk of genetic disease unless, "at the same time, there was widespread introduction of novel designer synthetic genes catering to idiosyncratic choices." (Baylis, 2019, p. 92 f.)

7.3   Discussion

In this chapter, we examined various arguments for and against germline editing based on its potential consequences. The first of these arguments is based on concerns about the safety of the technology itself. If there is consensus about anything in this debate, it seems to be, as mentioned earlier, that we ought not to edit the germline until the technology is sufficiently precise, efficient, and safe, which is not currently the case.

Beyond this, there is a wide scope for very different kinds of moral conclusions based on consequences. In order to draw any conclusions at all, there are

---

[11] Although, earlier in the same paper, they suggest that "which intervention we ought to choose—modifying the biological, psychological, social or natural environment—depends on the costs and benefits of the particular interventions, and relevant moral values" (Gyngell et al., 2019, p. 522).

four relevant factors: *the framing* of the moral situation and the options and consequences, as well as the time frame for relevant consequences; *the moral logic* one departs from and to what extent the consequences alone are understood to settle the moral issue; *the assessment of the nature and value* of the possible consequences of germline editing; and lastly, the degree to which we can presume to have *reliable knowledge* of the above to make informed decisions.

To draw any moral conclusion based on consequences, we must have some idea about what consequences to consider, both in terms of how far into the future the relevant consequences extend and how indirect those consequences can be. Furthermore, we need to be able to say something about how the action and its consequences compare to other alternative courses of action, including no action at all. This means that we must also have some idea about what these alternative actions are and how positive or negative their expected consequences are.

In short, the consequences of germline editing differ greatly depending on how the matter is framed. The relevant consequences and alternatives will differ greatly, should we frame it as a question of a private choice in the context of IVF, as a policy decision about population health, or as a democratic decision of a global nature that could determine the social relations and dynamics of future societies. The alternatives for addressing population health are not the same as those that can enable a couple to have a genetically related child. Furthermore, the full scope of options is not likely to be considered in most cases. For instance, if one considers germline editing primarily as a medical matter framed by the doctor–patient perspective with the addition of parental autonomy and a desire for a genetically related child as given values, then this way of framing the ethical matter limits the options to those of germline editing and PGD. Thus, for those cases where PGD is not an option, germline editing would not just be the only available option, but also the morally preferred option. However, the robustness of such a conclusion is weak; it depends on the soundness of the original framing. The overall balance of consequences that supports that conclusion could lean the other way and support a different conclusion with the addition of other kinds of concerns, such as indirect suffering or social costs. Perhaps fewer children in need of adoptive or foster parents could find new homes if germline editing would offer genetically related offspring to parents who carry genetic disease. Perhaps, inevitable slippery slopes and increased intolerance for difference would have great negative effects for those currently living with various kinds of genetic diseases and functional variations. Thus, any conclusion based on consequences alone will depend on how narrow and how broadly one casts the net.

Furthermore, the moral weight of consequences differs between the different kinds of moral logic discussed earlier. All moral logic attaches some weight to potential outcomes. It is worth noting that some of the strongest arguments against germline editing, in general or for a particular purpose, as well as the strongest arguments for germline editing, are based on consequences. It is important to note two things here. First, the value promotion logic allows consequences to fully determine the moral conclusions. We referred to this as the Strong Consequence Claim in the introduction to this chapter. On this view, that which brings about most value as a consequence is the right thing to do. Second, almost all of the arguments for germline editing, from the more narrowly drawn medical or IVF-based arguments to the more radical arguments that lean towards enhancement or population-wide benefits, are heavily based on the value maximization logic. Some combine these arguments with liberalism (as we shall see in the next chapter) to some extent.

The Strong Consequence Claim takes consequences to be the decisive moral factor. In other words, there is nothing beyond consequences that could decide what is morally right or wrong. What disappears, then, are various moral principles that draw lines in a moral space not reducible to an increase or decrease of overall benefits or harm, but whether autonomy, liberty, human rights, justice, fairness, reciprocity, dignity, and the like are promoted or undermined.[12] Furthermore, what also disappears are changes that are neither increases nor decreases, but of a more qualitative kind that instantiate or work towards particular ideals. According to value maximization logic, the right moral conclusion ought to follow from the most accurate calculation we can make of all the relevant positive and negative outcomes.

Again, how good or bad the consequences are, depends on *the measure for such goodness or badness* and on what constitutes a benefit or a drawback, respectively. Furthermore, at least from a value maximization perspective, different benefits need to be translated into the same currency or unit of measurement so that we can compare their relative "size" and weight. However, beyond very basic assumptions about benefits and drawbacks, the moral issues are too complex to determine what is and what is not an all-things-considered improvement. For example, it seems reasonable to assume that, all else equal, it would be an improvement if a childless couple who desired a genetically related child were able to fulfill such a desire. Similarly, it seems reasonable to assume that, that all else equal, it would be a drawback to be born with a severe genetic disease that caused a lot of suffering and shortened one's life expectancy. However,

---

[12] We have used the term "overall" benefit or harm here to highlight that it is not meant to be measured on an individual level but as an average or a total. Both views are defended in the consequentialism literature.

even these kinds of seemingly plausible assumptions have been questioned. For example, the presumption that being born genetically "normal" would be an indisputable benefit, has been questioned by members of the disability community. For example, Sufian and Garland-Thomson (2021) argue that the kinds of attitudes that a germline gene editing practice would underscore would make life much more difficult for people with functional variations (see also Garland-Thomson, 2019, 2020). Abstract philosophical reasoning occasionally assumes that there are unambiguous concepts of a "life not worth living." However, what is easy in hypothetical cases often becomes extremely difficult in practice. Additionally, in any actual scenario where basic and plausible assumptions about benefits and harms may hold true, such benefits and harms could be outweighed by other kinds of harms and benefits pertinent to the situation.

Lastly, drawing any kind of reliable conclusion based on the comparative advantages of overall consequences is *epistemically demanding*. In other words, to know what is morally best, we must know many things with a sufficient degree of certainty. This problem becomes particularly challenging for value maximization logic, given that in order to do the right thing, we must do *the best* thing; that is, the action that increases value *the most*. To know which action that would be, we must know: (a) what the available options are; (b) what the relevant outcomes for each option are and how probable they are; (c) what the relevant side effects and unwanted consequences are and how likely they are; and (d) how good or bad each of those potential outcomes would be. For new and emerging technologies adopted on a large scale, it may be impossible to reliably predict all consequences and their impact. In the context of germline editing, we also need to add the fact that many of the consequences may only be known after several generations. This raises serious epistemic concerns. Any conclusion to the effect that the benefits will be such and such and the negative consequences such and such, and hence the benefits outweigh the risks, will be premature unless we know with sufficient certainty that we are not overlooking whole sets of potential consequences that could turn that balance on its head, and that we are not overlooking superior alternatives. Such alternatives may not exist yet, but could tip the balance later.

Many of the techno-optimists count on the risks being overcome and the benefits being unequivocally positive, to such an extent as to tip the balance. One kind of argument is to compare the potential risks with those of previous reproductive technologies that were later proven safe and ultimately became popular (Harris, 2015; Charo, 2020). Here, the expectation is that germline editing will also prove to be safe and popular once its benefits have been demonstrated. Another kind of argument is to compare the risks of harm of germline editing with the risks of harm associated with *not pursuing* germline editing, particularly risks arising from increased dependency on medicine due to a deteriorating gene pool, increased medical costs, and possible loss of opportunity in terms of improved genetic health and capacity (Koplin et al., 2019). They argue that it is an open question whether the precautionary principle would support or oppose germline editing with the aim of improving the population's genetic health, on the assumption that there are risks on both sides: risks from using the technology and risks from foregoing the benefits, as well as vulnerabilities from increased dependence on medical remedies for genetic ailments (Koplin et al., 2019).

However, before we start measuring risks against benefits and draw moral conclusions based on the overall balance, we need to consider to what degree epistemic prerequisites for drawing such conclusions are satisfied. We need to be sufficiently certain that we are not underestimating the likelihood, frequency, or severity of the potential risks or overlooking certain risks or consequences entirely. It has been argued that we ought to assess the risks of pursuing germline editing against those of not pursing germline editing, and that the risks of either course of action are equally problematic (in that both are expected to cause harm). However, epistemically they are not on a par. We know of the expected benefits; indeed, these are what motivated the development of the technology in the first place and what they are tested for. The broader impact on norms and values remains speculation. It might be that all such concerns are overblown; however, we do not know this. By contrast, the benefits are less likely to have been underestimated. Thus, we are asked to weigh anticipated and studied benefits up against unknown consequences and conclude that the balance leans in favor of the former. We can see that it makes sense from this perspective to brush off arguments about harmful future outcomes of a social kind as mere speculation (which, indeed, they are and cannot be much else at this point): they do seem more abstract and improbable than the more realistic benefits much closer at hand. This need not indicate that the estimated benefits will be as anticipated, or that the negative outcomes will not outweigh the benefits—whether they are ultimately what we feared, entirely different, or something in between (see Hayenhjelm 2024, for discussion).

We need to be sufficiently certain that the benefits we count on will be as beneficial and likely to occur as we predict them to be. When it comes to well-established technologies, these kinds of epistemic risks are relatively small: if it has been in use long enough, it will most likely not give rise to unexpected consequences, and the known consequences are well-studied. However, when it comes to new technologies, new applications of technology, or potentially pervasive societal and cultural effects, these epistemic risks are likely to be substantive. This may mean that it will not be possible to ensure "safe and efficient" germline inter-vention through biological (whether in the laboratory or clinic) research alone. Such research could inform us about the technical safety (off-target risks, risks for mosaicism, and so on), but not about psychological, political, and social con-sequences—or even multigenerational medical consequences. It cannot tell us whether eugenics programs will arise or whether the child–parent relationship will change due to enhancement. If the degree of unknown risks is large, then we might not have an adequate level of preparation for negative consequences or developed strategies to counteract them.

Thus far, we have pointed out difficulties for any kind of conclusion based on consequences alone. Does this mean that we cannot say anything about where a consequences-based calculus might land when it comes to germline editing?

As long as the technology is not safe to subject a person to, it does not seem morally responsible to subject anyone to it. The differences arise once we set that concern aside and ask what the moral concern would be *on the assumption that it should become sufficiently safe,* assuming that this is possible, and that we at some point would have good reason to believe it to be safe. From the Technical View, this safety aspect concludes the matter: if it is safe, then there is nothing more to be concerned about. However, the Technical View constitutes a greatly reduced version of value promotion, in that it only takes one value (safety or lack thereof) into account, almost as a side-constraint, in a pursuit of value (medical or procreative intervention motivated by health) as an uncontroversial given.

From a more comprehensive view of value promotion logic, safety can only be one part of the matter. Equally important, or even more so, is the potential to increase well-being or overall value. The morality of germline editing, here, depends on how much well-being or value it could be expected to create and how big the net increase would be after any expected harm or risk of harm is subtracted. The range of potential benefit is impressive in scope. At the one end, we have benefits for parents carrying genetic disease being able to choose to have a genetically related child who does not carry a genetic disease over PGD, adoption or other options, such as not having a child. This includes benefits for the child born with edited genes and the benefit of being born without a genetic disease or the risk of developing a disease later in life, and without having to depend on somatic gene therapy or other treatment, or being concerned about passing the condition on to their offspring. It also includes the benefit of having been born at all rather than having not been selected as an embryo. It includes the possibilities of removing the genetic prerequisites for various kinds of medical harm or suffering. On a societal level, it includes financial gains from saving on treatment for genetic disease, as well as overall improved genetic health, which has all kinds of societal knock-on effects. It is not unlikely that this could collectively increase productivity and material welfare, leading to greater resources that could be spent on those that require medical treatments for ailments. From this perspective, the benefits seem quite tangible, and societal norms, like cultural concerns, are always shifting, and could be influenced to ensure a just and fair society—but with better genes.

Once we add all kinds of enhancement possibilities to this, the potential magnitude and scope of possible benefits become significantly greater. So much so that there is some ground for arguments that such benefits would be so decisive that they would swing the balance greatly in favor of using such techniques once one accepts the value maximization logic. If we, for instance, could add 15 years to our overall lifespan, globally and equally, and ensure good health until the end of our lives, then it would be hard to argue that this would not benefit humanity as a whole.

However, just as safety does not settle the matter, neither do benefits or well-being. We must take both direct and indirect negative outcomes into account as well. Side effects of the technology would be direct negative consequences. This includes off-target effects or unwanted on-target mutations, as well as other unintended outcomes due to the multiple functions of genes. We could imagine something like an increase of certain kinds of cancer, should the technology not be as safe as presumed. We also need to consider additional "costs" that could come with a germline intervention, such as increased medical monitoring and check-ups if medical uncertainties linger. Although, such costs would presumably subsume after the first generation or so. There could be other kinds of drawbacks that reveal themselves later, such as increased vulnerabilities or unexpected reactions to other interventions or medicines. Such drawbacks are, however, likely to affect only the first generations and might cease to be an issue of concern once knowledge improves. Thus, if we could conclude at some point that the technology would be safe enough, then the direct negative consequences may be fully manageable.

It is worth pointing out that, should a first generation of genetically edited individuals come to harm, this might be heavily outweighed by all the generations they would have paved the way for; and, thus, when adding up all the benefits and risks over all future generations, it could tip the balance in the favor of germline editing, even at the cost of a guinea pig generation. The same would hold for a generation of currently existing individuals with disability suffering from discrimination from being the last generation with such functional variations. From a value maximization perspective, the only moral question is whether the overall outcome in the end is better than the alternatives. These alternatives need not use germline editing at all; they could, for instance, include further development of the technology with plans to have an even stronger case two generations into the future with only clinical tests until then. According to permissibility logic, however, consequences are not the only thing to consider, and it may be impermissible to use one generation as a means for the benefit of another: Who reaps the benefits and who is faced with risks matter, and there are certain things we must not do to others regardless of how beneficial it may be overall.

The indirect consequences are probably more worrisome and harder to predict, as they depend on much more than the technology itself. These indirect consequences are those of norm-shifting and attitude changes to difference, diversity, disability, justice and access to "good genes" as a token of privilege, medicalization of reproduction, and general societal changes that would create and solidify an unjust society.

Beyond matters of safety and societal effects in terms of injustice, intolerance, and shifts in norms, the moral question seems largely to depend on two things: slippery slopes to more serious outcomes and the degree of uncertainty and epistemic unknowns involved. That said, safety is not a small matter, nor is injustice, intolerance, or shifts in norms. However, should the technology prove to be safe and in line with justice, fairness, and tolerance for difference, and rolled out together with a firm global stance against more experimental applications, and a limit to our practices such that the risks imposed would not exceed what we could repair, then there does not seem to be much ground for objection to germline editing for medical and reproductive purposes or the elimination of uncontroversially bad genetic disadvantages. The issue is, of course, that it is hard to guarantee that our interventions would not affect values and norms and consequently justice in some way. It is also unclear to what extent we can reach an agreement on what kinds of genetic variations could be considered unwanted and thus eliminated without controversy. However, this depends on how narrow or broad the set of possible germline interventions are. Then again, morality may not be limited to a calculation of consequences, but rather ideals worth pursuing along lines of permissibility and obligations.

In this chapter, we have examined various arguments on the possible consequences of germline editing and, to some extent, genetic enhancement. Although there are arguments both for and against germline editing, *the matter of time* is essential. Many of the least controversial benefits lie in a future realistically very close to our own. We can thus easily imagine and realistically predict some of these benefits, such as preventing various cases of genetic disease. By contrast, many of the more serious moral concerns are based on what might happen when the technology is applied on a broad scale in the distant future and has consequences that we cannot yet foresee. There is thus an obvious asymmetry when it comes to the kinds of arguments that could be brought forward. Not surprisingly, many of the concerns about future consequences are viewed as speculative, emotional, vague, and unrealistic by optimists. It seems improbable to oppose an obviously beneficial technology based on what might occur in the distant future. It seems irresponsible to let people suffer now because of what could possibly hurt others in the distant future. Furthermore, the risks that lie in the near future seem more realistic and thereby easier to address with proper research, responsibility, regulation, and control.

Thus, from one perspective, there are valid risks and benefits in the near term. Furthermore, the near-term risks may be controllable and the benefits would apply to many generations beyond our own. From this, there may appear to be a certain arrogance: some waive simplistic, unconvincing arguments based on fear and speculation for realistic propositions of great gain. But just because something is in the distant future and hard to imagine, and all such imaginings are speculative, does not mean that it does not warrant concern, even if we may only know the particulars much later on. Thus, there is an obvious epistemic asymmetry when it comes to near-future risks and benefits that we are already well-acquainted with, and distant-future risks and benefits that we are not yet acquainted with. We will return to the topic of risk and worst-case scenarios in Chap. 9.

Enhancement Arguments

8

In this chapter, we will continue to analyze consequence arguments for and against germline editing, with the focus on more speculative kinds of interventions that go beyond the prevention of disease and seek to *improve* the genetic prospects of individuals and humanity as a whole. Many of the core arguments in the debate on enhancement predate, and are thus not specific to, germline gene editing and CRISPR, but the main concerns and hopes are largely the same. Using germline editing for enhancement purposes significantly raises the stakes: the potential gains are much greater, as are risks and the things we could stand to lose.

8.1   Improving the Human Gene Pool

Germline gene editing might enable us to prevent genetic disease and improve the overall state of the population's genetic health. But it could also probably be used to "improve" upon our genetic heritage and add traits or seek to extend existing human limits. Or, as Baylis (2019, p. 87) sums it up, "The idea is that, in the future, this technology could be used to correct 'bad' versions of a gene, introduce 'good' versions of a gene, or add new 'good' genes—as a way of increasing the prevalence of desirable traits, and reducing the prevalence of undesirable traits." Some scholars hope to employ germline gene editing, not just to maintain current levels of genetic health, but to *improve* upon the capacities of humanity. Germline editing, then, is viewed as a way to eventually control evolution. Harris (2015), for instance, argues that compared to natural evolution, technological enhancement is much more superior, since natural evolution is both slow and

© The Author(s) 2025   153
M. Hayenhjelm and C. Nordlund, *The Risks and Ethics of Human Gene Editing*,
Technikzukünfte, Wissenschaft und Gesellschaft / Futures of Technology, Science
and Society, https://doi.org/10.1007/978-3-658-46979-5_8

not geared towards improvement but only survival and reproduction.[1] He writes, "[w]hat human reproduction does not do very well is improve it," and elaborates as follows:

> The problem is that progress via Darwinian evolution is extremely slow and the direction unpredictable, save only that it will facilitate gene survival (Dawkins, 1976). We surely need to accelerate either the development of better resistance to bacteria, disease, viruses, or hostile environments, or of the technologies that will be eventually necessary to find, and travel to, habitats alternative to Earth. (Harris, 2015a, p. 31)[2]

Powell and Buchanan (2011) have made a similar point and argued that deliberate and intentional improvement must be better than one that happens merely by chance. They open their paper with the following grand statement:

> Only quite recently in the history of life has nature produced a species whose understanding of evolution makes possible the intentional modification of its own genome. There is mounting evidence, including successful genetic modifications of laboratory animals, that human beings will eventually be able to change their physical, cognitive, and emotional capacities by modifying their genes. To an extent that it is now impossible to gauge, human beings will be able to take charge of their own biological development and evolution. Evolutionary theory is becoming self-reflexive: Understanding how evolution works is enabling us to modify the course of our own evolution—if we choose to do so. (Powell & Buchanan, 2011, p. 7)

In other words, if we are not bound by what we happen to be and the capacities that we happen to have, but instead are free to develop adequate and safe technologies to this end, there are no limits, beyond those of technology, to what we could do and what we could be.

Some arguments in this debate put forward relatively bold claims about *the urgency* of enhancement based on the idea that the possible positive outcomes

---

[1] See also Buchanan (2011) for a similar point. He distinguishes between IGM and UGM (intentional genetic modification and unintentional genetic modification) and argues specifically against notions of some master engineer or wisdom in nature aspect of evolution. Deliberate modification, by contrast, would have a specific purpose and be controlled.

[2] Part of Harris' argument seems to be less about improvements than risk prevention. In the same paper, he writes, "We will at some point have to escape beyond both our fragile planet and our fragile nature. One way to enhance our capacity to do both these things is by improving on human nature where we can do so in ways that are 'safe enough'." (Harris, 2015, p. 33) He clarifies, "An over-precautionary approach may stifle the science that we need to make us safe; a reckless approach will be equally disastrous." (p. 33). Buchanan (2011) also alludes to the possibility that certain challenges might require the matter of enhancement, such as cognitive enhancement, to be solved.

are so considerable as to clearly outweigh the possible drawbacks. Thus, Bostrom (2003), in a paper defending transhumanism, reasons as follows:

> Every day that the introduction of effective human genetic enhancement is delayed is a day of lost individual and cultural potential, and a day of torment for many unfortunate sufferers of diseases that could have been prevented. Seen in this light, proponents of a ban or a moratorium on human genetic modifications must take on a heavy burden of proof in order to have the balance of reason tilt in their favor. Transhumanists conclude that the challenge has not been met. (Bostrom, 2003, p. 11)

Savulescu (2019) similarly argues, under a section aptly named "The Harm of Not Enhancing," that a person could be wronged if they were not genetically enhanced by their parents when they had the opportunity. He asks, "How will people feel if their parents don't enhance them, when they could have?" He imagines a case where he could have lived to be 160 had he been modified, but where his parents chose not to and argues that he would have been "furious" if he had been denied an additional 80 years of a good, healthy life. Prior to this, Savulescu had argued that there is a moral obligation to enhance one's children's "lives and opportunities" (Savulescu 2005, p. 37):

> Once technology affords us with the power to enhance our and our children's lives, to fail to do so will be to be responsible for the consequences. To fail to treat our children's disease is to harm them. To fail to prevent them getting depression is to harm them. To fail to improve their physical, musical, psychological and other capacities is to harm them, just as it would be to harm them if we gave them a toxic substance that stunted or reduced these capacities. (Savulescu 2005, p. 38)[3]

In addition to arguments for enhancement based on additional well-being, there are also arguments that suggest that enhancement is necessary to maintain current levels of well-being.

All of the above arguments follow quite naturally from the value maximization logic discussed earlier (see Sect. 5.2). According to the value maximization logic, morality does not merely require us to refrain from not doing harm or actively do what is good, but *to maximize* what is good. In other words: it is *obligatory to do what is morally best*.

Thus, if (a) morality is about maximizing the good, and (b) the good is whatever increases well-being, then (c) if germline gene editing could increase an individual's chances for well-being more efficiently than comparable options,

---

[3] One can see how he would reach this conclusion based on the status quo bias test.

then this is what morality requires us to do. Furthermore, if going beyond normal human functioning or expected capacities were to increase our chances for well-being even more, then this is what morality demands. This argument could be elucidated as follows:

1. The Value Maximization Premise: An action is only morally permissible if that action maximizes that which is of value for its own sake (has final value).
2. The Well-Being Premise: The only thing of value for its own sake (has final value) is well-being.
3. The Efficiency Premise: If two actions maximize well-being equally, then only the action that achieves that maximization *most efficiently* is morally permissible.[4]
4. The Imperative to Enhance: If genetic enhancement is the most efficient option to maximally increase well-being, then it is morally required to genetically enhance.

The imperative follows from the three premises. The point here is that none of the three premises is particularly unusual or implausible, even if the conclusion is. That is not to say that there is any kind of consensus of the premises or that they would not be contested.

The first premise is simply the value maximization logic restated as a premise: What determines what is morally right and wrong is only a matter of what action brings about the greatest amount of value. Nothing else matters morally. This is standard consequentialism.

The second premise proposes a currency for such increases and decreases, namely that of *well-being*. This is simply welfarism restated as a premise. It narrows down the possible candidates of what ultimately matters to just one: well-being. Monism and welfarism as theories about value are not the only ones, but, again, out of a handful of dominant theories about value, this combined view is a very influential one. In fact, the combination of value maximization and welfarism constitutes one of the most influential versions of consequentialism in

---

[4] This premise may be entirely superfluous, since most ways that one action would be more efficient than another would, presumably, mean that it would entail greater well-being. But this is not necessarily the case, especially if we take time into account. Imagine that a particular desired outcome could either be achieved by natural evolution in another 200.000 years from now, or in 50 years with enhancement; imagine also that both scenarios would entail the same level of well-being and that this "era" would last the same number of years. Then, without the efficiency clause, these would be equally valuable. Here, the efficiency premise would suggest that we ought to prefer the more direct route.

moral theory. Furthermore, the idea of maximizing welfare is the dominant logic in cost–benefit analysis.

The third premise is also a normative principle, but more one of rationality than ethics. If there are two means to the same end, then we must prefer the "better" means. On many interpretations, a means is better in terms of its *efficiency* in bringing about the desired end. This occurs in two ways. If there is a choice between two means and one has a higher success rate than the other, then that means would clearly be better, because it is more efficient. However, if, in a choice between two means, one has a faster or some other more direct way of bringing about the desired end, then this would be better in terms of efficiency as well. It could perhaps be assumed that the more indirect the means, the more chances of additional and unforeseen costs (and thus less well-being) or the more delayed the desired outcome, the less time that it could be enjoyed (it may even lose its value over time).[5] Thus, it would not be an uncommon position to be favorable towards all three: consequentialism, welfarism, and efficiency. If so, the morality of genetic enhancement depends on whether genetic enhancement does, in fact, maximize well-being.

All of these arguments point towards some kind of moral imperative for germline editing and tend to rely on some version of *the efficiency premise*. In other words, germline editing would be *right* (if sufficiently safe), because it would be *better*. But how compelling are the arguments that some kind of enhancement scheme would be the overall most beneficial option compared to the alternatives?[6] Before we take a closer look at what the exact benefit of enhancement is, we will address the charge that all calls for improving the human gene pool are essentially inviting back eugenics.

---

[5] Especially in more financially influenced reasoning one may presume that there is discount of value over time, such that a gain next year is worth less than a gain tomorrow, and so on.

[6] It is worth noting here that the set of options differ greatly if we look at germline editing as a form of medical treatment (to prevent disease in a future child), as a form of IVF treatment enabling parents to have a healthy child, and as a technology that, in addition to all the above, can also improve upon humanity. In the first case, the comparison must be between no treatment and alternative treatments: such as somatic gene therapy and other medical treatments. In the second case, the alternatives include having no child, having a genetically unrelated child (via adoption, surrogacy, donorship, etc.), embryo testing and abortion, PGD, and embryo selection. In the third case, the alternatives are no enhancements, letting nature run its course, and various non-genetic enhancements, such as education or improvements of social and environmental factors, but also enhancing drugs and non-heritable genetic enhancements. Most enhancement enthusiasts are pro enhancement, but not committed to any one particular means of achieving this.

8.2   Back Door Eugenics?[7]

Is what is currently proposed as "enhancement" in any relevant sense different
from early eugenics? As MacKellar and Bechtel (2016, p. 10) put it: "Eugenics
is driven by this impulse to maximize what is good, as seen in the relentless
quest for health and the avoidance of suffering." In that sense, what has been
described above as enhancement could equally well be *called* eugenics. Is it also
morally problematic in the same sense? Or does this new kind of eugenics in any
significant sense avoid the severe moral concerns and objections associated with
the old one?

Many scholars have argued that there is, indeed, a significant difference
between the two and that this largely has to do with *liberty*. The new kind of
eugenics or enhancement is thus of *a liberal* kind: it is meant to be an opportunity
that could be chosen voluntarily, which is far from any state-imposed eugenics
programs of the past. As Agar puts it: "While old fashioned authoritarian eugeni-
cists sought to produce citizens out of a single centrally designed mould, the
distinguishing mark of the new liberal eugenics is state neutrality" (Agar, 1998,
p. 137). More than that, enhancement could be viewed as an extension of procreative freedoms: the prospective parents would be able to review "the full range of
genetic therapies" and could "look to their own values in selecting improvements
for future children" (Agar, 1998, p. 137).

In this way, the advocates for enhancement distance themselves from the
eugenics of the past: it is not the eugenics of an ideologically driven state, but
eugenics offered as a free choice and as an extension of reproductive liberty.
Instead, it is a voluntary kind of eugenics, if that is what we ought to call it, based
on personal choice in a free market. The free reproductive choices of parents
would have the benefit of avoiding some fixed and centralized idea determining
what kinds of future persons there should be (Nozick, 2006, p. 315n).

However, a liberal "free market eugenics" gives rise to different kinds of concerns. In particular, there are concerns about the resulting societal impact of
such free choices in terms of societal justice and deepening division (Paul, 2005,
p. 124). Paul argues that "what critics primarily fear is 'back-door' eugenics—
the collective impact of practices voluntarily chosen by consumers (especially in
the context of largely unregulated fertility industry), rather than those mandated
by governments" (Paul, 2005, p. 124). Condit (1999) cited in Baylis (2019, p. 74)
makes a similar claim: "the entry of eugenics by the front door at the beginning of

---

[7] *Backdoor to Eugenics* is also a book by Troy Duster (1990). The notion first appeared
in an essay by Rollin Hotchkiss, see Paul (2005, p. n3).

the twentieth century may have been repudiated, … It has now firmly entrenched itself in our national homes via the back door of parental choice and medical manipulation." In other words, the free choices by many consumers on a market may also drive progress in a particular direction and speed up enhancement via social pressures and shifting norms.

Some are unconvinced that there is much that is "new" about "liberal eugenics" at all. There are two parts to this. The "new eugenics" may not be as free as thought, given the social pressures likely to arise as norms change. Furthermore, the "new eugenics" may not be that distant from the old eugenics, which had ideals of a favored race, skin color, sex, sexuality, functionality, and so on. Here, the concern is that the outcome of the new eugenics may not be all that different.

Buchanan (2011) states that there are two distinct concerns about the "new eugenics." The previous concern about state-driven coercive eugenic programs, and the concern about a "laissez-faire eugenics" and that "private choices in a market for enhancements will lead to the same attitudes and results that characterized the old, state-driven eugenics" (Buchanan, 2011, p. 22). Rather than focusing on the latter issue alone, he suggests that we ought not to entirely dismiss the possibility of state influence, even in liberal democratic societies.

"The state may take an interest in the development and diffusion of those enhancements that promise greater productivity" Buchanan (2011, p. 22) suggests, and thereby use softer measures to encourage such choices by means of, for instance, subsidies. Such softer measures could work in conjunction with other social pressures and market forces. "The combination of state encouragement, vigorous private marketing, and the herd-like impetus of popular culture might result in a situation in which individuals had more choices, but were worse off" (Buchanan, 2011, p. 22). In particular, it could lead to social pressures to enhance one's future offspring so that it would not fall behind its peers. If so, the number of choices would have increased in a formal sense, yet social pressures would make only one choice attractive. Buchanan himself views such scenarios as extremely speculative, but as worth taking note of and possibly preventing.

Comfort (2015) argues in an article in *The Nation* that "neoliberal eugenics is the same old eugenics we've always known:"

> When it comes to controlling our evolution, individualism and choice point toward the same outcomes as authoritarian collectivism: a genetically stratified society resistant to social change—one that places the blame for society's ills on individuals rather than corporations or the government. (Comfort, 2015)

He is not alone in this view. Sparrow (2011) similarly argues that there is nothing particularly new about the "new" eugenics and agrees that the outcomes may be remarkably similar. He writes, "Many of the implications of the new eugenics are genetic interventions that in substance—if not in motivation—look very much like those advocated by the 'old' eugenics" (Sparrow, 2011, p. 34). Sparrow also argues that the kind of prejudices and discrimination that informed the old eugenics are likely to influence the new kind of eugenics as well. Given that parents will want to improve their children's prospects and given that the societal context attaches higher status and more privilege to certain properties, then parents are likely to want to use their reproductive liberty to produce those properties attached to societal privilege. Thus, free parental choices aiming for the best possible prospects for their children in a sexist, racist and homophobic society may lead to outcomes that are not that dissimilar from the eugenics ideals of the past:

> Thus, for instance, in a racist society, where children born with particular racial markers—skin color, hair type, shape of nose and lips, presence or absence of an epicanthic fold, and so on—will have reduced life prospects, a proper concern for their children's well-being requires that parents work to mitigate the impact of racism by altering the child's environment, or by manipulating the genes associated with these markers, or both. (Sparrow, 2011, p. 35)

It is not merely an empirical point, according to Sparrow, that parents are *likely* to act in this way. It is also how they *ought* to act if we follow the implications of the reasoning of the new liberal eugenics, such as Savulescu and Harris, according to Sparrow (2011, p. 35; see also e.g. Savulescu, 2008; Harris, 2001; Quigley & Harris, 2009).[8] In short, if each parent has an obligation to ensure that their offspring has the best possible prospects for a good life and such prospects depend on genetics as well as on environmental and social aspects, then given that "it will often be much easier to alter a child's genetics than the social conditions that will shape the ultimate impact of their genetics" (Sparrow, 2011, p. 35), they ought to enhance their children in order to achieve that end. Thus, if one takes seriously the arguments that parents have an obligation to bring about the child with best chances for the best possible life in terms of well-being, then this seems to follow. "The new eugenics is, after all, supposed to be concerned with individual well-being—and, as we have seen, it will always be to an individual's benefit to be born with the genetic markers of social privilege" (Sparrow, 2011, p. 35).

---

[8] Sparrow discusses various sources of both writers, in particular Savulescu 2001, 2005, 2006, 2007, 2008 and Harris 1998, 2007.

Free choices to edit one's future offspring could lead to a society where only the rich have access to germline editing for their children and the poor do not. This is one of the recurring objections to germline editing (see Sect. 6.2). To combat this concern, some advocates point out that germline editing could also be used to address the already existing inequality and unfairness in the natural genetic lottery (see also Savulescu, 2006; Singer, 2009).[9] Gyngell et al. (2019) make such a claim with respect to intelligence and the possibilities to even out existing inequalities. Speculating that it could become theoretically possible to "use HGE to shift individuals from the low or medium predisposition groups [to high intelligence], into high predisposition groups" they argue that employed in this way, germline editing might decrease injustice and improve equality (Gyngell et al., 2019, p. 521). The biological lottery is already deeply unfair when it comes to talents, pain, disability, and lifespan, they reason. Furthermore, we already seek to address this unfairness in various ways. "Genome editing could be used as part of public health care for egalitarian reasons" (Gyngell et al., 2019, p. 521). This, they argue, would have "the additional benefit of being passed to future generations" (Gyngell et al., 2019, p. 521).[10]

Singer (2009) argues that even if it is possible to make enhancement accessible only to those worst-off and not those at the top, "unless we take a gloomy view of human nature, there seems a fair chance that enhancement for all, including those at the top, will eventually improve the situation for everyone, including the worst-off" (Singer, 2009, p. 286). Of course, even if equality was achieved by means of germline editing on the national level, it may still increase a divide between rich nations with access to such enhancement and poor nations without such access (Singer, 2009, p. 286).

8.3 The Liberty Versus Well-Being Dilemma

There is an underlying tension in the debate on enhancement between two partially conflicting values: that of *maximizing well-being* and that of *promoting and protecting liberty*. Thus, some of the pro-enhancement arguments defend

---

[9] Although, as Savulescu (2006, p. 332) notes, on a libertarian view, it would not necessarily be *unfair* that the rich had access to buy genetic advantages for their children.

[10] Gray and Gorin (2019, p. 27) suggest that inequalities could be combatted via the tax system, and a special "enhancement tax" such that those not enhanced could benefit from the economic advantages from enhancement. They are also hopeful that once enhancement becomes reality, if it does, it could be met with a parallel improvement of moral capacities such that arising moral problems could be met.

enhancement on the grounds of liberty—in terms of the reproductive liberty of parents, and possibly also greater liberties for enhanced individuals. Others defend enhancement on the grounds of well-being, either to combat a decline in well-being or as a means to increase individual or collective well-being.

The concern that enhancement would let eugenics in through the back door has been, as we saw in the previous section, addressed by appeals to *liberty*. What is advocated is a new "liberal eugenics" that is distinct from the old coercive kind of eugenics in the form of state programs (Agar, 2004; see also MacKellar & Bechtel, 2016, p. 7 f.). It is argued that this "new eugenics" would be voluntary and compatible with individual freedom and rights. It would increase the number of options for parents and increase parental reproductive freedoms. Critics, by contrast, argue that there is nothing "new" about so-called new or liberal eugenics at all (Sparrow, 2011). Furthermore, it is unclear how the appeal to liberty can be reconciled with the value maximization logic that underpins some of the motivations and rationale for enhancement. There is tension between the idea of enhancement as part of *parental autonomy and liberty* and the idea of enhancement as an efficient means to *increase or maximize well-being*. This tension is twofold.

The first tension brings us back to the moral logics introduced earlier (Chap. 5). There is a tension in terms of *moral demand*. What a liberty-based argument demands and what a well-being maximization argument demands are very different. In the first case, we would be free to do whatever we choose to, as long as it falls within what is morally permissible and refrains from what is morally impermissible. In the second case, we must in each action seek to bring about as much moral value as possible and avoid any action that aims for less than that. It is this kind of logic that underscores the various suggestions that there are moral imperatives to pursue enhancement or that parents have an obligation to create the best possible child, or the child with the best chances for the best life, and so on. In short, if we truly want to put forward parental liberties, this must come with no strings attached or an implication that they have a moral obligation to choose one particular alternative. Anything less would dilute the value of liberty. Conversely, if we want to truly put enhancement forward on the grounds of the levels of well-being it could create, then liberty disappears: The fact that certain acts will increase well-being is enough to suggest that those acts are morally right.

The first tension comes down to this: When it comes to enhancement, are we obliged to do what is morally best or are we free to do whatever we wish, as long as we do not mitigate the liberties of others? As Sparrow (2011, p. 33) points out, consequentialism does not speak against authoritarian interventions for effective enhancement programs but rather for it. It is only by seeking to combine liberty with consequentialist reasoning that Harris and Savulescu can even suggest the idea of a moral imperative (to enhance) and avoid the natural conclusion that we must take the most effective route towards enhancement, even if that means state intervention. As Sparrow puts it:

> Given the notoriously demanding nature of consequentialism and its lineage as a philosophy of radical social reform, one might expect that their conclusions would include a strong role for the state in encouraging or even requiring people to meet their obligations to have better babies. Instead, both Harris and Savulescu deny that the state should pursue eugenic goals and insist that the decision about whether to pursue enhancement (and which enhancements to pursue) should be left up to individuals. There is, therefore, a tension between their consequentialism and their (apparent) libertarianism when it comes to the rights of individuals to use—or not use—enhancement technologies as they see fit. (Sparrow, 2011, p. 33)

Savulescu downplays this tension by using moral imperatives in a much weaker sense than normal, meaning nothing more than that there are moral reasons to that effect, and although acting on the imperative would be the right thing to do, we would not be legally required or coerced to do so. The latter is, however, beside the point. In addition, if there is a moral obligation to enhance future individuals, then there is nothing to suggest that it would be wrong to make it a legal requirement.

The question is this: Would parents who do not enhance their offspring when they have the option to be acting in a morally impermissible manner? Whether they are legally free not to enhance does not answer the question. If they are not morally free to do this, then enhancement is not morally optional but required. There is not much moral space left for autonomy or liberty in this line of reasoning. Furthermore, Savulescu suggests that we could avoid injustice through subsidies, and generally make enhancement more easily accessible to all. If so, then shifting norms and social pressures may not leave much social space for autonomy and liberty either. In fact, parents choosing not to use germline editing to correct their children, were it to become a widespread, safe, and acceptable practice, could come to face social sanctions and even be viewed as bad parents (Baylis, 2019, p. 90).

The second tension is about *final values*, what is valuable in itself. Liberty and well-being are different values and pull in different directions. What creates this tension is that they attach to different parts of moral actions. Liberty is about protecting a space free from interference or dominance for an individual to make their own decisions or actions, whatever they might be and whatever the outcomes may be within the limits of moral permissibility. Part of such a liberty is the freedom to select one's own ends and pursue projects that one considers worthwhile for personal reasons. The value of liberty comes from the value attached to this space of non-interference and the idea that its value is not merely instrumental but intrinsic. The outcomes are not the morally defining aspect here, since that would narrow the freedom.

Well-being, on the other hand, is a value that is attached to outcomes. It is about discerning what outcomes are best. It is neutral about how those outcomes came about and by whom they were decided; in fact, whatever means brings about the best outcomes is preferable and right. This means that if coercion is more efficient and achieves better outcomes, then it is also morally better. Thus, there is little room for liberty here, unless it is reduced to a choice between options that are all roughly equally efficient or, at least, all produce well-being to a particular threshold. Instead, it is assumed that well-being has intrinsic value and makes everything else worthwhile. Well-being in the philosophical literature is a common measure of final value; that is, moral goodness. One need not be monist about such values, and well-being could be made compatible with other outcome values, but if one takes the outcomes to be what determines moral rightness, then values attached to processes must weigh less.

It seems that if we take liberty to be the primary value that motivates enhancement, then we cannot guarantee that this will lead to more well-being overall or is compatible with any notions of a just and fair society. If we take well-being to be the primary value that motivates enhancement, we cannot argue that this will be fully compatible with liberty. In other words, it is difficult to see how the joint project of arguing for a moral imperative to pursue enhancement based on the expected increase in well-being can be combined with the insistence that this is a new liberal kind of eugenics that will not impose a particular notion of the ideal human being upon everyone.

At one end of the dilemma, we could say that there are good arguments for population well-being to pursue enhancement, but we need to admit that this will come at the cost of individual liberty. At the other end, we could argue that there are good liberty arguments for viewing enhancement as different form the old kind of eugenics, but if true to that commitment, we would not make any assurances about well-being increases, nor could we guarantee that this would not come with great moral costs in terms of genetically informed inequality and injustice.

The second tension comes from the internal conflict between liberty as a driver for whatever outcomes individuals choose and where that liberty constitutes an intrinsic value to be protected, and the idea that well-being is the driving moral value, and we have a moral obligation to increase what is good and decrease what is bad (in terms of consequences). We can justify enhancement by appealing to the fact that this would provide parents with an additional reproductive option, and furthermore, potentially provide their child with more options, given their new or improved capacities. Then, overall, enhancement would add more freedom to the world for those individuals who can access it. But, if this is our line of argument, we cannot simultaneously argue that enhancement is good because it would improve the human gene pool, since this would be to preempt the result of free choice, and in any case, clearly exaggerate the affordability and accessibility of the technology. Thus, those who want to point to the advantages that could be achieved on a population level by means of enhancement, whether merely to protect current levels of genetic health or achieve radical improvements, cannot do so by appealing to liberty, since this would not have the kind of population-wide effects sought. On an individual level, these are less in conflict: A person may choose to enhance their offspring as an expression of reproductive liberty motivated by prospective well-being benefits.

However, in the individual case, liberties are in conflict with equality. Now, such inequality could be explained in terms of inequality, liberty, or inequality of well-being. If one is concerned about the options not being available to all, we could increase tax funding, among other things, to make it widely accessible. But this would also increase pressures and reduce liberty along another dimension: the possible ways of being in the world. Furthermore, this could accelerate development and avail more radical options for those who are wealthier and willing to pay more for additional genetic advantages. If one is concerned about inequality as a result of well-being, then this would most likely lead to a more interventionist program for enhancement for all at the cost of liberty.

One cannot both argue that enhancement is nothing like the old kind of eugenics on the basis of it being liberal in nature and would have many population-wide benefits in terms of well-being and health, and that it could even out the odds in the genetic lottery. Nor could one convincingly defend new eugenics as a fundamentally liberal project without thereby generating warranted concerns about genetic and social injustice. This, of course, does not exclude that some kind of balance can be struck—by means of regulation or subsidies (to enable equal access), while keeping it a free choice, perhaps as part of some kind of persuasive effort. Nor can enhancement be defended on grounds of significant increases in population well-being, while at the same time being framed as an individual choice. In the end, both values cannot carry the same moral weight: When they are in conflict, it must either be that freedom trumps the moral imperative to maximize well-being or the other way around.

8.4   The Good of Enhancement

What is it that makes the prospects of genetic enhancement so attractive? A common view, at least among its proponents, is that enhancement is valuable because *to enhance* means *to improve*. Thus, to enhance something is to take what is valuable and make it more valuable (cf. Savulescu, 2006, p. 325). Harris (2009, p. 131) argues that enhancement is *per definition* improvement, and thus, on the assumption that it would be of obvious benefit to a person to be improved, *not* enhancing someone who could have been enhanced is to harm that person.

On this view, enhancement is *a broad concept* in that it could include almost anything that is considered an improvement. Below, for instance, Savulescu includes ordinary medical therapy and treatment as a kind of "enhancement":

> Enhancement is, indeed, a wide concept. In the broadest sense, it means "increase" or "improvement." For example, a doctor may *enhance* his patient's chance of survival by giving the patient a drug. Or a doctor may enhance the functioning of a person's immune system or memory (the functionalist account). These are no doubt enhancements of a sort—enhancements in an attributive sense. (Savulescu, 2006, p. 324, italics in the original)

Furthermore, it is *an evaluative concept* in that a positive change of some sort is already implicit. We can refer to this view on enhancement, that it is equivalent to improvement in an evaluative sense, as the *Improvement View*.

Two things follow from this kind of view. First, such a broad definition of enhancement undermines any sharp distinction between therapy and enhancement. Consequently, it also weakens any moral significance attached to such a distinction and effectively passes the moral burden of proof to those skeptical of enhancement: If there is something morally objectionable about enhancement as opposed to therapy, then there must be some *morally relevant difference* between the two.[11] Notably, Savulescu (2006, p. 325), after defining human enhancement in terms of increasing the value of a life, lists the following as examples of enhancements:

---

[11] Cf. Gyngell, Douglas, and Savulescu (2017, p. 509): "We have argued elsewhere that arguments against human enhancement face conceptual challenges. There are several different ways to understand the term 'enhancement', which are often only imprecisely communicated by opponents of enhancement. No commonly offered definitions describe something clearly morally problematic. Further difficulties arise when considering how biological enhancement can be differentiated from non-biological enhancements, which are nearly universally celebrated.".

(i) Medical Treatment of Disease
(ii) Increasing Natural Human Potential—increasing a person's own natural
     endowments of capabilities within the range typical of the species *home
     sapiens*, for example, raising a person's IQ from 100 to 140.
(iii) Superhuman Enhancements (sometimes called posthuman or transhuman)—
     increasing a person's capabilities beyond the range typical for the species
     homo sapiens, for example, giving humans bat sonar or the capacity to read
     minds. (Savulescu, 2006, p. 326)

Others would refer to the first category as treatment and the other two as enhancement. Some might also refer to the last category as "radical enhancement"
(Agar, 2010; Savulescu, 2009). The point, here, is that if enhancement means
improvement, then they are all enhancements. Many use this line of argument to
demonstrate that we already accept enhancement in other forms than germline
editing, specifically biotechnological enhancements: we use glasses, enroll our
children in schools, and so on. Even though Buchanan resists the idea of equat-
ing enhancement with what per definition makes someone *better off*, enhancement
is better understood as the improvement of an existing, or the creating of a new,
capacity. The broad notion of enhancement thus means that literacy, even though
it is not a biomedical intervention, counts as a form of enhancement (Buchanan,
2011, p. 23 ff.):

> Human beings have always tried to enhance themselves—to improve their mental,
> physical, and emotional capacities. The invention of writing, for example, was a dra-
> matic enhancement of our cognitive powers: the development of the method and
> practices of science was another. But for the first time we have scientific knowl-
> edge that has the potential for transforming ourselves perhaps more profoundly—and
> certainly more deliberately—than ever before. (Buchanan, 2011, p. xi)

Thus, for the purposes of the relevant bioethical debate, enhancement is narrowed
down to specifically address *biomedical enhancement*. This is defined as "improvements in our capacities by working directly on the brain or body," including
"the administration of drugs, implants using genetically engineered tissue, direct
brain-computer interface technologies, and insertion of our genes into human
embryos" (Buchanan, 2011, p. ix).

Second, the *normative conclusions* about the value of enhancement are already
implicit in the concept itself: if it is a case of enhancement, then it is good,
and if it is not good, then it is not enhancement. This line of reasoning thus
undermines moral objections to the idea of enhancement. Who could possibly
object to making things better? If good is good, then surely better is even better?

Here, we can recall Foot's (1985, p. 198) argument that "it can never be right to prefer a worse state of affairs to a better" as the key notion of consequentialism (but also what made utilitarianism problematic, since the whole notion of total outcomes in a non-moral sense is a problematic measure of right and wrong in a moral sense).

The *Improvement View* thus differs from another common view on enhancement that we could refer to as the *Beyond Therapy View*. On this view, any intervention *that goes beyond treatment and prevention of disease*, or that seeks to alter a person's genetic traits in a way that goes beyond what is "normal," is to be considered a case of enhancement. Consider how Juengst explains the term: "The term enhancement is usually used in bioethics to characterize interventions designed to improve human form or functioning beyond what is necessary to sustain or restore good health" (Juengst, 1998, cited in Savulescu, 2006, p. 322). Such a definition avoids the normative implicature: Something that is an enhancement could be good or bad, but it needs to rely on some notion of "health," "disease," or "normality" to distinguish between what is and is not enhancement.[12] "Enhancement" understood in this way in the context of gene therapy and gene editing thus refers to genetic interventions that go beyond what is needed from the perspective of medicine or health to what is desired (on some aspirational view of humankind).

Let us return to the *Improvement View*. What exactly is it that is improved upon? There are largely two views on this that dominate the debate. We could refer to these two as the *Improved Function* and the *Improved Well-Being View*, respectively. The first view, the *Improved Function View*, understands the relevant improvements in terms of increased *functioning* of humans. Particularly those that go beyond normal human capacities. Buchanan, as an example of the first,

---

[12] Such a distinction is notoriously difficult to make and there is bound to be some gray area between more definitive outcomes. Consider, for instance, what Singer wrote about selection (2009): "Many people say that they accept selection against serious diseases and disabilities, but not for enhancement beyond what is normal. There is, however, no bright line between selection against disabilities and selection for positive characteristics. From selecting against Huntington's Disease it is no great step to selecting against genes that carry a significantly elevated risk of breast or colon cancer, and from there it is easy to move to giving one's child a better than average genetic health profile" (Singer, 2009, p. 278). Singer adds that even if we were able to distinguish between the two, this still does not explain why there would be a moral difference between them. The same point has been made by several others. This "beyond therapy" view has the advantage that it leaves the moral question open: enhancement is not per definition an improvement, but something that adds some genetic property beyond what is medically motivated and/or beyond what is "normal." But it has the drawback that it must be able to make sense of the therapy-enhancement distinction.

describes enhancement in the following way: "to enhance human beings is to expand their capabilities—to enable them to do what normal human beings have hitherto not been able to do" (Buchanan, 2011, p. 38). Earlier in the same book, he defined it as a deliberate intervention "which aims to improve an existing capacity that more or all normal human beings typically have, or to create a new capacity" (p. 23). The functional definition thus defines enhancement as improvements of a relatively descriptive kind. Buchanan provides the following indicative list: "improvements in physical characteristics such as speed, strength, and endurance; improvements in cognitive capacities, such as various aspects of memory, information-processing, and reasoning; improvements in affect, emotion, motivation, or temperament; improvements in immunity or resistance to diseases; and increased longevity" (p. 25).[13] What is improved upon, then, is what humans are, can be, and can do. This view aligns well with the idea that humanity is a work in progress (Bostrom, 2005, p. 4) and that enhancement is a way to take charge of our own evolution (Buchanan, 2011; Powell & Buchanan, 2011).

However, not all cases of enhancement need to be in the person's own best interest. For this reason, some want to reserve the term 'enhancement' for interventions that benefit the individual:

> What is enhancement? Surely it is a procedure that improves our functioning: any intervention which increases our general capabilities for human flourishing. We exclude from consideration those procedures often termed "enhancements" that are of dubious overall benefit (for example breast or penis augmentation, or the taking of anabolic steroids to increase muscle mass). Equally we are not talking of "designer" modifications which are more akin to aesthetic or fashion preferences than to improvements: hair colour, eye colour, or physique. An enhancement (as we are using the term) is something of benefit to the individual. (Chan & Harris, 2007, p. 1)

Savulescu holds a similar view. He argues that not all cases of improved functioning are relevant enhancements: "It might not constitute *human* enhancement. It might not enhance intrinsic good" (Savulescu, 2006, p. 324). For this reason, he favors an account of enhancement that limits enhancement to what promotes *the well-being* for the person whose life it is:

---

[13] These areas of enhancement could be improved by various means. Buchanan lists the following five: embryo selection, genetic engineering, administration of drugs, implantation of genetically engineered tissues or organs, and brain-computer interface technologies (Buchanan, 2011, p. 25).

The term *human enhancement* is itself ambiguous. It might mean enhancement of functioning as a member of the species *homo sapiens*. This would be a functionalist definition. But when we are considering human enhancement, we are considering improvement of the person's life. The improvement is some change in state of the person—biological or psychological—which is good. Which changes are good depends on the value we are seeking to promote or maximize. In the context of human enhancement, the value in question is the goodness of a person's life, that is, his/her well-being. (Savulescu, 2006, p. 324)

This leads us to the second view of enhancement, the *Improved Well-Being View*. This view is perhaps the most explicitly stated in Savulescu's *Welfarist Definition of Human Enhancement*: "Any change in the biology or psychology of a person which increases the chances of leading a good life in circumstances C" (Savulescu, 2006, p. 324), where "C" refers to some particular set of circumstances.

There are important differences here between the functionalist and well-being view of the concept of 'enhancement'. Although both agree that all cases of functional improvements may not be to the benefit of the individual (or society), they draw different conceptual conclusions from this. Savulescu thus narrows down the relevant enhancements as those that are *improvements in well-being*. By doing so, anything that counts as enhancement will by definition also be a case of welfare improvement (in some sense), and thus, by consequence of the value maximization logic, makes all cases of enhancement morally warranted. Buchanan takes the other path; because not every case of functional improvement is a case of welfare improvement, he defines 'enhancement' in a more descriptive way. His definition, according to him, thus has the advantage of avoiding "a simple mistake," namely, "thinking that an enhancement by definition makes one better off" (Buchanan, 2011, p. 23). He provides two vivid examples to illustrate this point: enhanced hearing in a noisy environment and enhanced memory without the ability to control when memories arise or manage the emotions they give rise to. In other words, on Savulescu's account, we first need to know whether some act will be an improvement in terms of well-being in order to know whether it is a case of enhancement. On Buchanan's account, we only need to know what kind of action is involved and to what kind of end in order to know whether or not it is an act of enhancement in the relevant sense.

The latter kind of approach has the benefit that it needs not simplify the relevant reasons for and against an act of enhancement: We could all agree that some act is an act of enhancement without agreeing that it is morally good. Defining "enhancement" in such a non-evaluative and descriptive way leaves the moral question open—as in, not already determined conceptually—and could thus be settled in view of all the moral reasons for and against it. On a well-being account, by contrast, it might be tempting to prematurely assume that some act does or does not improve welfare before all the facts are in, so to speak. In fact, Savulescu and Kahane (2009, p. 278) seem to favor an expected outcome view on welfare maximization, which measures well-being *ex ante*, rather than an actualist view, which measures well-being *post ante*.

8.5 The Moral Obligation to Enhance

From the notion that *enhancement is improvement*, or increases well-being, together with the notion that *morality's primary demand is to promote well-being* as far as possible, the step to the notion that we have *strong moral reasons to enhance* is very short. Consequently, some argue that we have *a moral obligation* to promote enhancement (see, e.g., Savulescu, 2006; Harris, 2009):

> When enhancement is understood as an intervention which increases the chances of a person having a good life, it is hard to see how there could be any objections to trying to make people's lives go better. Indeed, the fact that enhancements increase well-being provides a strong moral obligation based on beneficence to provide them. (Savulescu, 2006, p. 326)

How strong is this line of thought that there might be something like a moral obligation to enhance, given that enhancement means improvement, and on the assumption that morality (on the value promotion logic) asks us to increase well-being? Recall the consequentialist line of argument discussed in the previous chapter:

1. *The Maximization Premise*: Morality requires that we only perform that action that maximizes intrinsic value (here: final value) compared to all comparable alternative actions.
2. *The Well-Being Premise*: The only thing of intrinsic value (here: final value) is *well-being*.
3. *The Efficiency Premise*: If two actions maximize well-being equally in terms of outcomes, then we ought to perform the action that achieves that maximization *most efficiently*.
4. Thus: *If* genetic enhancement is the most efficient way to maximally increase well-being, *then* we ought to genetically enhance.

On the one hand, the idea of a moral imperative to enhance follows the above premises in a fairly straightforward manner. In fact, as we shall see, several writers do argue that there is a moral imperative to enhance for reasons of well-being. However, the conclusion in number 4 above is stated in the conditional tense: It merely states that *if* it is the case that genetic enhancement was to maximize well-being more than the alternatives, *then* it would be morally obligatory. This, of course, leaves it open whether or not enhancement actually maximizes well-being more than the alternatives, and also whether it would do so more efficiently than the available alternatives.

However, several of the key terms in the above argument remain open. It could thus be read to imply very different kinds of moral obligations, depending on what kinds of actions we are contemplating, who is thought to benefit, and who is thought to be obligated, and how we interpret maximizing well-being. To give some idea of the scope of possible implied moral imperatives here, compare the following three:

> *Good for All Policy*: It is morally imperative that governments promote genetic enhancement for the welfare benefits for the wider population and society.

> *Good for Child Parental Duty*: It is morally imperative that parents genetically enhance their future offspring for the welfare benefits of that child.

> *Good for All Parental Duty*: It is morally imperative that parents genetically enhance their future offspring for the welfare of society.

All three suggest that there are arguments of maximizing well-being that lead to some kind of moral imperative to enhance, but distinct ones. However, a number of the variables have been changed: who it is that is supposedly obligated to act, what it is that they are supposed to do (in relation to enhancement), who is supposed to benefit, and what the relevant and efficient maximizing action is considered to be.

The first claim, the *Good for All Policy*, focuses on large-scale societal benefits of enhancement and, consequently, on moral actions in terms of policy implications. The moral work is done by *maximizing overall well-being*. Of course, this could also lead to individual obligations to enhance, and encourage others to do so, for the good of the many, giving rise to something like the *Good for All Parental Duty*, or a collective duty not limited to government policy in the form of the *Good for All Collective Duty*.

Buchanan's (2011) argument for enhancement is not too far from this kind of reasoning. In his 2011 book *Beyond Humanity?*, he presented what he termed a *pro tanto* case for enhancement (p. 35). He argues:

> ... (a) that some enhancements will increase human productivity broadly conceived and thereby create the potential for large-scale increases in human well-being, and (b) that the enhancements that are most likely to attract sufficient resources to become widespread will be those that promise to increase productivity and will often exhibit what economists call network effects: the benefit to an individual of being enhanced will depend upon, or at least be greatly augmented by others having the enhancement as well. When these two points are appreciated, it becomes clear that we must take the potential social benefits of enhancements—and hence the social costs of forgoing enhancements—very seriously. (Buchanan, 2011, p. 36 f.)

In this context, Buchanan makes a very interesting productivity argument for the effectiveness of enhancement in terms of well-being. First, "productivity" on his account, means "how good we are at using existing resources to create things we value." Although increased productivity cannot guarantee increased well-being, it has historically been a "precondition of major gains in human well-being," and such increases have been the result of what we could take as enhancements of human capabilities in the broad sense. In other words, on a broad definition of enhancement as improved capacities, together with the fact that we would only improve capacities that could promote what we value, there is a strong connection between enhancement and well-being: we would only enhance what we believe will, in fact, improve our well-being. Furthermore, given that some of the benefits depend on the collective effect of many being so enhanced, there are moral reasons to make enhancement widely accessible to all. Buchanan writes, "The potential of cognitive enhancements for increasing productivity is straightforward," and "other things being equal, with enhanced cognitive abilities we will be able to do what we now do more quickly and efficiently, and we also may be able to do some new things we will value" (Buchanan, 2011, p. 45).[14]

The second claim, *Good for Child Parental Duty*, differs from the first claim in that it focuses on well-being benefits *for a particular individual*: the future child of prospective parents. This might seem like the standard value maximization logic applied to the singular case: If we ought to always maximize overall well-being, then, by extension we ought to, in each individual case, also maximize well-being

---

[14] Cognitive enhancements are, however, only one of several kinds of "biomedical enhancements" that Buchanan lists as potentially instrumental in large-scale well-being increases. The others mentioned relate to longevity, improved health at the end of life, and enhancements of the immune system.

for those involved in that case. However, that only follows straightforwardly for cases where we can safely assume that the contemplated action would lead to more overall well-being. In Singer's (1972) famous case of the drowning child or contributing to world poverty, it is hard to see that such acts could diminish overall well-being and not contribute to it. However, when applied to private cases of enhancement, this assumption is not as plausible: We could well imagine that promoting one's own child's above-average capacities would not contribute to raising overall levels of well-being but instead increase injustice, discrimination, or undermine resources and priorities needed elsewhere. The problem is that, according to value maximization logic, parents have no special obligations to their own children. This is actually one of the implications in Singer's text: If we could help someone in great need on the other side of the world instead of increasing our own child's well-being a little, then we ought to do the former.

By contrast, from deontological views based on the permissibility logic, we would wrong our children by not caring sufficiently for them—in other words, we have special obligations to our children in our role as parents (such rights and duties would only apply once there is a child). However, on this view, maximization does not really have a moral role to play.

Savulescu wants to combine both: Parents have an obligation to act in the interest of maximization for their own future offspring. He has argued that prospective parents have a moral obligation, in the case of embryo selection, to select *the best* possible child (2001), or to create a child with *the best chance* for the best life (2008), where the "best life" is to be understood as "the life with the most well-being" (Savulescu, 2001, p. 419). This moral obligation is summed up in *the Principle of Procreative Beneficence (PB)*:

> … couples (or single reproducers) should select the child, of the possible children they could have, who is expected to have the best life, or at least as good a life as the others, based on the relevant, available information. (Savulescu, 2001, p. 415)

In a later version, the same principle is stated as follows:

> If couples (or single reproducers) have decided to have a child, and selection is possible, then they have a significant moral reason to select the child, of the possible children they could have, whose life can be expected, in light of the relevant available information, to go best or at least not worse than any of the others. (Savulescu & Kahane, 2009, p. 274)

Originally, the arguments for *the Principle of Procreative Beneficence* were aimed at embryo *selection* and the obligation to select the best embryo. How far could this principle be extended to apply to germline *editing* as well? There is nothing in the inherent logic that seems to restrict it to selection cases only. In fact, should editing provide even greater chances, or chances for an even better life, than the best unedited embryo, then it would seem that we ought to edit the embryo.

There are, however, some morally interesting differences between editing and selection. One of these differences has to do with the *non-identity problem* (Parfit, 1986) and the fact that, in selection, our decision is not about what will happen to one embryo/person, but what will happen to one embryo/person rather than another (related to the discussion in Sect. 7.2.1). Thus, according to Savulescu, there is a difference in that, in germline editing, on the assumption that such editing benefits a person, the benefit for the editing could be outweighed later if risks materialize as harm that exceeds the benefit. If so, we would have committed a wrong to that person. In other words, there is a moral risk in editing that is different from the case of selection.[15] In the selection case, we could cause one embryo to come into being over another; thus, the harms and benefits are only those attached to existence itself.

There is another difference. On the maximization logic, we must do what is *best*. However, the achievable level of "best" differs when it comes to embryo selection and embryo editing. In the case of selection, "the best embryo" is simply the best among an actual existing set of healthy embryos. In other words, it is a selection within the realm of natural human potential. To put it differently, to maximize well-being by means of embryo selection; that is, to select the child with *the best chances* for "the life with the most well-being" (Savulescu, 2001, p. 419) could never bring about enhancement beyond improvement of natural human potential.

Once we move over to germline editing and add the same kind of maximization logic there, *there is no upper limit for what is best*. If there is a superhuman improvement that could increase the chances for well-being ever so slightly, then this is what we must do if we are to maximize well-being. The only limits to chasing further enhancements seem to be temporary and contingent: limits set by what the best technology can achieve at that point in time, limits of opportunity costs and financial resources of the parents, and limits that well-being itself

---

[15] Here, a problem crops up with the welfarist notion of "enhancement" based on *expected* well-being. Given that Savulescu takes enhancement to imply improvement in terms of *expected* well-being (such that it is conceived initially), rather than the actual well-being, any act of enhancement could, in fact, turn out to be more harmful than beneficial. A welfarist notion of enhancement based on actual well-being would always, per definition, outweigh any risk and harm. The trouble with such a definition is that we would never know whether something, in fact, was a case of enhancement or not until after the intervention.

imposes in that context (diminishing marginal utility, improvements that only add value if shared with others). An obligation to maximize could rapidly become an obligation to push the boundaries towards more and more extreme human and superhuman capacities.

The third claim, *Good for All Parental Duty*, is merely added here to highlight the available differences. This is not a position defended in the current debate for obvious reasons: The claim is that parents have a moral obligation to enhance their children, irrespective of the children's best interest, solely based on its contribution to overall well-being. Thus, if society needs some of its future citizens to have some particular capacity, parents would be obliged to enhance their children accordingly. This would run counter to any notion of liberty and parental autonomy, but it reveals the inherent value conflict between a liberty-based framework on the one hand and well-being maximization on the other.

8.6 Lost in Enhancement

Just as there are arguments highlighting anticipated benefits of germline editing, there are arguments highlighting anticipated losses or harms from such interventions. Here, the focus is not so much on risks in terms of safety or concerns that things may go wrong in a technical or medical sense. Rather, these arguments suggest that once parents seek to alter the germline of their prospective children, *something changes* in their expectations towards such children and *something changes* in the child–parent relationship; and, possibly, something of fundamental value might be lost. This loss has been framed in different ways.

One greatly influential argument against enhancement based on what might be lost is Sandel's argument that enhancement involves a loss of a sense of "giftedness" towards life, replaced with "a drive for mastery" where everything is under our control. The argument was introduced in a short paper by Sandel (2004, republished in 2007, and expanded upon in 2007):

> The deeper danger is that they (i.e., enhancement and genetic engineering) represent a kind of hyperagency, a Promethean aspiration to remake nature, including human nature, to serve our purposes and satisfy our desires. The problem is not the drift to mechanism but the drive to mastery. And what the drive to mastery misses, and may even destroy, is an appreciation of the gifted character of human powers and achievements. To acknowledge the giftedness of life is to recognize that our talents and powers are not wholly our own doing, nor even fully ours, despite the efforts we expect to develop and to exercise them. It is also to recognize that not everything in the world is open to any use we may desire or devise. An appreciation of the giftedness

of life constrains the Promethean project and conduces to a certain humility. (Sandel, 2007, pp. 26–27, cited in Hauskeller, 2011, p. 56)

The problem, according to Sandel (2004, p. 57; 2007, p. 46), lies "in the hubris of the designing parents, in their drive to master the mystery of birth. ... it would disfigure the relation between parent and child, and deprive the parents of the humility and enlarged sympathies that an openness to the unbidden can cultivate." The key concern is that parents, in seeking to enhance their children, change the relationship between parent and child, and replace the sense of being gifted with a child, come as they may, with something planned and designed. There is a loss here: an openness to the unbidden and the humility that comes from one's owns limits is replaced with hubris.

This argument has been greatly criticized and almost ridiculed. First, there are obviously many aspects to human life and human nature that do not warrant any gratitude and that we would rather not be "gifted"; some unbidden outcomes for which we have every reason to be ungrateful. Caplan has also questioned whether gratitude makes sense without a giver (Caplan, 2009, p. 208). Buchanan is skeptical of the extent to which it is possible to avoid the unbidden in any case. He states, "Only a genetic determinist on steroids (so to speak) would think that even the most thorough-going pursuit of perfection through biotechnology could banish contingency from human life and rob us of ample opportunities for exhibiting the sense of 'giftedness'" (Buchanan, 2011, p. 81).

Second, striving to enhance the chances for one's children seems more part of the parent–child relationship than in opposition to it. Caplan (2009, p. 207) asks rhetorically whether there is "value to be found in accepting the random draw of the genetic lottery with respect to one's own children?" To the contrary, he suggests that "[m]uch of what parents try to do is shape and control their children" (Caplan, 2009, p. 208). "The fact that there are some neurotic parents around should not be enough to prohibit the use of biological engineering to improve eyesight, enhance memory, or allow a child to learn languages with greater facility. The problem is bad parenting, not bad technology," Caplan concludes (p. 208).

Hauskeller (2011), in a particularly charitable attempt at engaging with Sandel's argument, suggests that there is a difference between what is merely given (and therefore the case) and what is gifted (and thereby warrants gratitude). Departing from a quote from Voltaire, that "the better is the enemy of the good," Hauskeller (2011, p. 71) argues that there is in enhancement a risk that we undermine what is good in pursuit of what we consider to be better, only to find that, whatever that better state, it is worse than some other better state. The point is that if everything is only relatively valuable, then nothing is valuable in itself:

> The worth of what has been given to us is here acknowledged as an absolute value in the Kantian sense, that is, a value that allows for no comparison. It is not good merely in the absence of something better or in comparison with what is worse. Rather, it is good in itself [sic], absolutely. The better is the enemy of the good in the sense that by confronting the good with the 'better,' the good changes its appearance and re-emerges as the 'worse.' When we focus on the better that we might achieve, we tend to forget what is good about what we have already got. It is, in other words, an act of conceptual devaluation, which in turn justifies the demand for improvement. Optimism regarding the future has as its flipside pessimism regarding the present. This pessimism may or may not be justified. It all depends on whether we set our hopes on the future because the present actually is found deficient, or we judge it deficient merely because we envisage a (largely imaginary) future that is (in some unspecified sense) better. The way calls for human enhancement are framed often suggests the latter. (Hauskeller, 2011, p. 71 f.)

We thus come up against two very different readings of the same argument: one about a slippery slope towards a situation where there is no room left for contingency, and one about undermining the very foundation for our capacity for gratitude and satisfaction with what is the case, in a constant chase for improvement, and the concern for how that might affect the bond between parent and child.

Another greatly influential argument is that of Habermas (2003). He points to a significant and fundamental shift in the parent–child relationship and our self-understanding when we start designing the nature of other persons and can hold others responsible for our own nature. "A previously unheard-of interpersonal relationship arises when a person makes an irreversible decision about the natural traits of another person," he writes (Habermas, 2003, p. 14). The concern is undermining the moral symmetry between each one of us as equals. In the traditional case, a child grows to become their own person and own their developmental history, and become an equal to their adult peers and also to their parental generation. This is what is undermined when a person is a product of someone else's mind; symmetry can never arise. "Rather, the adult would remain blindingly dependent on the nonrevisable decision of another person, without any opportunity to establish the symmetrical responsibility required if one is to enter into a retroactive ethical self-reflection as a process among peers. For this poor soul there are only two alternatives, fatalism and resentment" (Habermas, 2003, p. 14).

Why would this be the case? We assume that the point is one of principle rather than prediction of a particular outcome; it is about the nature of the kind of action that designing the nature of another person is, and the centrality that the moral axiom that each person is born free and equal occupies in our modern ethical worldview. Instead of each person having equal standing with all other persons, we will now have persons whose very nature was predetermined by the choices of others before they were born, and those who have predetermined the nature of others and are thus responsible for their nature:

> This new type of relationship offends our moral sensibility because it constitutes a foreign body in the legally institutionalized relations of recognition in modern societies. When one person makes an irreversible decision that deeply intervenes in another's organic disposition, the fundamental symmetry of responsibility that exists among free and equal persons is restricted. We have a fundamentally different kind of freedom toward the fare produced through the contingencies of our socialization than we would have toward the prenatal production of our genome. (Habermas, 2003, p. 14)

Why would this matter? One interpretation, given the centrality of modernity and universal postenlightenment in Habermas' philosophy, would be that symmetry lies at the heart of the moral frameworks of modernity, including universal rights, equal freedoms, democracy itself as a project of reciprocity, and the equal standing of all persons and people, regardless of religion, culture, gender, ethnicity, and so on. Or, to put it differently, all modern ethical systems and all democratic political systems depart from the idea that we are born free and equal as a point of departure. It is the core value on top of which everything else rests and what has made criticism against discrimination, exploitation, colonialism, servitude, genocide, and the like possible: they are morally wrong because they violate the notion of everyone having the same moral standing.

A fundamental tenet in the modern postenlightenment worldview is that *we are all born free and equal*. This is the notion that enabled modern democracy, criticism against racism, sexism, colonialism, and everyone being equal before the law:

> For as soon as adults treat the desirable genetic traits of their descendants as a product they can shape according to a design of their own liking, they are exercising a kind of control over their genetically manipulated offspring that intervenes in the somatic bases of another person's spontaneous relation-to-self and ethical freedom. This kind of intervention should only be exercised over things, not persons. (Habermas, 2003, p. 13)

Without going too far into Habermas' argument (and its critics), we can take note of two things here: there is a concern that something fundamental changes in terms of who we are and who we can be when our nature has been determined by choices of other persons who ought to be our equals and peers as persons. This is not about psychological effects on the child born or what they can do as much as a metaphysical concern about the kinds of beings we are and will become and the kind of political society and ethical relations we can have when that becomes the norm. How can we be a society of equals and autonomous persons when our very nature is determined by others by choice? In reality, that power may only be carried out in insignificant ways, but a person could potentially be designed merely to be born to fulfill a particular function, such as an artistic one, a reproductive one, and so on. Whereas one can fight back against the given social odds, one is in a lesser position to change the genetic odds one was dealt. The argument makes more sense as violating a republican notion of freedom or dignity, rather than as one of predicting a particular kind of outcome: One is never free if one is under the arbitrary will of another—here, the potential realm of despotism is increased not only to apply to the political sphere but also our own genome.

Similar points have been defended by others in the earlier debate. The concern is that we might "commodify" life, or that the embryo becomes a "bio-fact" and an "object of technoscience" (Primc, 2018, p. 107 f.). Much more recently, Sparrow (2015, 2019) added an interesting new argument: Assuming that germline enhancement became widespread and continued to progress much as other kinds of technology, we should also assume that the various models would become obsolete and replaced with newer and better ones. Should the speed of such a "rat race" be fast enough, a child may be born and already obsolete; in essence, "yesterday's child" (Sparrow 2015, 2019).

8.7   Radical Enhancement, Transhumanism, and the Posthuman

"Enhancement" is, indeed, a very broad concept. It could apply to, at one end, any intervention that goes beyond treatment. Such interventions could largely play into a medical rationale, as in the case of boosting the immune system. At the other end, it could apply equally well to attempts to deliberately surpass our natural limitations and improve on the human model, as it were. At the farthest end of the enhancement project, we find the explicitly *transhumanist* aspirations.[16] Transhumanism can be described as a movement with the aim of radically enhancing humanity and, ultimately, overcoming human limitations and transcending humanity to the next evolutionary step that surpasses us: the posthuman.[17] Levin (2017, p. 278), for instance, describes the transhumanists as embracing "an extreme of enhancement advocacy." Bostrom, one of the key proponents of transhumanism, describes the transhumanist quest in the following way:

> Transhumanists hope that by responsible use of science, technology, and other rational means we shall eventually manage to become posthuman, beings with vastly greater capacities than present human beings have. (Bostrom, 2005, p. 4)

More (1990), another advocate for the transhumanist notion, describes transhumanism as "a class of philosophies that seek to guide us towards a posthuman condition." Porter, in a critical essay, sums up the core idea, in the following way:

> The core of transhumanism is to encourage the use of biotransformative technologies in order to "enhance" the human organism, with the ultimate aim being to modify the human organism so radically as to "overcome fundamental human limitations" and thereby the "human" as such. (Porter, 2017, p. 237 f.)

The focus has thus shifted from improvements within the limits and normal expectations of what humans can be, to transcending those limits and expectations and "become posthuman." The goal is to take on evolution as a deliberate project, but not to improve upon our species as much as to transcend the limits of humanity. One of the key ideas is that "human nature is a work-in-progress, a half-baked beginning that we can learn to remold in desirable ways" (Bostrom, 2005, p. 4). Key terms within this framework are "transhumans" and "posthumans," where the former refers to "transitional humans" who have greater capacities than normal humans, but not yet fully those of the posthuman. The posthuman is no longer

---

[16] According to Porter, "Long a fairly small or even fringe movement in philosophy and futurology, transhumanism is gaining steam as a cultural and intellectual movement, and it is increasingly becoming a global force" (Porter, 2017, p. 239).

[17] There are also other aspirations that are less relevant to the topic of germline gene editing: space colonization, creation of superintelligent machines, the possibility of uploading human minds electronically to avoid physical decay and enable a virtual existence and various incarnations, etc.

human, but has become something altogether better, a new kind of being, as it were. Or, as Porter, sums it up:

> According to transhumanists, a "transhuman" is a "transitional human" who aims at becoming posthuman and takes appropriate steps (e.g., technological enhancement) toward that end—whereas a "posthuman," the ideal for and goal of transhumanists, is becoming so radically different in physical, cognitive, and emotional capacities from normal or current humans as to be no longer unambiguously human. (Porter, 2017, p. 238)

Who, then, is this posthuman? What can they be and do that is sufficiently different from us to be *post*human, yet, so magnificent as to come with its own imperative to fast-forward their arrival? First, a point of caution: Although the end in the abstract is largely the same—to bring forward a new kind of human that is much improved and without any of our current weaknesses but with our strengths developed beyond what we can currently imagine—not all, or even most, routes go through genetic engineering specifically. Some look instead towards AI and the merging of humans and machines or even the idea of virtual existence of "uploaded minds" that can live various virtual realities without limits. More (1990) mentions "neuroscience, neuropharmacology, life extension, nanotechnology, artificial ultraintelligence, and space habitation, combined with a rational philosophy and value system" (cited in Aydin, 2017, p. 49). Aydin (2017, p. 4) adds "genetic engineering, prosthetics and powered exoskeletons, and tissue engineering" to these.

Bostrom in his *Letter from Utopia* (2008b) imagines what a future self might write to us mere humans in a plea to approach a path that would enable the existence of such a future self. There are three necessary transformations we need to embark upon to achieve this future: combat death, expand mind and intelligence, and increase well-being. The implied notion is that mortality is to be avoided or at least delayed as much as possible:

> Your body is a death trap ... You be lucky to get seven decades ...

> ... Take aim at the causes of early death—infection, violence, malnutrition, heart failure, cancer. Turn your biggest gun on aging, and fire. You must seize control of the biochemical processes in your body in order to vanquish, by and by, illness and senescence. In time, you will discover ways to move your mind to more durable media. Then continue to improve the system, so that the risks of death and disease keep receding. Any death prior to the heat death of the universe is premature if your life is good. (Bostrom, 2008b)

Furthermore, the values to be promoted are joys that mental capacities can bring. "Your brain's special faculties: music, humor, spirituality, mathematics, eroticism, art, nurturing, narration, gossip! There are fine spirits to pour into the cup of life and greater realms of well-being." (Bostrom, 2008b) But, again, it is what we could have, beyond the human limits, that we ought to pursue: "Your brain must grow beyond the bounds of any genius of humankind, in its special faculties as well as its general intelligence, so that you may better learn, remember, understand, and so that you may apprehend your own beatitude" (Bostrom, 2008b). The mind is both the means to the posthuman existence and an end—in that "it is in the spacetime of awareness that Utopia will exist" (Bostrom, 2008b) Finally, what makes the posthuman existence a utopia is the vast amount of pleasure. ("We have immense silos of it here in utopia. It pervades all that we do, everything that we experience."). Moreover, there is also a qualitative difference: "There is a beauty and joy here that you cannot fathom. It feels so good that if the sensation were translated into tears of gratitude, rivers would overflow" (Bostrom, 2008b). There are two parts to this, the increase of pleasure and the elimination of pain and misery, "in addition to the removal of the negative, there is also an upside imperative: to enable the full flourishing of enjoyments currently slumbering in their bulbs and buds, unknown to man and woman" (Bostrom, 2008b).

With all this in place, we can now revisit the question of possible benefits of germline gene editing. The kind of benefits transhumanists hope for are as radical as the future beings they envision. The benefits imagined are not just more of the same, but also beyond what we can currently imagine. Bostrom (2005) discusses the prospects of radical improvements across all of the following parameters: radical extension of lifespan and radical increase in intellectual capacity, body functionality, sensory modalities, special faculties, sensibilities, mood, energy, and self-control. "The range of thoughts, feelings, experiences, and activities accessible to human organisms presumably constitute only a tiny part of what is possible," writes Bostrom (2005, p. 4), with the implication that there is much more that we could potentially experience and be beyond our current limits. These radically improved capacities are thought to lead to a superior kind of existence and a superior quality of life, as described above in the excerpts from the *Letter from Utopia*. Between here and there, there is the transhuman that is more than we currently are, not quite posthuman yet, but on the right path. Bostrom adds:

> You have just celebrated your 170th birthday and you feel stronger than ever. Each day is a joy. You have invented entirely new art forms, which exploit the new kinds of

cognitive capacities and sensibilities you have developed. You still listen to music—music that is to Mozart what Mozart is to bad Muzak. You are communicating with your contemporaries using a language that has grown out of English over the past century and that has a vocabulary and expressive power that enables you to share and discuss thoughts and feelings that unaugmented humans could not think or experience. (Bostrom, 2008b, p. 5)

At this point, we can begin to anticipate a potentially forceful argument that could be made for germline editing: If transhumanism can deliver what it seeks to achieve, namely to eradicate major sources of suffering, radically extend life expectancy, and radically enhance our capacities for well-being, then this could indicate that such interventions, if safe and successful, could increase human well-being more than any of the alternatives. We will, for now, set aside, concerns about what is practically achievable and at what risks and costs, and focus on the ideal itself. To what extent is the ideal imagined a coherent and desirable one?

The first line of objection challenges the coherence of the proposed ideal. Specifically, the idea that we can do away with the negative aspects of the human experience while maintaining the positive aspects presumes that the latter does not depend on the former. This runs counter to how philosophers and scholars have believed values work since antiquity, and the contrast-dependency has been taken for granted—it is not clear that happiness, pleasure, bliss, and so on hold any meaning in a world where its contrary does not exist. This is at least what Levin (2017) and Porter (2017) argue. Essentially, we are promised strength, success, talent, genius, bliss, beauty, and so on in a world where no one is weak, no one is mediocre, no one without talent or genius, and there is no source of suffering, sadness, grief or regret, and everyone is beautiful, and so on.

The second question relates to the first: Who is it that is supposed to benefit from the posthuman quest exactly? If the posthuman is truly beyond human, then it could not be said that this would necessarily be in the interest of humans, and, as has been previously argued, we cannot be said to benefit someone who does not yet exist. It is not even clear that it would on the whole be an improvement to add posthumans to our mix, even less to replace us with them. The former, because this is bound to raise issues of justice, access, fairness, discrimination, and shifted notions of normality, and so on. The latter, because it would result in a permanent loss and destruction of what we have up until now placed at the heart of all our moralities: the preservation and well-being of humanity.

8.7.1   The Value Challenge

Porter argues that transhumanism faces a *value challenge*. The question is whether the transhumanist ideal is conceptually coherent (Porter, 2017, p. 245). Transhumanists "want to 'have it all' without any sacrifices or downsides—a life of perpetual bliss untarnished by suffering, a happy life without any (involuntary) experience of unhappiness, etc.," Porter writes (Porter, 2017, p. 245). However, according to Porter, such a position may be conceptually incoherent. Porter points to two different kinds of concerns. Both stem in part from the ambitions of transhumanism to abolish human pain, suffering and boredom, combined with the equally ambitious quest to enable bliss beyond what we can currently imagine.

The first concern is that all of the positive states the transhumanist seeks to establish in the posthuman condition might necessarily depend on the negative states they also seek to abolish. For instance, should ambition and aspiration require necessity and desire as motivation, then we could not achieve new heights in the former while rooting out the latter. Should health and well-being require illness and suffering to hold value or be experienced, then we could not reach new heights in the former while abolishing the latter. Should prosperity require necessity and lack to hold value, then we could not find new heights in the former while seeking to abolish the latter. Levin (2017, p. 286, p. 289) argues that "contrast-dependency" is intrinsic to experience or motivation. Thus, the very project that the transhumanist seeks to achieve, one where all suffering is abolished, or merely optional for the posthuman, and such posthumans are thought to "continue to have all matters of desires" is inconceivable, given what we know of aspiration as a response to a lack of something. Thus, Levin argues, "transhumanists elude contrast-dependency neither between human and posthuman modalities nor within posthuman existence itself." The posthuman existence is constantly described as better than ours. Yet, as Levin points out, "posthumans are the telos now but are likely not the best simpliciter. How do we know that having eliminated restrictions under which we currently chafe, posthumans would not construct—literally or interpretively—another set of adversaries? If as transhumanists imply, contrast-dependency remains, whatever is opposed to the 'good' prong must bear the weight of negativity. In that case, bliss would be if not utterly fragile then unreliable because not wholly regulable" (Levin, 2017, p. 288).

The second concern is that the transhumanist vision of the posthuman condition is not a coherent notion in that it essentially seeks to maximize conflicting values that cannot simultaneously be maximized. As Porter observes, the transhumanist ideal "tends to be hyperbolically optimistic" (Porter, 2017, p. 244).

Porter writes that one might get the impression that "transhumanists think that posthumans can 'have it all,' or even perhaps that the term 'posthuman' merely names a particular techno-fantasy of 'having it all'—a life pervaded by pleasure and unsullied by suffering" (p. 244 f.). Porter's concern is that when maximizing one value, we might undermine another value we also seek to maximize, or vice versa: "what if it is, in some cases at least, impossible to have it all or maximize all values—and not due to any merely human limitations, such as could be overcome by technology, but because of the nature of the values involved?," Porter asks (p. 246). He takes the example of equality and beauty: "Is it possible—that is, is it conceptually coherent—to maximize both beauty and equality simultaneously? Can the beautiful exist if everything is equally beautiful, for example can human beauty still exist if everyone is equally beautiful?" His conclusion is that they cannot both be maximized, but they can be balanced (p. 255). The problem with transhumanism is that it is not looking for a balance between values, but wants it all: "But the transhumanists, with their goal of 'having it all,' do not wish to balance values that internally conflict or acknowledge the need to" (p. 255).

8.7.2 An Old Argument

Before we move on to the question of who benefits from the posthuman ideal, we need to address the view on limits and their perceived goodness and badness. A central part of the transhumanist project seems to be not accepting limits on human capacities, pursuits, or experiences of what is good and pleasurable. This comes in the starkest view in the reasoning around extending life. The assumption seems to be that living longer is good; hence, living for an infinite time, or as close to it as possible, would be ideal. The supposed value of living forever is not new but has, in fact, been discussed since antiquity as well as in the more recent meaning-of-life debate. Here, we will briefly visit what Nussbaum refers to as "an old argument," which consists in "pursuing seriously the thought that the structure of human experience, and therefore the empirical human sense of value, is inseparable from the finite temporal structure within which human life is actually lived" (Nussbaum, 1989, p. 336). According to this argument, it is our very finitude and mortality, "which conditions all our other awareness of limit, is a constitutive factor in all valuable things' having for us the value that in fact they have. In these constraints we live, and see whatever we see, cherish whatever we cherish, as beings moving in the way we actually move, from birth through time to a necessary death" (p. 336). Without mortality, many of the very things we value would lose their value. From this point of view, removing mortality from humanity would not constitute an improvement but their undoing: "the removal of all limit, of all constraint of finitude in general, mortality in particular, would not so much enable these values to survive eternally as bring about the death of all value as we know it" (p. 336).

What, then, is the exact problem with an unlimited or immortal existence, according to Nussbaum? As we have seen, according to the transhumanists, there is no problem at all. Harris for instance, suggests that "lifesaving is just death-postponing with a positive spin" and argues that if it is good to postpone death a little bit, then "it is difficult to see how it would not be better and more moral to postpone death for longer—even indefinitely." (Harris, 2007, p. 33) At first, one might think that whatever we value, the more of it the better: the greater the intensity, the greater the durability, and the greater the overall state of happiness, by some kind of simple happiness calculation. However, when we radically extend the span of a human life, other things may also change that could undermine the very values we seek to quantitatively extend.

The problem, according to this argument, is that when moving from a limited and mortal existence to one that is unlimited and immortal, the assumption that we will simply have more of what we currently value is false. This is because all, or at least most, of the things we currently value are not without context, but gain their value from the temporal structure and limits of a human life. Remove those limits and we will undermine the basis of those values. Nussbaum writes:

> The claim to be established is that, for many, if not for all, of the element of human life that we consider most valuable, the value they have cannot be fully explained without mentioning the circumstances of finite and mortal existence. They would not exist as they are, or have the value they have, in a life not structured by mortality. (Nussbaum, 1989, p. 337)

Agar (2010), an advocate of moderate enhancement and liberal eugenics, makes a similar point. He argues against any kind of enhancement that significantly goes beyond the maximum that could be achieved by current or past human beings, on the basis that it risks taking our humanity from us and eliminating what we value about being human.

According to Nussbaum, two things change when we move from the mortal case to the immortal one: the role of *risk (of death)* and of *time* (Nussbaum 1989, p. 338). This seems right; without the possibility of death, there will be no risk of death, and living forever alters the temporal aspect of a human life. Nussbaum's point is that nearly all human virtues and values depend in one way or another on either one of these two factors.

Without the risk of death, many human virtues and values fall away. Without the risk of dying, the notion of risking one's life for someone or something no longer makes any sense. To the immortal, nothing could be "worth" risking one's life. With the risk of death off the table, many of the virtues we value become senseless. Nussbaum specifically mentions courage, moderation, political justice and private generosity, and so on. "The profound seriousness and urgency of human thought about justice arises from the awareness that we all really need the things that justice distributes, and need them for life itself," Nussbaum writes. We have to imagine the immortal condition as a condition where courage has no place, since there is no sense in risking one's life for anything or anyone. We have to imagine the immortal condition as a condition where there is no room for protecting the weak, young and vulnerable from risk of death, no room for political justice in the sense of ensuring that each and every one has equal access to what is necessary for life. Furthermore, we have to imagine parenthood (if there is such a thing in the immortal condition) as a condition where there is no sense of protecting one's young from risks of dying. "If parents are not necessary to enable children to survive and grow, if a city is not necessary for the life of its citizens, if altruistic sacrifices of what one actually *needs* cannot be made, then human relationships would more and more take on the optional, playful character that Homer, depicting the gods so marvelously shows us" (p. 339). According to Nussbaum, "the further mortality is removed, the further they [human virtues and their importance] are" (p. 339).

Without time and temporality and a sense of finitude, many of the things we value most lose their meaning and significance. One part of this has to do with the temporality and fleetingness of opportunity. According to Nussbaum, "the intensity and dedication with which very many human activities are pursued cannot be explained without reference to the awareness that our opportunities are finite, that we cannot choose these activities indefinitely many times" (p. 339). She exemplifies by mentioning activities such as raising a child, "cherishing a lover," and performing various kinds of creative or otherwise challenging tasks (p. 339). While engaged in these kinds of activities we are "aware, at some level, of the thought that each of these efforts is structured and constrained by finite time" (p. 339.).

The general point is that two aspects are affected when we consider time and temporality for the immortal. First, we have this loss of value connected to the purpose and meaning that arises with the temporary, the fragile, the vulnerable, and that which could be lost: the beauty of a spring morning, the fragile life of a newborn, and so on. Second, there is the freezing of time when we imagine a life that goes on and on, and how it disrupts all values attached to multiple generations. If everyone who is currently alive lives on, there would be little need for new generation, and even if there was a new generation, it would soon become contemporary. All sense of learning from the previous generation, passing things on to a new generation, and so on disappears.

With the above "old argument" in mind, we can revisit the rosy picture that Bostrom painted earlier. Even if we celebrate our 170th birthday, for the immortal, this will not be a celebration with multiple generations of another year when death was beaten, but one in a never-ending line of birthdays celebrated among contemporaries who will all be around for every one of those countless birthdays. When we imagine the great musical genius able to compose greater masterpieces than Mozart, we have to imagine those conquests produced in a context where a million such pieces could be conducted every year, by everyone, for eternity. The peaking levels of bliss that far exceed anything a human has experienced will be much the same as the levels of bliss experienced yesterday, last week, last month, last year, last decade, last millennia, and so on. We have to imagine the cognitive mind far greater than any current mind, as a mind with no pressing problems to be solved, since there is no real risk of death—and if there were, it might already have been solved by the even greater artificial mind. Thus, there is nothing for the human mind to achieve, nothing to solve, nothing to salvage, and no reason to leave any legacy of any kind, since one will always be around and one has already met everyone in the future.

There are two conclusions that we could draw from the above. The conclusion that Nussbaum draws, from our perspective, is that there will not be much of our values left in the immortal condition. The other conclusion we can draw is that what might appear to be a case of radical enhancement from our perspective, is likely to be viewed as the norm to the posthuman. Thus, intelligence that far exceeds our own and bliss beyond what we can imagine will not count as enhancement *for the posthuman*. Thus, no matter how great their capacities and experiences may seem from our limited human perspective, it is unlikely to impress or satisfy the posthuman. Essentially, the ideal—a posthuman existence that both eliminates all sources of suffering, yet is exciting and stimulating in contrast to a flawed human one characterized by "rockiness and boredom"—does not exist (Levin, 2017, p. 288).

8.7.3   Beneficial for Whom?

But *who* exactly benefits from humans either being superseded or joined by posthumans? Consider the following claim by Bostrom (2005):

> Transhumanism does not require us to say that we should favor posthuman beings over human beings, but that the right way of favoring human beings is by enabling us to realize our ideals better and that some of our ideals may well be located outside the space of modes of being that are accessible to us with our current biological constitution. (Bostrom, 2005, p. 8)

Here, Bostrom suggests that promoting this cause is "the right way of favoring human beings."[18] In his *Letter from Utopia*, there is a plea from the posthuman writer to the human recipient to promote the kind of technology that would enable the posthuman to come to be (thus, in some sense, benefiting them), which is presented as something that would benefit the human in the sense that it would be their future. But how could the promotion of the posthuman benefit humanity? Given the lengths to which transhumanists go to stress *how far beyond us* their existence would be in terms of their experiences and way of being, it is difficult to see that it would be *us* who would benefit *as* posthumans. Much of the transhumanist argument for bringing about the posthuman seem to rely on the following two premises:

1. *The Radical Difference Claim [RD]*: The Posthuman *will be radically different* from us, no longer essentially human or bound by human limits—they are *post*human not human.
2. *The Radical Bliss Claim [RB]*: A posthuman future would essentially constitute a utopia and the experiences of a posthuman would surpass anything we have ever experienced in terms of greatness.

Against the background of the two premises above, it is argued that we must therefore promote the posthuman condition and realize this utopia. This leads us to the following:

3. *The Transhumanist Imperative [TI]*: We ought to promote the posthuman condition so that we can realize the posthuman utopia.

Let us consider three options: humanity will benefit, the posthumans will benefit, and some ideal will be realized (and those who value that ideal will in an abstract

---

[18] Elsewhere, Bostrom writes, "ideally, everybody should have the opportunity to *become posthuman*" (Bostrom, 2005, p. 10, italics added). However, the very notion of becoming posthuman makes no sense in the context of germline editing, even though it may carry greater plausibility within the broader context of enhancement technologies. Thus, whatever the benefits are, it cannot be that it would provide any opportunity to *become* posthuman.

way benefit). Undoubtedly, it seems that the transhumanists would benefit in that a cause they advocate strongly would be promoted. It is much less clear that it would be of benefit to humanity, who would either be replaced or attempt to peacefully co-exist with beings with certain capacities designed to surpass them. It is not even clear that the cause would benefit the posthumans.

First, if we accept the logic that we can only benefit someone that exists, we would not benefit posthumans by bringing them about. However, one could object that this seems a bit hasty. Clearly, it is better to be born into better circumstances than worse circumstances, and there could be good moral grounds to ensure that a future person is born into the former rather than the latter, and that is so *for the sake* of those born. On these grounds, it may be fair to say that for some individuals it would be beneficial to be born as a posthuman.

Would the posthuman existence be a better kind of existence? On the one hand, this seems plausible: the posthuman would have all the new capacities and improved ways of being. If we believe Bostrom, the posthuman existence would be a feast of genius, talent, and never-ending bliss that was devoid of pain, sorrow, and death. Yet, on the other hand, it is very likely that the posthuman would not view themselves as enhanced, but see their circumstances as the new normal and therefore not enjoy any greater levels of happiness or contentment than if they had not had those capacities. Beyond the specific value of particular enhancements, it is very difficult to draw any conclusions either way about the potential for a greater kind of existence. All relevant understanding of "better" refers to our perspectives and values. We can only speculate about what the posthuman values and does not value. In fact, all that we can say is that *whatever* the posthuman values, it is very likely *not* to be the same as what we value and may even run counter to what we value. Furthermore, if the posthuman is a product of our invention more than one of natural evolution, it is not even certain that the correlation that seems to hold for all other species that what they value are things they can actually achieve or gain; the posthuman may not achieve what they value, and they may not value what they achieve.

8.8 Status Quo Bias and the Reversal Test

One of the recurring arguments for enhancement is that the benefits are so significant that the burden of proof must fall on those that object to opportunities for improvement. Bostrom confidently writes that "the potential gains" of germline enhancement are "enormous" (Bostrom, 2003, p. 498):

But if we think about it, we recognize that the promise of genetic enhancements is anything but insignificant. Being free from severe genetic diseases would be good, as would having a mind that can learn more quickly or having a more robust immune system. Healthier, wittier, happier people may be able to reach new levels culturally. To achieve a significant enhancement of human capacities would be to embark on the transhuman journey of exploration of some of the modes of being that are not accessible to us as we are currently constituted, possibly to discover and to instantiate important new values. (Bostrom, 2003, p. 498 f.)

Furthermore, should we accept the magnitude of the potential benefits, and still advise against enhancement, it could be argued that this must be due to some kind of irrational bias, such as risk aversion or familiarity bias, and so on. The status quo bias is an example of shifting the burden of proof. Essentially, it is irrational to prefer the status quo over a future state that is better. Bostrom and Ord (2006) suggest that one can test for such bias by "reversing the perspective" and asking whether one would be equally against using the technology to *lower* the same capacity as one is against using technology for enhancing it. Should it be the case that neither the improved state nor the deprived state is preferred over the status quo, then unless there are rational reasons to prefer the status quo, this would constitute a case of "status quo bias." This led them to propose a reversal test to test for such bias:

> Reversal Test. When a proposal to change a certain parameter is thought to have bad overall consequences, consider a change to the same parameter in the opposite direction. If this is also thought to have bad overall consequences, then the onus is on those who reach these conclusions to explain why our position cannot be improved through changes to this parameter. If they are unable to do so, then we have reason to suspect that they suffer from status quo bias. (Bostrom & Ord, 2006, p. 664)

It is not difficult to see where this line of argument is heading: Unless we can come up with compelling reasons not to bring about the posthuman utopia or pursue the "transhumanist journey," we may simply be expressing an irrational preference for what *is* rather than what is *best*. What this line of reasoning suggests is that we could compare two outcomes: one of which is actual and one of which is hypothetical, and we ought to assess them merely in terms of goodness (presumably, with the addition of any transaction cost). The status quo comes with no additional cost or risk and its outcome is certain. The posthuman dream first needs to demonstrate that it is actually realizable, second, that it is accessible to humans, and third, that the transitional cost and risk from here to there is worth it. There is a considerable epistemic asymmetry between what is the case (our status quo) and any idealistic future based on technological advances that are still hypothetical, of which the full impact on a social scale remains merely speculative. We can add anything we want to a wish list and compare it with what currently is, but if the ideal outcome depends on new technology with a transformative element, it is highly likely that we are missing fundamental parts of what that future will actually be like.

The idea of a "status quo bias" is, of course, directed towards more bioconservative positions and is meant to demonstrate that it is irrational to prefer the current state of affairs merely on the grounds that it is what exists rather than on account of what is best and has more value (see Hayenhjelm, 2024 for discussion). Cohen (2011), however, has defended the idea that it might be rational to attach special value to what is valuable and actually exists. He refers to this as a "conservative attitude:"

> Conservatism: We have reason to preserve valuable things that currently exist, even when we could replace them with things of equal or greater value. (Cohen, 2011)

Such an attitude may make particular sense when it comes to our own existence. To illustrate, one could just replace "valuable things" with "our own existence" and "things" with "other beings" in the quote above:

> Conservatism about Humanity: We have reason to preserve our own existence, even when we could replace ourselves with other beings of equal or greater value.

This does not seem like an irrational position to take. Should we disagree with that claim, we would have no reason not to replace humanity with any being greater than us. Objectively, there might be a good case for such a replacement. However, from the subjective perspective of humanity, this is not a position we could adopt. Part of being human is to place value on our own existence and our own survival as a species. Basically, all morally dominant theories are premised on the value and moral priority of our own existence and would support that we ought to, in a situation of conflict, value humans over other beings when in direct conflict such that only one could survive. No one claims that we ought to favor the survival of viruses or bacteria over humans, or favor the flourishing of tigers at the expense of humans consumed, and so on. When put to the test, loyalty to our own species is a core moral value for us as humans. Often, we expand upon this to include and cover the best interest of other species, but not when the two are in conflict. We do not feed our own babies to the hungry wolf even if we defend the rights of wolves when our babies are safe from harm. It seems that the only way the transhumanist can get away with not favoring humanity is by giving the impression that the posthuman is our own future self, rather than as distinct from us as the hungry wolf. In short, the basic idea is confused: it cannot both be the case that the Radical Difference Claim is true, a claim on which the Radical Bliss Assumption rests, and that it is us who will benefit from such radical bliss.

8.9   Discussion

In the previous chapter, we looked at various arguments based on the consequences of germline editing, particularly arguments based on the value maximization logic. In this chapter, we looked at arguments specifically concerning enhancement. Most of the pro-enhancement arguments are based on an optimistic outlook of the benefits of such interventions and some notion of significant increase in terms of scope and magnitude. Thus, it is argued, should we enhance the population as a whole (even in a more "modest" way so that the whole population has been genetically improved, but is still within the range of normal human capacities), then this would increase well-being, productivity, and quality of life.

Furthermore, should one venture into more radical forms of enhancement, the very nature of well-being may be increased such that the levels of well-being will be improved beyond what could currently be experienced. Thus, it would seem that the enhancement case for benefits heavily tilting the balance has some merit.

Once we move from medical and more moderate kinds of enhancement, such as boosting the immune system and correcting for various biological disadvantages beyond disease, to deliberate measures for more radical enhancement, the stakes and the risks increase considerably. Although morally much more controversial, they also have a stronger theoretical case—given that their prospective benefits (if correctly projected) are so much greater.

When comparing our current state of affairs with an imaginary future alternative state of affairs, there are always transition costs from here to there. Here, this means the first generation of germline edits, the "guinea pig generation," will be the first to enjoy the benefits if all goes well and all promises are delivered upon, and the first to suffer the consequences, foreseen and unforeseen. It also means that the introduction of technology may come to harm those currently living with genetic variations that would be eradicated, as they now live lives that are deemed not worth living. It could also mean that resources would be allocated in one place rather than another, which could come at very real costs in a public healthcare system. In case of a private system, it could be the start of widening injustice. It could also mean costs in terms of suffering in the biological supply chain with regard to women delivering eggs and embryos for research. It would most certainly rely on animal lives in research. Of course, this latter point is not unique to germline editing, but needs to be factored into the overall calculus of well-being. All such costs will be temporary. At some point, further research may become redundant, the changes in society will already have taken effect, and, in certain circles, societies, or countries, there may not be anyone born with certain kinds of genetic variations to be concerned about discrimination.

Thus, if the risks become predictable and manageable and the benefits are as impressive as the enthusiasts hope, one could see the consequentialist argument take shape: Given the magnitude of benefits, the increased well-being over all future generations, and the longer lives lived, any transitional costs will soon be outweighed by the benefits. Of course, those who would take the risks would not be the ones who would reap the best benefits. In fact, this is one of the most common objections based on the permissibility logic: The harm done to them cannot be outweighed by the greater benefits to us; there are individual rights and things we must not do to others, including risks we must not expose them to.

The question is whether that society is worth the costs of getting there, even if it were as great as the optimists predict. In part, this question must be answered in terms of fairness and moral acceptability of those transitional risks and costs. Are such costs, for instance, compensable or are they problematic in a principled sense? This is a question that evokes the permissibility logic of morality. However, in part, this question must also be answered in terms of whether the future society imagined is one worth striving for and one that is genuinely better. This is a question that evokes the third moral logic, the question about what ideals we want to pursue and what ultimately matters.

Currently, all these more radical kinds of enhancements are merely speculative, and the risks are largely unknown. Thus, it is hard to make a robust case based on how the benefits would add up based on nothing but speculation. More concerning is that it is hard to assess what value more radical interventions would actually have. There are a number of interesting value challenges that must be met for enhancement arguments to be convincing. First, should we change human nature too much, then the values that we thereby hope to increase may no longer apply. Second, should we enhance human capacities, we may only push the scale and point of reference and establish a new normal rather than an experienced increase. Third, the kind of world we promote may not be aligned with what we value or what is in our interest, and, if so, it is unclear why we should promote it. In the end, the enhancement case seems to rest on a particular kind of ideal and the value that some attach to that ideal. Here, it seems that the arguments draw, in part, on the third kind of moral logic, the pursuit of ideals. It is a certain kind of human that is imagined in the transhumanist case, one that is better in ways that is appreciated now. A kind of ideal wish list with added imagined amplifications along a scale that shoots through the roof. As long as one shares the same outlook on what it means to be human and what makes it valuable, largely one of individual capacities, including high intelligence, this has a strong appeal, at least as an ideal.

It is, however, not a universally shared ideal and runs counter to other views on humanity that are rooted in more social and humanistic notions of what it means to be human, and departs from a view of humans as vulnerable, and a value of solidarity with others based on diversity. In the end, consequentialist arguments for enhancement are currently too speculative; we have to imagine the actual risks, and the impact—not only on society, but also on what it would mean for us as humans and our identity and relations. Here, the answers are not clear; the kinds of values that we are to assess such a course by are not clear, and the basis for the relevant values is the nature we seek to alter. In the end, it comes down to questions about what ultimately matters to us as humans.

Many of the objections to radical enhancement and transhumanist projects are concerns about what we could potentially lose, what is ultimately at stake, and what humanity means. These lead us to the next chapter and the question of risks and lingering concerns about germline editing in general, particularly when we extend the possible consequences further to investigate what is truly at stake. What weight we ought to attach to such concerns will depend not only on alternatives, but also on how likely such outcomes are in terms of probability, the case for some kind of slippery slope, the degree of reversibility and compensability of any risks, and ultimately what we value, who we would like to be, and what kind of society we would like to promote.

To conclude, once we move from germline editing as the only means of having a genetically related child for parents who otherwise would not be able to, to germline editing as a means to improve upon the human model, whether this be as an available option for parents, as an obligation to future individuals, or as a means to take control over human evolution, the nature of the rationale and the relevant arguments change. In the former case, the pro arguments depend on the parental desire for a genetically related child. It is this desire that germline editing can fulfill. It does not offer a treatment to an existing patient as such. Thus, the relevant alternatives are other reproductive options, such as those based on donorship, embryo selection, adoption, or refraining from having a child of one's own, and so on. The cases for and against enhancement are different. Here, there is no need for an embryo to be at risk of any genetic disease. Instead, the embryo is seen as something that could be improved upon. This means that women without any genetic disease or fertility challenges would need to turn to some kind of IVF clinic or something similar to ensure that embryos or eggs are released and edited before being transferred. It would mean that parents would alter the genes of their child upon recommendation (from the clinic or provider of the technology) or by their own initiative or out of social pressures, or some combination of these, to fit some projection of what kinds of capacities would be desirable in their offspring for their own well-being, or according to their values or those of society. The point is that whereas the first scenario is motivated by a wish to avoid a genetic disease and have a genetically related child, the second would be motivated by placing a higher value on what could be—on what we could make a human person to be—over what the person would otherwise be. It is important to see that these distinct rationales are not underscored by the same kinds of values, but one just more radical than the other. In fact, the value placed on genetic relatedness stems from a value of connection, similarity, and reflection in the parent–child relationship. By contrast, in the case of radical enhancement, similarity is not the primary value. Instead, it would be much better if the child were drastically different from their parents if this meant that the future person was drastically improved or had better chances for a good life. Here, it is closeness to an ideal that is of value, rather than closeness to the parents.[19]

However, if the benefits are on a scale of their own, so are the risks. If all is staked on bets of increased benefits, then what we presume to be beneficial for the future human must also be just that from their perspective. If all is staked on some vision of a better future or a better kind of being, it must also turn out to be a valuable ideal to pursue in the first place. Rather than being a rational pursuit for us based on our current values, it seems that the pursuit of enhancement is

---

[19] Different scholars seem to have different kinds of aims in mind. Savulescu and others seem to specifically have increased well-being and chances of a good life in mind. In other words, enhancement is motivated from value maximization, but on an individual level rather than a collective one. Bostrom and other transhumanists, by contrast, seem to be motivated by an ideal and the allure of a much different kind of being that is in all respects better than humans. Agar (2010, 2013) is motivated by large-scale benefits from modest enhancements, such that overall welfare and well-being is increased. Agar, on the other hand, opposes any enhancement that goes beyond what falls within our normal human span of capacities; the key drivers in his reasoning is entirely an evening out of the odds (on an individual level), improved productivity, and increased welfare in society as a whole.

about the promotion of a particular kind of ideal—one that is far from shared by everyone as the ideal kind of future we desire. To this, we must add all the uncertainties, risks and costs of transition, as well as the fact that all of this may be fully unrealistic.

Lingering Concerns

In this chapter, we will look specifically at the question of whether there is something *particularly morally problematic* with human germline gene editing. What, if anything, is it that warrants serious moral hesitation towards germline editing? It might seem as if this question has already been answered, in that we have looked at both categorical arguments and consequentialist arguments. Here we will, however, reframe the questions in terms of ethics of *risk*.

If we ignore the optimists and the equanimous voices and focus on those raised against taking germline editing lightly, these divide roughly along the same parameters as our three moral views. There are technical reasons to be seriously concerned based on technical risks. There are social reasons to be seriously concerned based on social and societal risks. And there are moral reasons to be seriously concerned based on moral and metaphysical risks.[1] These kinds of risks and their possible remedies are very different.

Furthermore, there is a common notion associated with value maximization logic, that any kind of risk is, in principle, compensable. Thus, there is nothing that we ought never to do because of its risk per se, but only relative to, and conditional on, there being no amount of benefit that could compensate for such risks. This notion could be challenged in two ways. First, all risks might not be compensable, because the outcomes might not be commensurable or comparable in the relative sense. If so, it would at least be difficult to tell what, if anything, would compensate for the potential losses. Second, from the moral permissibility

---

[1] Moral risk in this context refers to the risk of acting morally wrong, especially in light of moral uncertainty. Metaphysical risk refers to risk of existential losses and potential losses of whole kinds (of things or beings). See Sect. 9.1.3.

© The Author(s) 2025
M. Hayenhjelm and C. Nordlund, *The Risks and Ethics of Human Gene Editing*,
Technikzukünfte, Wissenschaft und Gesellschaft / Futures of Technology, Science
and Society, https://doi.org/10.1007/978-3-658-46979-5_9

logic, morality is not about the final sums of consequences, but about whether the acts concord with core moral values, such as dignity, rights, consent, and so on. Thus, an act that is not particularly risky might still violate fundamental moral principles. For instance, it might be fully safe to make one's children fluorescent, but it would hardly be morally defensible in terms of dignity and consent. Here, however, the main idea will be a different one: Is there anything that speaks to the claim that at least some of the potential acts of human germline editing, or at least some of the consequences such edits might lead to, belong to a different moral level of risk-taking than ordinary violations of rights or impositions of risk of harm?

We will first briefly review the various worst-case scenarios that each moral view highlights and then divide these risks into two categories, quantitative and qualitative, after which we will finally explore the idea of "metaphysical risk." If germline editing could be taken as a form of metaphysical risk, then this could speak in favor of a more cautious approach, since such risk could not be properly compensated for. Instead, any losses resulting from such risk would need to be replaced with something else. This need not make such risks inherently wrong but may move them up a notch to a more severe kind of moral risk-taking. This is what we will explore in this chapter.

9.1   What Are We Concerned About?

What, if anything, is it that we are really concerned about when it comes to human germline gene editing? Recall Church's question presented earlier (Sect. 7.1.2): "What is the scenario that we're actually worried about? That it won't work well enough? Or that it will work too well?" (Vogel, 2015, p. 1301). The kinds of concerns that underscore objections to germline gene editing are largely arguments based on risks, but the kind of risk that underwrites such objections are very different. In the above quote, such risks are divided into two categories: those that are related to risks from the technology itself, presumably off-target risks, mosaicism, and so on, and those that are related to concerns about its potential social and psychological costs in terms of discrimination, injustice, and effects on human relations. Notably, the three views introduced earlier, the Technical View, Democratic View, and Moral View, could be employed to highlight distinct risks. We could refer to them as technical risks, societal and social risks, and moral risks. These are all concerns about unwanted outcomes that may or may not come about as a result of germline editing as a single act or widespread practice.

9.1.1   Technical Risks

From a technical perspective, the focus lies on what we could refer to as technical risks. Thus, from this perspective, the most serious concerns about germline editing are related to the act of editing genes in a way that are heritable and will affect all the cells of the future person. From a very narrow perspective, it is clear what those risks are: the edit not being as precise as intended, not having the intended effects, being in the wrong place, being incomplete, and so on. From the same narrow perspective, the remedy is obvious: to ensure that the technology is as precise, efficient, and safe as required. From a broader perspective—or rather, if we ask precisely how such unsuccessful gene edits would be harmful to a person inheriting them—it becomes clear that the kinds of risks involved here are as much epistemic as they are technical. If the scientific knowledge of the gene that we edit, and the relationship between that gene and other genes is incomplete, the outcome may be different than intended, and in unforeseen ways. The fact that we do not know enough to know what will result if things go wrong (or if they go right) makes the technology unsafe and morally unjustified as long as there are safer options. This could eventually be overcome with more research. Even if such research might harm those who partake in it, the risk of harm is limited to those persons (unless made widely available) and could potentially be reversed or remedied.

9.1.2   Social Risks

From the perspective of social risks, the focus is less on technical harm, and more on what happens once germline gene editing becomes common enough to have a wide societal and potentially global impact. Again, there is no obvious single answer to what would happen to a society or humanity, should it become a widespread common practice to edit the genes of future persons. The concerns here seem to roughly divide into what we could consider near-future risks, distant-future risks (as a result of large-scale implementation), and those that are time independent.

The near-future risks are those we could imagine might result once germline editing takes hold. In the very first instance, issues are raised about how this might affect women who would be part of research or IVF treatment to enable germline editing. We also have the first generation of individuals who would be germline edited, perhaps when most effects are still unknown. These need not be negative. For instance, there has been some suggestion that the edited Chinese twin girls,

Nana and Lulu, could have benefited a cognitive enhancement (Regalado, 2019). Here, we also have the concerns about currently existing individuals and groups with disabilities that could face increased discrimination. After a generation or two of such germline editing, other kinds of risks come to the fore. Here, we might have concerns about equal access to germline editing, should such editing at that point have become safe and attached to privilege. Here, there are also concerns about deeper divisions between those who are edited and those who are not. Furthermore, there would be concerns about obsolescence as a result of fast-paced progress of the technology (Sparrow, 2015, 2019).

Further ahead, there are different kinds of questions to be asked and different kinds of concerns to be raised, should germline editing become a widespread phenomenon and used on a large scale. Here, we are left more to speculation. Some of the concerns are about what a totalitarian regime might do with such a technology, some about what a genetically vastly superior class would do to a genetically inferior one, and some about what humans would do to various new kings of beings that might not fit the mold of rights-bearing humans. In general, there is concern that germline editing would open Pandora's box or lead down a slippery slope to a grossly unpleasant society of our own making. These kinds of concerns hinge on what humans can do with a particular technology and how that could play out in society. The causal routes to any kind of unwanted society are many, but none of them is likely to be determined or, strictly speaking, unavoidable.

These concerns are thus causally much different from the technical risks. The technical risks would occur with a certain degree of probability if the technology used is not sufficiently safe. The societal risks could occur if many interactive turns of events lead to such outcomes. At the same time, there are various ways in which all risky trajectories might be stopped, since they hinge on what we as humans value, believe, can do, and would want to do at any given time. Much of which depends on constantly changing ideas due to trends, opinions of influential bodies and people, education, regulation, religion, pop culture, the wishes of parents, and so on. While we can currently imagine that this first step of germline editing will not likely lead to the worst-case scenario, we cannot confidently say that it will not eventually with global reach, in some future society and in some social context, be either largely misused or lead to very unpleasant consequences. Furthermore, it is not likely that a consensus now will capture all that is relevant in the broad perspective. Nor does our responsibility necessarily extend that far.

In any case, the far-end societal risks do not seem to kick in as soon as we start to edit the germline, but only as feared outcomes at the end of a slippery slope. Should the slope not be quite so slippery, or could the slope have various outcomes, some good and some bad, then these kinds of risks might be avoidable, even if germline editing is embraced in some form and for some purpose. Here, it seems as if the main concerns are about what kinds of regulations, restrictions and precautionary measures of a more social kind would be called for so that all individuals maintain their equal standing and we do not increase societal tensions or pave the way to societies we would rather not want.

9.1.3 Moral and Metaphysical Risks

From the Moral View, other kinds of risks could be highlighted and added to the above categories. Thus, apart from concrete risks for individuals or society, there are also more abstract risks, which could be referred to as "moral risks" and "metaphysical risks" respectively. The former refers to the risk of moral wrongdoing, the latter to bringing about ontological losses of kinds, properties, or potentialities, such that the fabric of reality is altered in some fundamental way.

Moral risk in this context denotes the risk that we may do what turns out to be deeply morally wrong. It would suggest moral precaution, such that we "err" on the safe side, morally speaking. It is in this light that we can view the various objections about dignity, hubris, playing God, naturalness, injustice, and so on. The bottom line is that there is a concern that we may do the wrong thing. Now, to err on the side of moral rightness involves a degree of epistemic risk-taking as well, given that we do not know for certain what the correct moral theory is and what the correct criterion of rightness is. This relates to the concept of "moral uncertainty" and the fact that we do not yet have all the moral answers or know which, if any, moral theory is the right one. Previously, one of us (Hayenhjelm, 2018) has argued that we take greater risks when we impose risks that could not even in principle be repaired, replaced, or compensated for, and that by avoiding staking what could never even in principle be replaced and only staking what could be compensated for, replaced, or repaired would be to err on the safe side.

Metaphysical risks highlight the concern that we might change reality in fundamental ways that could not be undone, which risks undoing exactly what it means to be human, what it means to be good, and the very meaning of a good society, such that something fundamentally human is lost. The metaphysical risks could be viewed as a special category of risks that may warrant a concern about moral risks: Should we cause a fundamental loss of a whole kind, and that loss turns out to be irreversible, irreparable, and incompensable, then there would be something unforgiving about it. Thus, it does not seem too farfetched to conjecture that when it comes to moral risking, such metaphysical risk belongs to the gravest kind of moral risks. Whether there is such a risk element to human germline editing depends on (a) whether there is a risk that something could be permanently lost (such as some part of human nature or humanity as a whole); (b) the value of such losses; and (c) whether the losses could, in fact, be irreversible, irreplaceable, or incompensable. Should the transhumanists be right, then a transhumanist replacement of humanity might be something to embrace. However, unless we know what makes us human and what is valuable about humanity, the risk exists that we might undo our humanity in ways that could not be repaired later.

9.2   Greater and Smaller Risks

The notion of "risk" is often used in a comparative way, such that one risk is taken to be greater or smaller than another risk. Such comparative moral risk could be captured in three different ways: as *a quantitative measure* of risk (more likely or more severe outcomes); as *a qualitative measure* of risk (the stakes are on a different level of value or moral significance); and as an *absolute risk* (more likely to bring about a metaphysical loss, such that the number of substantive things that exist or are made possible is permanently reduced).

It is common in the risk literature to distinguish between *objective* and *subjective* measures of risk. The objective measure overlaps with the quantitative measure above and the subjective measure overlaps partially with the qualitative measure. The objective and quantitative measures compare risks in terms of probability and/or severity of outcomes, both of which are measured numerically. Thus, one risk would be greater than another if the probability of it occurring is higher than the other, or if the severity is assessed to be worse, perhaps measured in mortality, or a combined measure of the two: expected number of negative outcomes where the severity of the outcome is adjusted by its probability. This is the *quantitative measure of risk*. The subjective risk measure has dominated the risk perception research (Slovic, 2000). In this context, one risk is greater than another if it is perceived to be worse. Such perceived risk could be the result of a number of factors, such as whether or not it is perceived as more "catastrophic," "familiar," "in one's control," and so on. On Slovic et al.'s account (2000), risk is a subjective notion and comparisons between more or less risk thus refer to psychological parameters and a subjective rationale rather than objective features of the world. Such risk perception studies are typically studied through quantitative psychometric studies in which comparative risk is a function of subjective evaluation. This is quite different from what we refer to as qualitative risk measures. On the contrary, qualitative measures pertain to objective properties of a certain kind of risk that could provide reasons for objectively viewing it as more or less risky than another risk. A risk would be greater than another risk in a *qualitative sense* if the potential losses of that risk are different, such that it is the kind of loss that makes the risk seem greater than it actually is. Such properties could very well overlap with those listed by Slovic et al. (2000). For instance, we may have objective reasons to consider catastrophic risks as greater risks than non-catastrophic risks, even if the latter had a higher probability of occurring or a higher expected disutility.

Here, we will also add a third measure of risk. A risk would be greater than another risk in *an absolute sense* if that risk, in contrast to the other risk, could bring about a permanent rupture in what exists or not and what is possible and not, and thus could permanently undermine the foundation for some kind of existence or possibility that is deemed valuable.

These three measures—quantitative, qualitative, and absolute—partially overlap with the most intuitive measures for the three kinds of risks—technical, social, and moral—discussed in the previous section. This is an oversimplification, of course, but it may make the overall picture clearer. The very worst category of technical risks is that with the greatest degree of harm (greatest impact and scope) and the highest probability, such as the late discovery of, say, infertility, or cancer risks as a result of germline gene editing affecting a whole generation of edited children. Similarly, the worst category of social risks would be those that represent the qualitatively most severe kinds of risk, such as a dystopia of extreme class societies divided into genetic groups. The worst kinds of risks on the absolute measure would be the loss of fundamental categories of possibilities for value such that they could neither be retrieved nor replaced. Such losses do not occur in degrees, but the kind of loss could, of course, be fundamental, having greater or less impact on the world that remains as a whole. Thus, should germline editing come to pose a risk for the survival of the human race, or constitute species suicide, then this would constitute a risk of this kind.

The Moral View is, however, not limited to the absolute measure. When applying the value promotion logic, we would compare risks in a quantitative sense based on how much they promote different values. Conversely, when comparing risks based on whether they might violate rights or not or based on whom they might affect, we compare them in a qualitative sense.)

These three notions of relative risk also have implications for how comparable they are to other risks, and thereby how compensable or replaceable they are. The relative risk in a quantitative sense could generally be fully compared to other risks that could be measured in the same way. In simple terms, it is more rational to prefer what is less risky to what is more risky in quantitative terms when we stand to gain the same kind of benefit. This is not the case with qualitative risk. We may assess two different qualitative risky actions very differently; how a qualitative risk is measured depends on how that particular unwanted outcome or risk exposure is valued. Furthermore, there is no straightforward way to compare quantitative risk with qualitative risk: one qualitatively risky act may be deemed much riskier than some relatively high risks in a quantitative sense. For instance, we may view the prospects of our life partner becoming senile as a much greater risk than being hit by a meteor. However, the qualitative risks need not be incommensurable compared to other risks, but they do require some external ranking of values that affect what is deemed risky. Absolute risks point to permanent and objective losses so substantive that they cannot be retrieved or repaired.

9.2.1 Quantitative Risk

From the Technical View, all risks tend to be understood in a predominantly quantitative sense. This means that all risky options are more or less comparable. If risky action A is riskier than risky action B, but it has a much greater prospect of bringing about the desired benefits, then the moral question is reduced to the following: Which of the two actions have the greater expected utility when taking both the expected benefits and expected risks into account?

Consequently, there is little grounds for a principled position against germline editing on this perspective of risks. The fact that it is risky to conduct germline editing would only speak against it if there existed some alternative action that could bring about the same kind of benefits in a less risky way, an equally risky action would bring about greater rewards, or a much safer option would offer good enough rewards.

On a quantitative reading, any moral reason against something could be reversed when the balance between benefits and harms changes: in principle, any kind of harm or risk could be outweighed by a greater benefit. When the expected benefits are, comparatively speaking, too small, or the risks are, comparatively speaking, too high, or there is too much uncertainty to know either way, then there are good reasons not to take those risks. However, such a conclusion is sensitive to rapid change: what was once comparatively risky may become comparatively safe, either because of increased safety of the action in question or increased riskiness of the alternatives. What was once comparatively promising in terms of prospective benefits could become comparatively worthless, either because of decreased value, or because of improved alternatives, or because values change overall. What was deemed epistemically uncertain could become known. Many of the aspects that we have discussed in this book suggest that germline editing involves a high degree of quantitative risk.

Furthermore, germline editing may be particularly challenging in *an epistemic sense*, given the heritability aspect, the gaps in genetic knowledge, and the complexity and multifunctionality of genes, as well as the irreversible nature of such interventions suggesting that the degree of risk is significant: We could unknowingly cause a great deal of harm and suffering to future individuals who have not consented to being genetically experimented upon. This seems to be reason enough to advocate great caution. However, such concerns could, in principle, be overcome, given that they are relative.

Over time, we could become increasingly knowledgeable about how our genes work and what they do, and what we can edit. We may also learn to re-edit and correct for later generations and thus control the degree of heritability, and the fact that someone is born with edited genes (on the initiative of one's own parents or those of a previous generation) may be an advantage if the risks are reduced and the benefits are substantial. In the case of disease prevention, such risks may sometimes be worthwhile, given the gains and the suffering it aims to prevent.

In short, to whatever extent germline gene editing could be viewed as particularly risky in a quantitative sense, such riskiness could largely be a temporary feature of the epistemic and moral situation.

9.2.2 Qualitative Risk

Both the Democratic View and the Moral View highlight risk in a more qualitative sense. What makes germline editing different from other interventions is its potential to change who we are, change the kinds of relationships we would be able to have, and change the kinds of societies that could be developed. Thus, the risks are less about losses and gains and more about morally significant changes. This raises moral questions that cannot simply be reduced to questions about the overall balance of costs and benefits, but qualitative questions about the kinds of beings we want to be and the kinds of societies worth promoting. Consider this passage from Hurlbut et al. (2018):

> Even if long-term side effects were wholly predictable, editorial interventions into human biology would not occur only at the level of individual bodies and physical health. Any editing, especially of the human germline, represents an act of intentional design. While the biological effects on edited individuals might be beneficial, the social meanings of departing from an order in which all persons come into being with equally unique and unplanned genetic futures—and thus are equally subservient to the hazards of being born—are significant. Even minor edits to the DNA of a developing human embryo would, in the view of many, redefine fundamental social relationships (between parents and children, individuals and communities, citizens, and states), and associated notions of responsibility and care. Put differently, what is at stake is not only the biological future of edited children, but potentially, the meaning of broader norms and legal rights and duties that unpin society. (Hurlbut et al., 2018, p. 640)

There are two ways to read the above passage: as being about qualitative risk and fundamental changes or about fundamental losses. But let us first focus on the former and return to the latter in the next section.

Germline editing could be regarded as risky in the qualitative sense because it could fundamentally change our identity, nature, and social fabric. Furthermore, it might affect the very meaning of being human and undermine the premises upon which equal human rights and other norms are founded. A recurring concern about germline editing is that it would create division and hierarchy along genetic lines. Social mobility could become a thing of the past, replaced only by genetic mobility, if any mobility at all. Germline editing could open doors to some while closing them to others before they are born as a result of deliberate action. Germline editing might even pave the way for a somewhat permanent genetic elite and underclass.

However, even such injustices would not strictly speaking be permanent in a metaphysical sense, given that even those born into "genetic poverty" could at least theoretically ensure that the next generation benefited from "genetic improvements." In a social sense, this might not be possible at all, should the privileged classes closely guard the source of their privilege. In either case, it could be argued, for instance, that the risk for such a divide in society is of such significance that it outweighs all potential benefits, no matter how great. If so, this argument would be based on a qualitative notion of comparative riskiness.

9.2.3 Metaphysical Risk

A risk could be considered great not only because of its likelihood or the severity of the outcomes in a quantitative sense, but because it would risk bringing about an irreversible change to what exists and what is possible. In one sense, every loss constitutes a change in the fabric of reality and alters what is and what is not. Some alterations, however, leave gaping holes and remove a whole kind of possible existence. It is in the latter sense that metaphysical risk should be understood. Many of our greatest leaps of progress may be of this kind, as well as many of the things we fear most. In either case, these kinds of fundamental changes seem to add a different tier of risking that suggests that more careful consideration is needed in such cases, so that we know whether we might change things in fundamental ways and whether such changes are desirable and wise or not. In this sense, one risk is greater than another when that risk could fundamentally change reality, such that a whole group of things that used to exist no longer does and no longer will.

Some point to the fact that germline editing, much like other disruptive technologies such as more radical applications of AI, might pose a threat to human nature or humanity itself. There are, in fact, several arguments that seem to point to the metaphysical risk of germline editing. All of them suggest that germline editing might, in one way or another, put humanity itself at stake, as a species, as a kind of existence and being, as a kind of nature, and/or certain kinds of values that are premised on the existence of such beings or a community among them. The moral implications of such a risk depends, as mentioned earlier, on the value of what is lost and to what extent it would constitute a replaceable loss.

9.3 "A Most Serious Kind of Risk"

Does human germline editing pose *a most serious kind of risk*? Not all morally bad outcomes are the same and not all risks are equal. Some are more serious than others. Some moral outcomes are reversible, replaceable, reparable, or compensable. Others are not. The same goes for wrongs: some wrongs may be forgivable, even if the losses are incompensable. Wrongs could, perhaps, be rectified on the promise of not being repeated and if there was some kind of compensation (Hayenhjelm, 2018). Are there certain things that we ought never to do to our own germline, at least unless very special circumstances apply, because of the risk of irreversible losses or potentially unforgivable wrongs?

We could think of risks on three levels of severity based on their hypothetical reparability. The first kind of risk would be that which could result in losses and harms that are, in principle, reparable, replaceable, or compensable. They would not typically be categorically impermissible, but rather permissible on condition that they will be fully repaired or compensated for, should harm arise. The second kind of risk would be that which could result in an irreparable loss or harm to an individual or particular member of a species. Such risks might very well be permissible on the condition of appropriate precautionary measures to make the frequency as low as possible and with due measures to mitigate any harm or loss. Both would, in principle, be forgivable if the purposes and intentions were appropriate and all appropriate precautionary were measures taken, as well as full responsibility for the consequences.

The third kind is different in that it could result in the losses of a complete *kind* or the very basis of something or other. This is what we have referred to above as metaphysical risk. The morality of such risk depends on the value of what is at stake. Some kinds cause suffering and harm and would be good to permanently outroot. Others would bring about a loss that could never be repaired or compensated for and they would not provide any second chance to make things right, since what was permanently lost as a kind could never again exist. Such risks seem to require very strong epistemic foundations; we must safely know what we are doing and what it would result in, and be certain about the right kind of motivations.

Here, we can see a first draft for a claim that germline editing may not be like other kinds of risks—even in a medical context. Given what we are tampering with, it could be argued that if there is even a miniscule probability that we could harm or lose humanity itself in some important sense, then we must have the highest level of certainty about what we are doing and all possible consequences (including relatively remote side effects, knock-on effects, and systemic effects on a global scale). In other words, in many contexts, it may be very important to be able to stake and risk a whole kind, but in all such cases, we must know what we are doing, and if not, whenever possible, exchange such risks for more reversible kinds.

The notion here is that for all cases of metaphysical risk, the epistemic obligations increase. The trouble is that when it comes to new and emerging technologies, the epistemic situation is much weaker than for established practices. Thus, even if one can argue that previous concerns about IVF were exaggerated on the grounds that the kinds of worst-case scenarios imagined never came to pass, *we did not know that* at the time. It could thus be considered a case of luck rather than a morally sound risk. The logic is simple, if we do not know that it is safe and if we do not know for sure that we can fix things if they go wrong, we ought not to do it. Most things we need not know how to fix ahead of time, and we can fix them once they occur. But metaphysical losses of kinds are different; they can never be fixed, and one can never promise to do things better next time around.

There are three kinds of arguments regarding the higher stakes in risking kinds.

A Metaphysical Argument based on the fact that we stand to lose a whole kind qua kind in losing humanity. Thus, human germline editing would be a more serious kind of risk, should it pose a risk to humanity as a kind.

An Existential Argument based on the fact that we will not just lose any kind but our own kind and our own way of being, and essentially everything that is us and everything that is the world from our perspective. Thus, human germline editing would be a more serious kind of risk, should it risk our own existence.

A Value Argument based on the fact that we stand to lose the basis for all human values along with human nature and human experience: Our whole horizon of values, sense of beauty, morality, and so on are risked becoming nonsensical and losing importance. Thus, human germline editing would be a more serious kind of risk, should it pose a risk to the very basis of our entire set of values.

None of the above arguments may appear very compelling at first glance.

What is so special about whole kinds that we could not risk them, at least for the greater good? We have eradicated disease, mammoths have become extinct, and we have eliminated evil practices like headhunting and slavery. That a kind is at a risk of being lost cannot be a reason in itself.

What is so special about *our own* existence in particular that we could not risk it if there was something else that came after us that was, in some sense, even better? How can this be defended without slipping into either a defense for a fixed idea about human nature or a case of blatant self-interest? How could that hold moral weight? That something exists does not provide us with any reasons in this regard, unless we view the values as being realized by their existence. If so, there is no obvious reason why we should not want to promote what does not yet exist if it is better than what does. Furthermore, that something is us or about our own existence would provide strong prudential reasons, but the moral weight is less clear. Especially if what is lost is a certain way of being rather than humanity as a whole. That a certain way of being is our way of being is no reason to inflict that way of being on future generations. What would be so bad about *changing our nature* in such a way that we become better than we currently are?

What is so special about our set of values that they could not be replaced with different ones? Values, if anything, seem to be adjusted to what is, and therefore it only makes sense if they change when nature changes. How would the risk that future generations value other things than we do have any moral significance for us now? Why should our values matter to future generations? Why assume that there is anything special about human values at all? Are the preferences and moral interests of other species not equally valid? What is the point of our values after humanity has expired?

The above arguments all seem relatively weak at this point. First, we will need to elaborate on each one.

9.3.1 A Metaphysical Argument: The Potential Loss of Humankind

Let us first take a closer look at the metaphysical argument. The basic notion, here, is that germline editing could pose the risk of a permanent loss of humankind, such that we could never, even in principle, repair the harm or compensate for or replace such a loss. It would constitute a permanent loss of humanity from the metaphysical fabric of the world. We would risk removing the possibility of being human from the total set of possibilities. Is this possible as a result of germline editing and, if so, would it necessarily be a bad thing?

Of course, the very notion of a loss of humanity is ambiguous. By this, we could refer to the extinction of humanity. Meteorites, warfare, and even conflict between humans and posthumans could, of course, bring about such an extinction. However, the risking of humanity by germline editing would most likely be of a different kind. We could imagine this assuming two different forms. First, alterations to the germline would be such that the resulting beings were no longer able to procreate with humans and would thus either replace us as a species or simply end our lineage. Agar (2010, p. 19) uses this kind of biological definition of membership to the human species based on the ability to procreate with humans and have live offspring. Thus, should germline editing lead the way to a new kind of species that were no longer able to procreate with us, this could, theoretically, lead to the end of humanity. In such a scenario, it is not obvious that all of humanity would be at risk; rather, a new species might be introduced alongside us.

The other possibility would be that alterations to the human germline would result in the end of "humanity" in a more abstract sense. It could be that these posthumans were so different from us that they would no longer be recognizable as humans. Or, it could be that the variety of genetically edited beings would collectively be so different from one another that there was no longer a shared experience of being human. This would be the case even if these beings were able to procreate with humans and thus did not technically belong to a different biological species. If humanity refers to a certain set of, partially socially defined, characteristics, and ways of being that depend on social facts, the alteration of some might suffice to undermine, and possibly even quash, the human way of life and human values. If humanity is replaced by such a motley mix of beings that we could no longer recognize ourselves in the other, this could potentially mean the end of humanity as a community; and thus, even if it did not end our lineage, would still put a definitive end to being human as we know it. What it *means* to be human would have permanently changed. Interestingly, Agar observes that the transhumanists are divided on whether or not radically enhanced beings could be human or not (Agar, 2010, p. 18).

Would either of these possibilities be so bad? The answer to this question naturally depends on the value of humankind as a shared experience. What constitutes the loss here exactly? In all of the above cases, we have not simply erased humans or humanity from the world, but effectively either replaced us with posthumans or added posthumans in our midst. Some argue that whether we remain human or not cannot hold any moral significance by itself. The argument here is that whether our descendants are human or not is not significant, but only whether their lives would be better or more joyful than ours.

To Harris (2009), what matters is whether the benefits are great enough and the risks low enough. What is not of relevance, in his view, is whether we achieve such benefits by changing human nature or replacing humanity as we know it with a new breed of humans:

> … whether any proposed changes amount to changes in human nature, or to involve future evolution, seem ethically uninteresting. In particular whether the enhancement might be judged to involve creating a new species, "a new breed", or amount to "self-evolution", or "posthumanism" are semantic rather than moral issues. (Harris, 2009, p. 136)

Most arguments against the notion of attaching any moral significance to humanity as a species come down to some version of Harris' argument: what matters is whether we improve upon the world, increase what is good (such as well-being), and decrease what is negative (such as suffering). From this perspective, well-being—not what species we belong to—is what is morally relevant (cf. value maximization logic, Sect. 5.2.), and moral questions about threats to humanity are the wrong kinds of questions. Munson and Davis (1992, p. 150) take the argument of humanity's moral irrelevance one step further: "From the fact that we are human, it does not follow that we have an interest in our survival as humans, nor that we have any interest in survival at all."[2] This may follow if

---

[2] It is, however, not entirely clear what Munson and Davis (1992) had in mind; the arguments in support of the above claim suggest something less dramatic than the irrelevance of human

one simply applies the value maximization logic objectively. However, it seems odd to take such an objective view on our own species and our own survival. Furthermore, we also care about humans not merely as abstract carriers of well-being but in themselves, and, quite possibly, we might care about humanity as such, and not merely as containers of value. As Cohen (2011, p. 206) describes it, "a person values something as the particular valuable thing that it is, and not merely for the value that resides in it."[3] This seems to hold not just for individual particulars but also to some extent to particular kinds as in the case of human nature. This brings us to the existential argument.

9.3.2 An Existential Argument: The Potential Loss of Ourselves

More than merely being a metaphysical risk in an objective way, the potential loss of humanity is *personal*. It is not about any kind of thing that we happen to value, but about *us*.[4] It seems odd, as we suggested above, to merely reduce our own continued existence to a mere calculation of benefits and risks. At some point, we must ask: for whom?

This particular point is somewhat obscured when it comes to the transhumanists. As Agar noted above, the transhumanists seem to have no consensus on whether the posthuman is human or not. On the one hand, they are what is meant

---

survival. They argue that a supposed threat to humanity is overstated and unrealistic and believe that there are obvious gains that could come from embracing germline alterations. However, that something is not likely to ever occur is something entirely different than the claim that we ought to be indifferent to it, should it occur.

[3] To destroy what has value for the potential greater gain of something else is, according to Cohen (2011), to misunderstand something about value (in the first sense): when we value something, we do not merely value it as an abstract container of value; we value the very thing that it is as a particular. Cohen defends what he refers to as a conservative bias for "retaining what is of value, even in the face of replacing it with something of greater value (though not, therefore, in the face of replacing it by something of greater value, no matter how much greater its value would be.)" (Cohen, 2011, p. 207).

[4] This also holds for increases in well-being to some extent: we care about well-being because we care about ourselves and our fellow humans, we do not care about well-being entirely detached from humanity. We would not agree to extinguish humanity on earth if it could be shown that this would massively increase well-being for aliens in a different galaxy. We also seem to value well-being for other species that we somehow empathise or sympathise with, such as pets and larger animals, but less so for insects, vermin, and bacteria. Thus, it seems that even when we value the well-being of other species, it seems to take on somewhat anthropocentric qualities.

to succeed us, the next better version of us, as it were. On the other hand, as in much of Bostrom's writings, it is presented as an opportunity for us and about our future (see, e.g., Bostrom, 2008b).

In any case, the idea that we could, or even should, be neutral towards the fate of humanity seems squarely at odds with some of the most fundamental assumptions of morality. We would not appreciate a person who judged objectively between an extraterrestrial and a human child, or between a tiger and a human, or bacteria and a human, and so on. When it comes to life and death, we always favor human life over non-human life; moreover, we view this as the indisputable moral priority. This does not mean that we think we do not need to treat other species with respect, only that when it comes to their lives or ours, we are always partial. The very first of the natural rights tends to be the right to life; all other rights are derived from that one. The greatest wrongs are most often those that involve deliberate execution of another member of our species. Even if maltreatment of animals counts as offenses, their mere killing does not. In fact, CRISPR's safety to humans presuppose clinical testing that so far includes harm and death caused to members of other species.[5]

Thus, when it comes to the potential end of humanity, we could not treat it merely as an objective loss of a kind, but as the end of us. Agar (2010) argues that we ought to compare the end of humanity with our own death. He ends his book against radical enhancement with the following:

> We should approach the seeming inevitability of our species' end much as we confront the prospect of our own personal demise. We know, pace de Grey, that our lives will end. When we die, many aspects of our lived experiences will be lost forever. The idiosyncratic combination of qualities, defects, and experiences that defines us will go out of existence, leaving to our loved ones only comparatively brief narrative outlines of our lives. ... The human species won't last forever, but that's no reason to either expedite its end or to remove ourselves from it. We should instead enjoy it while it lasts. (Agar, 2010, p. 198)

A universe without us is a universe a bit like the world after our own death: the end of our consciousness and our conscious perception is also the end of our world. On a collective level, we could argue that if humanity ceases to exist, then the entire universe as understood from the perspective of humans—all our values, relations, and so on—cease to exist with us. For us, it would be an existential threat and a loss of our very being. What it means to be human would be lost

---

[5] This might change in the near future since animal testing is rapidly being replaced by the use of cell lines.

forever. It is not just that we have to imagine the world without humans in it. The entire world *as perceived by humans* would also be gone. We could imagine a universe where there was no human consciousness to experience it. There might be dog consciousness, snail consciousness, cow consciousness, and the like, but no human thoughts, emotions, or perceptions. Such a universe appears, to us, as fundamentally deprived. There may be sublime sunrises and sunsets, but certainly no poetry or art to celebrate it.

However, in the case of transhumanism, the idea is not to remove human beings with nothing in our place, but to alter us in ways intended to improve on us individually and on humanity as a whole. The crucial question, then, is how we are to understand the loss of humanity and the rise of the posthuman in existential terms. Thus, a better comparison might be that between two breeds of the same species at different ends of an evolutionary path. Then, we are not at risk of extinguishing human nature as much as evolving it, much in the same way as birds are an evolution of flying dinosaurs, and the wolf ultimately led to the Chihuahua. Would the wolf still exist in an existential sense if all wolves were replaced by Chihuahuas? Would this matter if we learned that Chihuahuas were on average much happier than wolves? The existential argument would claim that the wolf would still not exist and that the well-being of Chihuahuas were neither here nor there from the existential perspective of wolves. We might be willing to replace things of value to us, but not when it comes to our own existence. We must assume that we are irreplaceable to ourselves.

Whether we view a new model of humans as a continuation of and improvement on us, or as the end of us and the beginning of something else, depends on what we consider to be essential or defining about ourselves. It seems that we could accept losses of what we consider inconsequential to our identity as long as we retain what is essential.

Thus, the transhumanist may not have any issues with radical alterations to body parts, and even with animal–man chimeras, or man–machine cyborgs, or even the idea of uploading the human mind to a computer for unending life, and have little concern for a loss of identity. This would be possible if one identifies humanity only with, say, its mental and cognitive capacities in a way that could be thought of as detached from its embodied experience. As long as the new kind of being is conscious and has advanced cognitive capacities and intelligence, possesses great talents and skills, has emotions and is able to perceive happiness and contentment, or something roughly along those lines, it would be no threat to our existence, according to this view. Replacing body parts would be inconsequential, since that is not what is essential to our kind of being.

The bioconservatives seem to favor a more relational concept of humanity; how we relate to others, parents, and children, but also ancestors, our past and nature as part of being human, and the ability to sympathize with others in need and weak and vulnerable (as well as strong and talented) beings. Some also seem to view humans as sexual and biological beings, where mortality and sexual reproduction are part of who we are.[6]

Thus, on the former view, if identity only pertains to our cerebral properties and some notion of autonomy, then one might see the posthuman as being more perfected versions *of us*. Especially if all the things we wish to overcome are attached to our biological nature: physical limitations, limitations of memory and computational capacities, limitations to talents, biologically affected mood and temperament, proneness to disease and death, and so on.

Thus, Cohen (2011, p. 208) uses the allegory of a man who gradually replaces each body part as it becomes worn with new things, and regards the image as "abhorrent," whereas Pugh et al. (2013, p. 338 ff., p. 351 f.), when discussing the same example, disagree with that value assessment. If the body is merely a vehicle for emotions, thoughts, and cognition, why should we not replace faulty parts? Especially if those parts are what limit us and make us mortal? To this, the conservative might respond: If our biological embodied nature is inseparable from ourselves as emotional and cognitive beings, then we cannot remove the body and still be the same kind of being.

It could be argued that even if the new model of humankind (or whatever it might be) were to fully replace the old one, and effectively bring about a loss of humanity, this might still not constitute a loss in value. In fact, if the new model is more valuable, then, perhaps, all losses attached to the end of humanity could be replaced by the new gains attached to the new model. Likewise, it would be argued, that edits that we come to later regret would constitute less of a risk to worry about should such regrettable edits be perfectly editable themselves. If so, then the stakes may not be worse than what we could deal with, and if the benefits are large enough, the risks could well be worth taking.

Given that germline gene editing is motivated by the prospects of increased benefits, it could be argued that we are, in fact, increasing value, not risking it. For all we know, we could lose humanity but gain new kinds of beings and ways of living that supersede us. Is there, then, any reason to lament a potential and permanent loss of human nature? Would it matter if humanity were replaced with

---

[6] Annas (2010) seems to imply such a concern with regard to cloning: "Cloning, for example, not only removes sexual reproduction from the definition of what it is to be human, but also seeks to eliminate human evolution by duplicating existing genomes" (Annas, 2010, p. 264).

a different species that descended from it, or whether it was so altered that we no longer recognized it as a human according to our current understanding of the term?

One could view such radical changes in a very different light, depending on whether one takes objective value or existential value as the primary value in this context. In other words, is what ultimately matters whether a potential loss is replaced by a greater gain, or is what ultimately matters partly a subjective matter, such that we cannot help but prioritize our own continued existence over any alternative, no matter how much objective value would be created thereby? One could, of course, consider humanity as morally irrelevant and insist that all that matters is whether some state of affairs is objectively better or not. Or, one might argue that, as humans, whether something is human or not can never be trivial or irrelevant to us: Our own survival is an existential matter, not a neutral one. How feasible is this latter position as a moral stance? Are there good moral arguments to favor our own continued existence as humans, such as we are, should it ever come to that?

Cohen (2011) raises two interesting points in this context. First, things matter to us because, irrespective of something else potentially holding greater value, we are personally attached to the former. Second, wanting to replace everything that we value with something else of potentially greater value leads to a devaluing of the former: everything becomes disposable and replaceable in a way that is counter to what it means to value something as a particular existing valuable thing.

If anything would hold personal value to us, it seems likely that our own existence and way of existing would be it. This, again, could find some support in Cohen's arguments about personal value: We value certain things because they matter to us personally (and are also reluctant to replace them with things of greater value). Here, one might argue that we happen to value our own existence in a way that makes its potential loss irreplaceable to us. For Cohen, this comes in a kind of "warts and all" package:

> … would not want to eliminate all of our bad features. I conjecture that that is partly because the negative traits are part of the package that makes human beings the particular valuable creatures that we personally cherish and are therefore worth preserving as part of the package, but it is also particular because we court vertigo if we seek to place everything within our control. (Cohen, 2011, p. 209)

In short, let us assume that we value the existence and experience of being human. Let us also assume that we have become quite personally attached to humanity as it is. It is thus not a case of rational preference for humanity after carefully comparing the pros and cons of all species, but a preference that has grown from a personal attachment and shared history. On those grounds, replacing too much of what humanity is with something new would not be "the same." Of course, it would not be "us" who experiences the replacement in the future, but we might still lament such a future now and all that is lost with it.

Furthermore, one could argue that we are mistaken when we think we ought to replace the human species with another species on the grounds of increased value if by doing so we devalue humanity. At least, it would go against the conservative attitude of valuing what already is valuable and what exists over what could exist (even if it is more valuable). Cohen writes:

> The conservative impulse is to conserve what is valuable, that is, the particular things that are valuable. I claim that we devalue the valuable things we have if we keep them only so long as nothing even slightly more valuable comes along. Valuable things command a certain loyalty. If an existing thing has intrinsic value, then we have reason to regret its destruction as such, a reason we would not have if we cared only about the value that the thing carries or instantiates. (Cohen, 2011, p. 210)

In short, to value something as intrinsically valuable is to appreciate it, be loyal to it, and to want to protect and keep it in some sense. This is what value entails. To wish to replace what is intrinsically valuable is to commit a rational mistake of sorts: to misunderstand what intrinsically valuable means. Thus, valuing humanity implies a desire to preserve it. By contrast, according to the value maximization logic, each valuable thing becomes a mere carrier for some abstract value, and it is this abstract value that counts, and a thing or being itself becomes valuable merely as a holder of this value.

To this, one might object along with Wiggins (discussed in Cohen, 2011, p. 216), that even if it is true that we value something as a particular and thereby have reason to regret its destruction, this need not entail that such particulars are irreplaceable. Wiggins' example is that of a beautiful rose bush that his gardener had cut down. A fact that had initially caused him grief, but he ultimately found perfect consolation in the promise of an even more beautiful rose bush to be planted in its place. The crucial point, here, does not seem to be whether that of intrinsic worth is valued as a particular in this case, but more a case of whether the loss would be replaceable or not. How far could we apply this example to the case of humanity? Would it merely be a case of a rose bush uprooted and replaced by a more beautiful one? It seems that there is both a metaphysical and personal value argument for why it would be different.

Let us imagine the gardener who just annihilated the very possibility of being or becoming a rose from the known universe. Here, we might agree that even though roses are not the only beautiful and sweet-smelling flower in the world, there is something tragic about the completeness of the loss here. It is not just this and that rose, or even all roses, but the very possibility of roses being grown, smelled, or viewed ever again. If nothing else, it would constitute a genuine loss (Hayenhjelm 2018). This seems to be true even if new flowers that were much more impressive in various ways came to supersede the short blooming history of the rose. Perhaps we can view the potential loss of the human species in much the same way. It may be true that an even better species were to replace us, but the fact that no new human could ever again be born is still some kind of tragic loss. This would be the metaphysical argument. In addition, one might argue that we value humanity not because we are the best species imaginable, but because we are an important part in a long history of things and events that we have come to love—our continued existence matters deeply *to us*. Whereas we might come to love a new kind of rose, we cannot adopt the same view on our own existence if it is at risk. (Yet, here it matters whether we are talking about a loss of existence or merely a change, and the line is anything but clear).

The potential loss of humanity is not just any kind of regrettable loss: it is personal. It is the loss of us. We have personal reasons to be attached to humanity, given that we are humans ourselves. We have personal reasons to favor the continued existence of humanity in that it is about our own continued existence. It is about a potential loss of ourselves.

It seems that the dismissal of concern about a potential loss of humanity hinges either on the assumption that the case is overstated or that no such risk actually exists. This, in turn, seems to depend to some degree on how quickly a change occurs. One change could be viewed as a destruction of what was if it happens very suddenly, and yet be viewed as a case of evolvement if it happens slowly. This brings us to the last argument about values and reference points.

9.3.3 The Value Argument: The Potential Loss of a Point of Reference

One of the main objections to fundamental changes to humanity is a concern about *alienation*.

Agar (2010) argues against radical enhancement beyond normal human capacities on the grounds that this would cause alienation, and with that an undermining of values. He compares this concern with the alienation feared with Alzheimer's disease:

One of the things people fear about disease such as Alzheimer's is the intellectual decline itself. It progressively robs its victims of their reasoning powers and destroys their memories. But there's something else they fear as much and perhaps more—this is the severing of connections with the people and things that they value. People with advanced Alzheimer's may no longer recognize their spouses. They may no longer understand the social and moral causes that were among their strongest commitments. They may no longer remember that they were once presidents of the United States of America. In Alzheimer's disease the severing of connections is closely linked with intellectual decline. *I think that significant intellectual growth may have a similar effect. It, like significant intellectual diminishment, has the propensity to sever your bonds with the things that really matter to you.* (Agar, 2010, p. 184, italics added.)

With radical enhancement we would face the same kind of potential losses of what we value, he argues. Agar reasons as follows: If Bostrom is right that a future posthuman would intellectually and cognitively be to us as we are to a child in terms of maturity, then it might also be the case that things that we think we would be able to do and enjoy as posthumans would no longer hold any allure to us; much the same as the kinds of things a child would want to accomplish is of no interest to an adult. In other words, this is the value challenge again (see Sect. 8.7.1). The posthuman may be entirely indifferent to everything that we value now. Thus, departing from our own values, as humans, we may have no reason to promote posthumanity: The thought that we would thereby increase our values may come at the cost of a being with no interest in those values or no ability to appreciate the value increase.

In a way, germline editing might not only affect what kind of beings future individuals could become, it might also, thereby, separate them from the larger unity of a shared humanity as well as from history. Perhaps there is something of this notion implicit in the UNESCO statement of humanity as a cultural heritage: Humanity is not merely about you and us and a long list of individuals; but to be human is to belong to a collective of humans, it is to understand one's own identity in relation to those of other humans and be part of that collective. It is to understand oneself as belonging to the history of humans and sharing the same kind of human nature and character; the very reason for all the greatness and horrors humanity has brought about, and the foundation for mutual respect, equal rights, reciprocity, justice, and fairness. If this is the case, it could be threatened in two ways: By the emergence of a new person or breed of humans too distant from us to be conceivable as a relatable cousin and by the dissolution of a human collective. The latter could, indeed, be achieved if humans were no longer similar enough to recognize each other as brothers and sisters.

Altering a future person so that they diverge too much from what humans have been in the past, risks bringing about a kind of alienation from human history, from humanity as collective, and from their own parents and family, should the changes occur from one generation to the next. Sagoff seems to allude to something along these lines:

> In a way, there is nothing new here. Since the medieval period, people have been liberating themselves—for better or worse—from their history. A half millennium ago, one did as one's parents did. One stayed put. One accepted the religion, beliefs, language, and so forth that came with one's heritage. Five hundred years later, individuals choose religions, careers, communities, and so on. They may soon be able to choose—to some extent—the genetic characteristics of their children as well. Not only does the individual not have a nature; the individual may no longer have a history. (Sagoff, 2005, p. 90)

Thus, there is a concern here that is less about losing a particular feature of human nature, and more about losing our frame of reference for our own person and kind of being and with a certain speed in that process become alienated from our human history. To Agar's (2010) mind, the risk of radical enhancement is not about the degree of change but the speed of such changes and the resulting alienation.

Whereas the old eugenics, proposed by Julian Huxley and others, were collective enterprises that would take many generations to deliver any radical result, the current advocates for radical enhancement envision far-reaching changes already in the next generation.[7] In contrast, according to Agar, the "technological transformations advocated by early twenty-first century defenders of radical enhancement differ in being abrupt" (Agar, 2010, p. 197). It is in this latter case that radical enhancement becomes a problem as it will cause alienation between our generation. The same would not apply when the changes are gradual: "But the gradual nature of this transformation wouldn't prevent us from relating to our former selves, our children, and our fellow citizens in ways compatible with our human values. We and they will be human" (Agar, 2010, p. 197).

Agar argues that there may be good reasons for preferring the posthuman existence to none at all, or as a natural consequence of evolution and/or catastrophe,

---

[7] According to Dunér (2024) it was Julian Huxley, a British evolutionary biologist, who in 1951 coined the term "transhumanism" in the English language. Huxley, who previously had called his view on post-Darwinian evolutionism "scientific humanism" or "evolutionary humanism," presented transhumanism as "a new religion for the future."

and that it would certainly be better than one not related to humanity at all, such as an alien civilization. However, he notes that there are very good reasons to want such a posthuman future to be a very distant one (Agar, 2010, p. 198).

The alienation argument is not merely about future individuals and their relation to others or their past and to what extent they would fit in and belong to the history of humanity. Yet we could alienate all of our moral concepts and all our values from the future being that continues our path, such that none of our values applies any longer. Or vice versa: we could alienate future beings from any preexisting moral or cultural tradition, without anything in its place (given that the new being has no other history than ours, and no shared experiences to build upon). Consider a being with no ability to experience pain or pleasure. For such a being, moral notions of harm may hold little weight or fail to make sense. Other notions such as promoting well-being or moral incentives or even virtues may make no sense. What, then, can guide moral choices? We should not underestimate the role and function that the concept of human nature has played in our moral concepts throughout the history of moral philosophy.

We could, of course, let the new beings develop a new morality and new moral concepts based on their superior cognitions and moral sentiments. But that would assume, besides time, that morality made sense to them at all, and there is no reason to assume this if they are radically different from us.

Morality is in some sense about priority: We protect what we value at the cost of what we do not value, whether the former is our own species and/or other species over other beings or inanimate things, or some more abstract ideal over things that contradict it. It is based on values widely shared and believed to align with what is objectively good, but it is also contrary to perfect impartiality between all events and all kinds of existences. We tend to value our own species and those we can relate to as things of value, or even intrinsic worth, and value abstract notions that make sense for the kinds of beings that we are, such as justice (among humans), fairness (between humans), reciprocity (among humans), rights (for all humans), respect for (human) persons, the promotion of well-being (of sentient beings of higher cognitive capacities) when not in direct opposition to the well-being of humans, and so on. We cannot assume that the posthuman will have any attachment to humanity. It is not even necessary that they particularly value the company of other posthumans. We have no reason to assume that genetically edited posthumans who were to trace their history back to genetic experiments of a totalitarian regime would have much in common with those that were the result of parental choices in a liberal society. We have no reason to think that posthumans who could trace their history to free choices and aesthetic preferences in a culture dominated by whimsical trends and pop culture would be very similar to those developed by scientists to withstand climate change and food shortages.

Currently, we are able to ponder questions such as whether germline editing violates human rights or goes against human dignity. But, alter human nature too much and the notions of rights and dignity may no longer make sense, and even less so serve as some moral guide. The question is not whether the future way of things would align with the morality of the new kinds of beings, but whether it agrees with or violates our own moral standards. Human rights are premised on all persons being born, in some relevant ways, similarly, such that they deserve the same universal rights. All the influential declarations on human rights from notions of enlightenment begin with the notion that we are all born "free and equal." That is, it is by virtue of being born as a human or similar, that we have certain rights.[8] Furthermore, it is against this notion of being born equal (in status, at least) that any social injustices are measured and deemed unjust. Although, the notion of being born equal can be given very inclusive interpretations, it would lose meaning unless there were some core of actual similarity that unified those it applied to. Should that similarity be dissolved, these rights may no longer extend to all of us, or all of the new kinds of beings. Should we extend them to all creatures, we might reduce our moral standing to nothing more than that of any creature, be it a mouse or a wasp. It might be more accurate morally, but it would certainly entail a radically different attitude to morality.

Furthermore, moral rights only make sense against a background of funda-mental vulnerabilities that necessitate protection. Remove those vulnerabilities and we remove the need for rights. Likewise, remove those vulnerabilities for some and the underlying assumptions of universality and reciprocity would also be undermined. In other words, rights are premised on a shared humanity and distinct human nature. For instance, were we to remove humanity's capacity to feel pain, the moral obligation not to harm others would no longer make sense. Similarly, in a future world of singularity, the respect for a person would carry little weight. Of course, this case may be overstated. Nussbaum (2011) has, for

---

[8] Lincoln's (1863) Gettysburg Address begins as follows: "Four score and seven years ago our fathers brought forth upon this continent, a new nation, conceived in Liberty, and ded-icated to the proposition that all men are created equal." The American Declaration of Independence (1776) follows similar lines: "We hold these truths to be self-evident, that all men are created equal, that they are endowed by their Creator with certain unalienable Rights, that among these are Life, Liberty and the pursuit of Happiness." Article 1 of the UN's Dec-laration of Human Rights, however, qualifies being born free and equal with "in dignity and right" but also declares that all humans are endowed with reason and conscience: "All human beings are born free and equal in dignity and rights. They are endowed with reason and conscience and should act towards one another in a spirit of brotherhood" (UN, 1948).

instance, defended an extension of her capability theory to cover the flourishing interests of non-human animals as well. Yet, this is not at the expense of humans.

9.3.4 A Combined Argument

Even if the three arguments above would fail to convince individually, a stronger case might be found in the combination of all three. Thus, the argument would be that a risk is of a most serious kind for us when one kind of action could risk (a) the loss of a *whole valuable ontological kind*; (b) that kind *is of existential and personal value* to us; and (c) *whole sets of deeply held values are premised on the existence and nature of that kind*. In short, if it were the case that some action, *a*, could bring on a complete loss of a whole kind, and that kind was our own kind (thus an end to our own existence), and that kind was the premise for our values, then we would have every reason to seek to prevent such a loss:

> A Most Serious Risk. If a risk is such that one of its potential outcomes would entail a permanent loss of a valuable kind (irreplaceable, incompensable, and irreparable) and if that loss amounts to the permanent loss of one's own species and continued existence and in a such a way that the foundation for entire sets of deeply held values are at risk of being undermined, then for any member of that species, these factors make it the case that such risks are of a most serious kind.

Should germline editing to some degree risk the foundation of our identity and distinct kind of being, our values and our societies, and should such a loss of humanity as a kind, and with it the foundation of all human values, not for reasons of superior value but because the values and this existence constitutes our existence and our values as we happen to be, then it would be hard to consider any stakes higher than that. Now it could, of course, be disputed if germline editing could put anything remotely like this at stake.

From an objective perspective, humanity does not seem irreplaceable. However, from our own humanistic perspective it does. In fact, in one sense, it seems that a partiality to our own species is the underlying value that underscores most of human morality. We are happy to extend moral status, at least in part, to other beings if they share whatever traits we view as most crucial (and defining). Thus, we might extend it to other intelligent or sentient life forms, but not to life forms that share neither the capacity to feel nor to think and are too alien from us or whose existence stand in direct opposition to our own survival interests (such as deadly bacteria). In fact, we tend to take it for granted that part of what it means to be human is to care for other humans at the expense of other species, but not vice versa: we can kill and eat pigs or cod and feed our starving children with their meat, but not vice versa.

As humans, we are seldom entirely neutral in the struggle between a human and their disease, and would never say that both life forms are equally valuable. In fact, it seems that animal rights and respect for nature most often applies when it is not a zero-sum situation, such that it is either them or us. No one celebrates the flourishing life of bacteria when it kills a human, or the full stomach of a tiger when a human was its last meal. The existential dimension means that we cannot remain neutral. To be human is to care about the destiny of humans and humanity. In fact, in this, the transhumanists and radical enhancers seem to be in agreement with the bioconservatives, among others. The different conclusions they draw stem not from one being partial to our own existence and the other indifferent, but rather in what is considered to be the defining characteristics of "us."

This fundamental value that we, rightly or wrongly, attach to our own survival is obscured in the transhumanist's writing by the use of first-person pronouns when describing the posthumanist condition. For instance, in Bostrom's *Letter from Utopia* (2008b), the letter is addressed to the reader in second person, written in the voice of the reader's possible future self: the "I," then, is the posthuman, and the "you," the person who could embrace a particular kind of future. Similarly, in "I want to be a posthuman when I grow up," Bostrom (2008c) wants us to think of the posthuman future as *our* possible future. These transhumanists' arguments would hold much less sway if described in terms of us and them.

The value dimension means that the only values we have at our disposal are not objective but founded upon our nature as it is. Thus, we can only assess any potential future against the values fit for our existence. Our moral horizon only makes sense to beings sufficiently similar to us. To some extent, it seems to end with us as well, unless superimposed onto a moral landscape it no longer fits. This implies that there are actually two and not just one metaphysical kind of risk at stake: We risk not only the loss of a whole kind (i.e., humans), but also a whole value system (i.e., human values). This means that, after humanity's demise, all our moral concepts could fail to have any meaning. There may not be anything we could refer to as "beauty" or "goodness" or "kindness" or "justice," and the like. Intelligent species that are sufficiently different may well have other kinds of concepts, but our moral horizon as we know it may no longer exist. This has the implication that we may not have sufficient knowledge to make sound decisions about the future on the basis of value, should we, or beings sufficiently similar to us, no longer exist in that future. It would be like the cat bringing freshly caught mice to the baby's crib. In other words, if we care about our own values (as we should, if we care about anything at all), then we ought to promote whatever promotes those values; beyond that, we would have nothing to navigate by.

9.4 How Much of a Risk?

In this chapter, we have examined various kinds of risks mentioned as a reason for concern about human germline gene editing. However, there are two aspects to a risk, both of which must apply for there to be any reason for concern. The first, as has been discussed above, is about the potential *outcomes* and the nature of those outcomes. The second is about *the likelihood* of those outcomes occurring, or, more broadly, to what extent those outcomes *are known to be realistically possible consequences* rather than merely speculative ones. Of course, if there is zero probability of an outcome occurring, then we need not be concerned about it. A low probability could still make an outcome morally relevant if the outcome is severe enough: we do not dismiss the possibility of nuclear power accidents, a third world war, or an airplane crash because the probability is low. In this case, at least two aspects are important: first, whether an outcome is a realistic concern—that is, something that we have reason to assume could occur—and secondly, whether the trajectory towards such an outcome allows us (easily or not) to deviate from that path once we have embarked on it. For the potential losses to warrant any conclusions about the ethics of human germline editing, we also need to address these aspects and ask other kinds of questions than merely what is potentially at stake:

1. Do such outcomes represent a *realistic possibility at all?*
2. If so, are they *probable enough* to warrant consideration?
3. If realistically possible and probable enough, do we have reason to believe that they will be difficult *to avoid and prevent?*

The first question is about modal assumptions and what results are, broadly speaking, possible or not possible. The second concerns likelihoods and the probability of something occurring. The third question, finally, deals with (practical) preventability and epistemic risks. It concerns what we can, in principle, prevent—even if possible and not entirely unlikely—or at least circumvent, mitigate, or adapt to so that the feared consequences do not arise, even if the risk materializes.

If the answer to any of the above questions is "no," then the risk arguments in the previous section are considerably weakened. No matter what is at stake, such stakes alone matter little if they do not actually constitute a realistic risk or if they could be easily avoided. Unless we can point to any reason that these kinds of outcomes pose any realistic threat, we are left with little more than a hypothetical: *if* we stand to lose *x*, *only then* would we be ill-advised to do *y*. Furthermore, we have no reason to avoid what could easily be prevented later on without significant costs or harm if the benefits are significant.

9.4.1 How Realistic and Probable Are the Risks Considered?

In the previous sections, we have described three different kinds of risks: technical risks, social risks, and moral and metaphysical risks. Some of these risks seem highly relevant to the moral picture, because they *are known to be risks*; that is, a particular kind of unwanted outcome is *known* to be a possible outcome of germline gene editing. This applies to the technical risks. In fact, the reason there is concern about these risks is that gene editing has already resulted in off-target effects, unwanted on-target effects, and, furthermore, there have been cases of mosaicism. The evidence for such risks is the very reason that they are part of the overall conception of the safety/risk of germline gene editing. Furthermore, by means of further research and development, the relative degree of risk of this nature can be reassessed. In short, we know that these outcomes are possible, and we could make some assessments about their frequency if given sufficient data. For obvious reasons, we will know less about the exact effects of these technical risks on a person, in terms of health and otherwise (QALYs, for instance).[9]

Technical risks are, however, not limited to direct impact, but include later side effects and knock-on effects as well as various effects that arise from more than one causal factor, whether they are exclusively chemical and biological or arise from an interplay with external factors. They would also include any effects, should there be any, for a person born from a long line of ancestors who had their germline edited in the same loci or across different ones. Currently, we do not know what happens when one gene is edited repeatedly in the same lineage. What was done in generation 1 may need to be re-edited in generation 2, only to be edited again in generation 3. There could be many reasons for such a development, not least of which a change in priorities, development in technology, or unknown side effects linked to a gene's multifunctionality. Furthermore, a person

---

[9] QALYs are "quality-adjusted life years," which is a measure in public policy where loss in life expectancy is adjusted according to quality of life.

may not know that their own germline has been edited—this seems increasingly likely for later generations. The further the risks in question are from what could be studied within the 14-day window of embryo research and animal studies, the less we know about them at present. Such epistemic gaps could presumably be bridged, and the more research executed on the matter, the better we might be able to assess the likelihood of various risks occurring.

The social and moral risks are by their nature more speculative in the sense that they predict possible scenarios from what we know about societies at present and in the past, as well as the kind of role that germline editing could play and how that might impact a future society. Of course, the more alien future societies and future persons are from our society and us, the less reliable such projections will be.

All social risks discussed must make a number of assumptions about the psychological and social aspects of future worlds and societies and about people thought to inhabit them. This includes assumptions about parental motivations, the social standing of people with disabilities, the possibilities of enforcing regulation and control, the future of IVF clinics, the value of genetic relatedness in children, the trajectory of somatic gene therapy, border control and travel, research, social classes, and overall priorities and values in the future.

The most common social risks all pertain to justice, particularly the concern that a world where germline gene editing plays a significant role would enforce and deepen social divisions between, for instance, rich and poor nations and classes. Of course, this is not the only possible outcome. Germline editing could, for instance, be made readily available and accessible to all—limited only to health disadvantages—and be sponsored by the state and tightly regulated. This could give rise to a diminishing disability community, but it need not. This would depend on what conditions were targeted and how this was agreed upon. Even in a society where enhancement is encouraged or even made obligatory, this need not lead to discrimination and social division. It could be part of a universal healthcare scheme and foreign aid. Wide access could give rise to other issues, such as social pressures that would infringe upon individual free choice, but it could become the new normal. What would happen after it had become the new normal? Would boundaries be pushed further ahead? Would there be a backlash? Or would it become a non-issue in due course? We do not know.

However, we cannot dismiss the scenario where germline editing enters IVF clinics as an option if made safe and legal. If so, this could be limited to a few couples who could not make use of PGD to have a healthy, genetically related child. Or it could become something of a trend, including all middle-class parents in richer nations and the elites in poorer ones. It could also gradually include more and more expansive edits that would eventually offer people different chances in life in terms of health, longevity, career choices, and other opportunities. The last scenario, at least, seems plausible in a society not too different from ours in a not-too-distant future.

What about that which we have referred to as the "most serious kind of risk"? We have talked about three parameters to such a risk: the loss of a whole kind (i.e., humanity as we know it), loss of ourselves (our own category, as it were), and a loss of intrinsic value that cannot be replaced. How likely such fundamental losses are to occur depends on how we specify the occurrence of such an outcome. For instance, if we define "loss of humanity" as a future state of the world where there is *no single member of the Homo sapiens species left* and define a "loss brought about by germline editing" as a loss that is directly caused by germline edits, then it would seem to be a very unlikely outcome. Even if germline gene editing became a widely adopted part of ordinary reproduction, there will always be those that would not be included. Thus, if that is the concern, then it does not seem to warrant much consideration. Similarly, should future generations of our descendants consist only of posthumans in no relevant sense similar to us, then this would qualify as a complete loss, but this seems even more unrealistic.

By contrast, should "loss of humanity" require nothing more than us in a not-too-distant future state of the world having *changed* what it means to be human by means of germline edits, such that the future human is in at least one respect different to what a human is today, then this seems more likely, but it need not necessarily be much of a concern either. We could, for instance, imagine humans in the future being just like us but with a much better sense of smell—perhaps to the extent that they could detect the first signs of disease this way. In such a scenario, humanity would very much exist, but it would be different to us in this one respect. This does not seem to warrant talk of a fundamental loss of humanity, but would genuinely be an improvement.

The more extreme or all-encompassing the nature of the loss, the less likely it becomes, and the more conservative we are in our view on what must remain, the more likely, but also more trivial, it becomes. Does this mean that any of the most serious risks are either highly unlikely or trivial?

The concern about metaphysical loss is less a concern about a particular outcome and more a concern that arises from the four specific aspects of germline gene editing: the fact that it is *pervasive* in that it affects all cells; the fact that it is *not limited to any particular gene as target*, but could be universally applied; the fact that *we do not know* what the precise effects of this will be in the long run; and the fact that human nature and values derived from it has served as a map for making these kinds of decisions. This means that any particular worst-case scenario we argue will be merely indicative. Any objection based on a concern about moral and metaphysical risk will actually be based on the nature of the stakes, the epistemic shortcomings, and the role genes play in our existence, nature, and identity. Should something go severely wrong, whatever it may be, it could—if we are unfortunate—harm us in our most constitutive parts.

There is a parallel here to how one reasons about risk in technical risk management. One can approach risks in a probabilistic manner. If so, one seeks to avoid particular identifiable outcomes, identify all the causal trajectories that could lead to that outcome, calculate the probability, and then implement safety measures to stop them from occurring. Here, the parallel would be to identify specific outcomes that we want to avoid, such as rogue experimentations by biohackers and terrorists, a free market for editing services, and social injustice, and then try to prevent these with the right kind of regulation and institutional measures.

The other way to approach risks is to address them in a worst-case scenario approach. Here, one looks at the potential source of the risk, such as the maximum amount of toxic substance kept at one site at any one time, and then calculate what could happen under the worst conditions and what it would take in terms of resources and preparation to deal with that outcome, regardless of the probability of it occurring. This would mean looking at the nature of our germline and considering what the worst thing is that could happen, should we mess up our own germline or should various alterations have unexpected outcomes in the long run, and to what extent such problems could be resolved.

This is the point: Even if we do not consider the genome of humanity as a shared cultural heritage, or as something to remain fixed, even if left to natural evolution, no one can deny that the overall state of the germline of an individual or the gene pool for a population matters. Changes to the germline will have consequences; otherwise, no one would have any interest in altering it. Being born with a severe genetic disease versus not being born with such a disease, being able to have children versus not being able to have them, and having the propensity for shortness, breast cancer, or musical and mathematical genius matters. We cannot change our germline and remain the same. Some alterations will be insignificant, while others will be considered medical "corrections." However, what happens to our germline is something that also happens to us. Thus, even if the metaphysical risks attached to germline editing are unlikely, they do reveal something about the stakes of the target of modification—they describe along what dimensions there will be a certain "trembling" if we start to experiment or make mistakes.

The germline serves as the basis for our existence, our identity, and our shared values. The moral risk concern is thus one of making informed decisions about altering the basis of our values, while being guided by those values. We cannot embark on making radical changes to human nature while navigating by the values of well-being, beneficence, autonomy, and justice—since the worth and importance of those values is based on human nature and what benefits a person on the grounds that they are a human being.

Of course, there is no (current) agenda to seek to remove our ability to suffer or experience pleasure, or to make rational decisions, or to separate what is just from what is unjust, and so on. Even so, and even if it is highly unlikely, the possibility of affecting what it means to be human could have severe consequences. For instance, what would someone like Pol Pot have done had he had access to germline gene editing and the same passion to erase the intelligentsia? Pol Pot is, of course, the result of many converging factors, one of which is the rise of a particular ideology. What the dominant ideologies of the future will be, we do not know. They may not be similar to the ones in the past. Furthermore, it does not seem entirely unlikely that many kinds of ideologies could make good use of germline editing as a tool towards their favored future. The point, here, is that such a tool *could* affect the grounds for our identity, our values, and our existence as humans—or at least set those dimensions trembling.

Most arguments in this context seem to presume some kind of *a slippery slope* to worst-case scenarios. Thus, we might imagine a psychological slippery slope, such that every step pushes forward what is socially accepted as "normal" in reproduction, such that eventually the most radical forms of enhancement will have become the norm, and at that point something fundamental would have been lost along the way.

Even if everyone were genetically edited as part of normal reproduction, this need not by itself involve a loss of humanity as a species, or a loss of our values. For one, if everyone moves in the same direction, humanity as a whole would be changed rather than lost. In such cases, we could seek to ensure that germline gene editing was only developed and embraced up to a particular point and not beyond that. Such safety measures, however, presume that the development is relatively predictable and linear.

However, some of the moral and metaphysical risks need not take that route. If the concern is about a loss of humanity as a *shared* community or family where we see each other as brothers and sisters in a relevant sense or as "neighbors" and as a unifying moral and existential concept, then the source of risk may be less about how radical interventions become, and more about how a new landscape of humans could undermine the degree to which we see each other as equals.

The "most serious kind of risk" need not arise along the standard formula for a slippery slope. It could occur along a more diffuse kind of path, where many small changes of different kinds, perhaps morally insignificant in themselves, lead to an unrecognizable whole. We might compare it with a thin piece of a very brittle vintage silk—there may not be any particular part of the cloth that is crucial to its integrity, it would be equally delicate all over, and one small tear may not be noticeable, nor a few of them even. However, should one continue to pull at certain threads, the whole cloth may unravel, and in the end, the whole fabric may be ruined without any particular tear being responsible; rather, it was the delicacy of the whole thing and the fact that it was put under strain. In the context of germline editing, it would be hard to allow for some wear and tear in the hope that we could still avoid the worst outcomes; instead, the most sensible approach would be to be very careful with the whole endeavor. If we have tampered in too many places, we may end up having replaced all that we currently consider to be essential to being human, without being able to point to any particular step as the one that has led to ruin.

The likelihood of a more serious kind of risk seems to depend on how we imagine a fundamentally altered humanity and how this may come about: *as a succession of changes* to the humanity in each person beyond recognition or as a kind of *undoing of humanity as a unifying concept*. The latter may have a higher probability, since the risks are not dependent on extreme alterations or any linear succession of interventions. "Humanity" in a universal sense is a relatively new notion; thus, the most severe risk posed by radical alterations may be the loss of humanity as a point of reference and something shared. We could, it seems, arrive at a place where there is no "we the people," since there is nothing that unites us and there is no basis for equality, since there is nothing that is the same about us, and I cannot understand you, nor you me, because we are not alike. Accidental birth has given us an abstract family to which we belong, based on the assumption that we are born equal and the same. Such a risk does not seem unlikely; however, it would presumably take a very long time to arrive at that point.

9.4.2 The Predictability, Avoidability, and Reversal of Severe Risk

What can we say about the question of *avoidability* of the risks discussed? To what degree would it be possible to mitigate risks and *reverse unwanted outcomes*? Again, the different kinds of risk present different routes and possibilities for reversal. Technical risks can be avoided by making the technology safer and more precise, and tightening regulation and control over who can use it. It could also presumably be reversed by a "re-edit" if this was possible without introducing new risks. A technical risk detected may be irreversible or irreparable for the person affected (or not), but once detected, it could be prevented from being passed on to further generations. Here, reversibility, or "un-editing" of what has been edited, would be key.

Societal changes and shifts in norms, on the other hand, are more complex and may thus be both harder to fully predict and avoid, as well as harder to reverse. Let us assume that the societal consequences of germline gene editing become problematic in the ways that have been suggested: that those without germline edits become an underclass. What would their demands be, should they rise up in revolt? Would they want to replace the edited elite? Would they demand the right to free germline edits for their children? Or would they call into question the kinds of traits favored and seek to steer the germline gene editing in a different direction? This we do not know. Germline gene editing could also become political. We can imagine that different political ideologies could favor different kinds of edits (and that societal advantages follow the preferences of those in power). There is much we do not know about the future world. To what extent are such developments avoidable? In one sense, it seems too late to protest being born to fulfill someone else's ideal, since one cannot undo one's own birth or what precedes it. Even if individual edits could be reversed, this would presumably affect the generation, and even if the genetic alternation could be reversed on an individual level, turning society back once such changes have become the norm and culturally influential would not be easy.

The main concern here is the unavoidability of unexpected outcomes on the one hand, and the potential for global and societal impact on the other. This concern is particularly warranted when it comes to new and evolving technology, especially when applied to something as complex and not yet fully understood as the human genome. We need to know more about which genes do what to expand the applications of germline editing, but many genes have more than one function and interact in various ways. It is thus unlikely that we will have the complete picture of biological or genetic effects until this has been fully studied, which seems hard to do without actually applying the technology in clinical studies.

Mariscal and Petropanagos (2016) draw an interesting parallel between CRISPR and the Ford Model T when it was new in the early twentieth century. They ponder what kinds of risks an imaginary Department of Transportation in the early years of this mass-produced car would have been able to predict, and what risks they would have overlooked? They speculate that:

Such a department would likely have foreseen some problems early on: traffic and city planning, collisions, car safety, and possibly the toxicity of lead in gasoline. Other problems may have been missed—air pollution, possibly climate change, and possibly oil demand as a driver of geopolitical strife. Such a department would also have focused on issues we no longer regard as problematic—the fate of the horse industry, the shift away from widespread public use of railroads, and the cost of redesigning cities and infrastructure. (Mariscal & Petropanagos, 2016, p. 11 f.)

This illustrates the difficulties in gaining a complete epistemic picture of the risks when it comes to emerging technologies that may have systemic effects. A moral assessment of germline editing under our current best understanding may be equivalent to assessing the Ford Model T, while only predicting its effects on city planning and the horse industry, and not anticipating its effects on oil as a geopolitical and global environmental factor.[10] For this reason, it might be too hasty to simply dismiss the more radical objections on the basis of improbability. First, they are not more improbable than any of the explicit aims proposed by transhumanist agendas. Second, we cannot limit the relevant risks to the kinds we normally consider when it comes to medical interventions. In those cases, we could cause great harm to an individual, but we do not risk altering or harming humanity as a concept or species. Perhaps we do not do this in the case of germline editing either, or at least not in more pervasive ways than evolution does or more than epigenetic changes would. The point is that we need to expand our imaginative horizon and think as broadly as possible in order to spot the blank spots where there could be hidden risks that we are currently not considering.

Of course, when it comes to CRISPR, this is not limited to the human germline or even human genes. Thus, we must consider a future scenario where we might *simultaneously* seek to genetically alter the food we eat (plants and animals), the organs and tissues we use for transplants and medicine (human, animal, or human-animal chimeras), the natural environment around us, as well as the human germline. We must situate this kind of experimentation in the context of rapid natural changes due to climate change (and possibly the effects of drastic measures to combat those changes), and we must consider the possibility of new and emerging political and ideological landscapes.

If the success of human evolution is measured in terms of "fit," then simultaneously altering both the environment into which we are supposed to fit and our own nature may risk making that fit weaker rather than stronger. We do not

---

[10] Mariscal and Petropanagos do not take this aspect as a reason to oppose germline edits categorically, but rather that CRISPR requires "continuous, interdisciplinary, and international oversight" consisting of various experts and stakeholders (2016, p. 13).

know what it would be like to grow up in a society where everyone who could afford it would have altered genes, and we know even less what it would be like to have one's genes altered and re-altered over multiple generations as genetic preferences and priorities came and went, or in a society where animals were altered as well. There is a concern, as mentioned in the previous section, about undoing all constants and replacing them with variables. To do this without a clear goal or plan seems unwise.

The unavoidability of risk does not end with the biological effects, but must include social effects. Here, the challenges seem to be this: If the major concern is about the totalitarian elements of genetic editing in the past and insistence on the fixed value of liberty, it seems hard to avoid concerns about genetic injustice. If, on the other hand, the major concern is about injustice and the risk of making class society more extreme, genetically based, and permanent, then one would wish to ensure equal access and wide programs. If enforced, however, even if voluntary, it could work against values of liberty due to social pressure making it socially impossible not to participate. Such a move, while avoiding the injustice charge, would then make any of the universal outcomes more realistic. Should anything go terribly wrong, or there are severe unanticipated effects—whether biological, psychological, or social—these would be much more damaging and likely to be irreparable.

In conclusion, there are two categories of severe risk to take into consideration. One is about *the fear of genuine losses and harm to humanity as a kind* (even if the technology is successful). The other is about *the fear of things going wrong*, either on a biological, natural, or social level. The former is about value and identity, and the latter about safety and epistemic risk.

9.4.3 Fairness, Risk, Liberty, and Progress

When it comes to human germline editing, there is tension between three different sets of moral values that pull in different directions: the values of fairness and justice, the value of safety and minimizing risk, and the value of progress and addressing existing harms and challenges. We seem to be able to easily combine two of the three, but we lose the third, whichever way we address it. We could potentially achieve progress, along with great medical and enhancement benefits and make this minimally risky, but not while also keeping research subjects safe and ensuring equal access. In general, the fewer people have access to experimental methods, the lower the risk for systemic risks. We could potentially seek to explore progress and equality, but then the risks would be higher, given the fact that, should anything go wrong, this could affect countless people and have broad, global, or even systemic effects. We could prioritize equality and safety, but then we might put a halt on progress.

9.5 Discussion

To sum up, what precisely is the lingering concern about editing the germline? There are three overlapping arguments: one involving the loss of humanity as a whole as a genuine loss, one about a loss of our kind of existence and experience, and one about alienation and a loss of value. Let us return to the question with which we began this chapter: Is there something particularly morally significant about germline editing?

The most prominent argument so far seems to relate to the fact that when editing the germline, we are not merely adding and subtracting values from the potential life of a person or to our lived world as humans, but tinkering with the foundations of such a life and world, and thereby also altering grounds for what counts as beneficial. There is a fine line between improving a recipe, altering a recipe, ruining a dish, and inventing a new dish. At the far end of possible uses of germline editing, difficult issues arise concerning the boundaries of our species and the value of appreciating what is over what could be when our own existence is at stake.

A natural question to raise at this point is: To what extent does any such concern affect the issues with germline editing in the near future in the more modest sense of preventing genetic disease and improving genetic prospects? There are three responses to this question. Thus, if we, for the sake of the argument, agree that risking the very existence of humanity would be a bad thing—on the grounds that it would not just constitute a genuine loss in an objective sense as a loss of species, but more importantly, it would pose a most existential threat to *us* in a collective and subjective way—how could this, admittedly rather remote, threat have any bearing on germline editing in general?

First, there is *the slippery slope argument:* Once we begin to edit the human germline at all, for whatever purpose, we open Pandora's box and start to edit for all other non-medical reasons as well; and with that we open up the possibilities for all kinds of ulterior motives: status, privilege, exploitation, fun, vainglory, and so on. This would push the boundaries, and, in the end, we will lose sight of what is human and what is not, and humanity as such might be lost forever.

This line of argument is not very convincing. It makes too many speculative causative assumptions. Furthermore, it makes strong presumptions about a leading to b leading to c, assuming that we could not halt at various stops in between. Even though the slippery slope argument is fairly plausible for the case that once we accept medical intervention, we will soon slip into some kind of enhancement or non-medical intervention, it is far less convincing that we would slip from moderate enhancement into more ambitious enhancement. Why? Germline editing, thus far, has really only emerged as an attractive option in the context of free parental decisions. While such free-market options would be problematic for a number of reasons, especially for reasons of risk (from a new technology and relatively little knowledge about genes) and for reasons of social stratification and discrimination (assuming that it will be something accessed only by already well-to-do parents wishing to further enhance their child's prospects), the concerns about abandoning humanity for posthumanity is not one of them.

The very rationale for parental interest in germline editing in the first place is the strong preference for a genetically related child. This preference could only be explained by the value of a strong connection with a biological child. Thus, there are reasons to suspect that if all germline editing choices are left to parents, they would not want to risk alienation or seek to promote an outcome where their children and grandchildren would not only belong to a different generation but also to a different species. (This does not exclude other interests in promoting such an outcome for ideological, aesthetic, or other reasons, presumably based on some kind of notion that the posthuman would either be us or our creation, and their imagined greatness would somehow reflect on us.)

Second, there is more of a definitional and ontological argument to the effect that when we edit the embryo of a future person, we *tinker with the possibilities* of what that person can and cannot be; thus, we experiment with the ontological variables of a future person, so to speak. Although this might be true, it is unclear what this argument actually claims other than stating the obvious. How would this be different from other kinds of decisions, such as deciding to procreate on a particular day rather than another? The point here might be less about the fact that we could affect what a person might and might not be, than that we could do so in radical and deliberate ways. This means that instead of a person being born as an outcome of chance and biology, it will be an outcome of the imagination and will of another person. Some argue that this makes us somehow responsible for the nature of another being, which is too much responsibility and reconstructs the relationship between persons to one of creator and creation, which risks making other beings objects or artifacts in a sense. This may be true, but unless we pair it with ill will or a lack of concern for the interest of the future person, it may not be anything problematic in and of itself.

Third, there is *the epistemic concern* that we may, in fact, have only a very fragmented picture of what the risks are. Thus, whatever we currently take to be the more concerning risks may actually be widely off the mark. There are three distinct areas of concern that could support this.

First, a technology such as CRISPR and other gene editing technologies are not limited to the human germline but are used in all parts of the natural living world. This means that if human success is measured in terms of "fit," the world to which we must "fit" may not be the slowly evolving "constant" that we may presume, but also rapidly change in fundamental ways. Thus, what might at present seem like a good idea in terms of improvement may turn out to be quite different in a new social and natural context. In any case, what we might consider to be improvements could turn out to be nothing of the sort.

Second, we may not know what the precise consequences of particular edits entail, given the many functions singular genes may have, the way they interact with each other, and the way that our lives and interactions with our worlds impose epigenetic changes.

Third, related to the issues raised above, we may not know enough about our future to predict what will be valuable or to exclude the worst-case scenarios we can imagine, even less so the ones we currently cannot imagine. Thus, it could be argued that unless we can confidently exclude the loss of humanity, irreversible changes to the detriment of humanity, or irreversible harms brought about by such changes, it would be unwise to take such risks.

To conclude: Morally speaking, human germline editing is a different kind of action than just about any other action we could perform. Why? Because no other kind of action is a case of deliberate manipulation of what it means to be human, and has the distinct possibility not only to drastically narrow or widen the scope of what a person can be, but also to drastically alter the inherent properties of that person, such that it is no longer a person or no longer a person in the same sense as everyone else that has gone before them or belongs to the same tribe, family, or community. In other words, with germline editing, we lay at some agent's hand a tool that could sever a person from all of humanity, construct their intrinsic properties such that it would be amusing to others, or experiment with their nature to fit some predesignated purpose that is not their own. Nature may not have intrinsic value, but evolution, chance, and nature do not treat single individuals as mere means for another individual's selfish interests; however, germline editing could enable a person to create another person to satisfy their whims. In short, we, in a sense, provide the despot with a new tool, and submit the republican notion of liberty to a new domain where it could be violated. Normally, there is a limit to what another person can manipulate and harm: at some point, there is dignity and integrity that could be maintained, even for the exploited person. This boundary could be violated, should someone wish to design future humans to suit their whims.

In terms of lingering concerns, three cases could be made that each give cause for caution and, when considered together, certainly do. The level of risk that comes with a new technology applied to such a complex system (which also interacts to such a high degree) provides plenty of opportunity for things to go wrong in many unexpected ways. The degree of uncertainty makes it difficult to predict what the actual risks and their full scope of consequences for individuals, relations, cultures, society and nature might actually be; and the fact that it is our own potentiality and nature that is the object of tinkering, beyond additions or removals of unwanted elements, could result in us compromising the very essence of who we are.

All three of the above arguments highlight genuine risks in the sense that the particular outcomes are not easily compensated for, replaced, or repaired: Should humanity be lost, or should we no longer fit into the world or no longer belong to our species, then there is no obvious way that we could reverse, repair, or compensate for that outcome—it would constitute a permanent loss, not just of something valuable (on some measure), but of the very foundation of our own kind of existence and our values.

But how likely is this result and can we avoid it? The epistemic risk could be reduced as we learn more. A cautious approach of oversight and various regulatory frameworks could limit the ways that things might go wrong. The existential risks do not seem to reside at the moderate end of interventions, only at the more radical end. Finally, until it is safer, it would be unwise to venture into germline editing too hastily. Should it ever become sufficiently safe and it is offered to well-to-do parents, it is likely to increase injustice, underscore privilege, and descend a slope to enhancement. However, the bottom of that slope is probably more likely confined to middle-class aspirational enhancement rather than the end of humanity—especially given that much of the interest in germline editing seems to be premised on the parental value of genetic relatedness. If that is the prerequisite for a broad interest in germline editing in the first place, then it seems unlikely that parents would want to venture past some point where their child may no longer belong to the same species as them. However, should the safety assessments be too limited and premature, and the epistemic gaps remain considerable, then the fact that what we are tinkering with is the human fabric could prove disastrous in that irreversible harm may be brought upon future individuals.

We draw two conclusions: Any kind of precaution must take a broad view on risk, such that it includes not merely those risks we are currently contemplating, but also the epistemic gaps that could hide from view much more serious risks that will become apparent at a later stage. Perhaps more than asking what the worst is that could happen, we ought to ask what we can be sure would be reversible, or in any other way possibly repairable, should it all go wrong. And, whom could we in good consciousness be comfortable exposing to such risks?

Human Germline as a Moral Boundary: Categorical, Conditional, or Precautionary?

10

What conclusions can be drawn about the human germline as a moral boundary? Is there a "red line" to be drawn at the germline? Interestingly, Resnik and Langer (2001) summarized the early debate on genetic engineering, long before CRISPR, into four key assumptions: that there is *a morally significant difference between germline therapy and enhancement*, that *enhancement is difficult to justify morally* (on grounds of eugenics, playing God, perfectionism, social justice, etc.), that *therapy can be justified* (on cost–benefit grounds when compared to alternatives), and that "*no human germline genetic experiment should be conducted until we have sufficient evidence concerning short-term and long-term safety and efficacy.*" (Resnik & Langer, 2001, p. 1449).

It would seem that in the over 20 years that have passed since, this still comes very close to what seems to be the dominant view. There is a broad agreement that germline editing and enhancement are morally different. Enhancement is definitely the most controversial issue. There is, at least on the scientific and medical side, much hope attached to the benefits of gene therapy—although there is also a discussion on how gene editing compares to PGD in terms of safety. As we have seen, the most unifying point of all is that it is currently not sufficiently safe, the risks are not fully known, and it would be irresponsible to proceed until it is sufficiently safe. However, some would not agree that we ought to conduct experiments on the germline at all and believe that we should rather focus on somatic gene therapy and basic research.

© The Author(s) 2025
M. Hayenhjelm and C. Nordlund, *The Risks and Ethics of Human Gene Editing*,
Technikzukünfte, Wissenschaft und Gesellschaft / Futures of Technology, Science
and Society, https://doi.org/10.1007/978-3-658-46979-5_10

Resnik and Langer challenged the first three of the four assumptions.[1] In short, they problematized the therapy/enhancement boundary on the grounds that it is vague and needs some kind of baseline for what is healthy or normal to operate; hence, they rejected the first two assumptions. Furthermore, they suggested that the latter two can be replaced with a concern about safety. Juengst (2017) has argued that the somatic/germline boundary, in contrast to the therapy/enhancement boundary, was always predominantly about safety. He writes:

> Of the two boundaries, the germ-line line has always been more dependent on safety and efficacy concerns than other ethical arguments. Beyond our ignorance of long-range consequences, and apart from enhancement worries, it has been hard to demonstrate why new genetic tools to treat and prevent disease in families would be in principle more problematic than any other biomedical and public health interventions. (Juengst, 2017, p. 18)

It is this thesis that will be investigated in this concluding chapter: Are there valid moral reasons not to ever edit the human germline and, hence, reasons to draw a line against such edits?

10.1   Four Steps and Two Directions

In this chapter, we will revisit the overall question about boundaries, and particularly the idea about a moral boundary at the germline. Is there a moral boundary to be drawn at the germline? If so, on what grounds? We will visit these questions in four steps.

The first step is about making sense of a distinction between germline gene editing and somatic gene editing and about identifying morally significant properties and morally relevant differences between germline editing and somatic gene editing.

---

[1] Resnik and Langer state them in the following words: "(A1) There is a medically and morally significant difference between therapeutic modifications of the germline, HGLGT, and nontherapeutic modifications of the germline, human germline genetic enhancement. (A2) Human germline genetic enhancement is very difficult to justify because it raises issues of eugenics, playing 'God,' perfectionism, social justice, etc. (A3) HGLGT, on the other hand, can be justified (in principle), because there are some situations where it would be the best (i.e., safest, most effective, and least expensive) method of treatment. (A4) No human germline genetic experiment should be conducted until we have sufficient evidence concerning short-term and long-term safety and efficacy." (Resnik & Langer, 2001, p. 1449).

The second step is about the case for a categorical boundary at the germline. It concerns questions about whether there are certain things we must never do and whether this applies to germline editing. It asks whether moral reasons support any notion of a "red line" in a moral sense. If we can reliably conclude that there is such a boundary, then our moral questions are largely already answered. If we cannot draw such a conclusion, we come to the third step.

The third step is about alternative moral lines that require a categorical boundary and includes conditional boundaries and categorical boundaries not drawn at the germline. There could be a morally relevant difference to germline editing as opposed to somatic editing without this implying a categorical moral line. Alternatively, some cases may be more serious than others, such that there is a categorical line to be drawn but not exactly at the germline. If we cannot reliably identify such an alternative categorical boundary or a reliable conditional boundary, we come to the fourth step.

This step is about what we morally ought to do when we do not have conclusive answers to the previous steps. It raises a more pragmatic question: If we do not know what is permissible, impermissible, or morally required, is there something about human germline editing that may suggest that it is morally safer to do one thing than another? When we are in a position to impose risks and benefits by altering the human germline for future individuals without the possibility of consent, what is the morally responsible thing to do? Is there a "wise line" to be drawn somewhere? If so, where and on what grounds?

The four steps can be approached from *two directions*, depending on whether we depart from germline editing and enquire about morality or if we begin from moral theory and enquire about germline editing. If we begin with germline editing and explore the four steps from this towards morality, we will arrive at something like the following:

1. Is there something distinct about germline editing that could be morally significant and that sets it apart from other medical or genetic interventions?
2. Does the germline mark out a moral boundary of impermissibility?
3. Is there another moral boundary that better marks out what we must never do when it comes to human gene editing? Is the moral difference between somatic and germline editing sufficient to draw a conditional line between the two, such that it can morally only be crossed if certain conditions are met?
4. Can the germline serve as a default boundary on the grounds of caution or responsibility?

This would be to pose the relevant questions from the position of germline editing towards moral answers. In these questions, we begin with that which is concrete, a medical genetic practice and a field of application, and turn to moral theory for answers. Here, germline editing is understood as part of a broader context of medical and genetic practices and compared with somatic gene editing and other boundaries in the debate, such as that between therapy and enhancement.

We can also ask the moral questions in the other direction: from moral theory towards the germline. Here, we begin with the abstract concepts and principles found in moral theory and ask if they overlap with boundaries found in the literature on germline editing and what they would imply when applied to these matters. From this direction, we would arrive at something like the following:

1. Is there something particularly morally significant about the germline when viewed from established moral theory?
2. Are there categorical moral principles that would make all cases of germline gene editing impermissible?
3. Are there moral properties that apply only to some cases of germline editing and not to others such that some cases of germline editing would be categorically impermissible and others permissible?
4. What is the morally responsible and wise thing to do should there not be clear categorical boundaries or conditional ones? Would refraining from germline gene editing be to err on the side of caution?

Here, moral theory is taken as primary and moral key concepts as a point of departure. It is not assumed that moral boundaries will overlap with any descriptive boundaries found in the debate, which remains to be seen. Instead, the questions are posed independently of preexisting boundaries: Are there descriptive differences such that they also constitute moral differences, do the distinctions established in the debate point to morally relevant differences? Or, would moral principles and concepts draw them in other ways and other places, and on other grounds than what has been discussed in the recent debate? Where would moral theory suggest we draw a line, if at all?

As can be seen from the two sets of questions, there is a great deal of overlap. We will address each of the four steps and, where appropriate, highlight the differences from the two positions.

10.2   First Direction: The Moral Significance of the "Germline"

What, if anything, makes the germline morally significant? For there to be a moral boundary at the germline, there needs to be something about germline editing that makes it different from other kinds of medical or genetic interventions thought to be less morally problematic. In this section, the question about relevant moral properties will be addressed from both directions. "Is there something distinct about germline editing that sets it apart from other medical or genetic interventions that could be morally significant?"; and "What is morally relevant in the case of germline gene editing when viewed from established moral theory?" The first is about salient features of germline editing that *could be of moral significance*. The second is about abstract morally significant features that *could coincide with the category of germline gene edits*.

10.2.1   Key Features: Heritability, Risk and Social Impact

What, if any, are the morally salient features of germline editing? By far the most dominant answer to this is *heritability*. In fact, many use the somatic/germline distinction as synonymous with heritable/non-heritable genetic interventions. In particular, three aspects have been suggested to make the case of germline editing more serious than somatic gene therapy. Apart from heritability, these include technological or medical risks, and concerns about the social and psychological impacts of genetic choices. Cwik summarizes these three kinds of concerns well as heritability, risk, and "downstream social impacts" (Cwik, 2020b, p. 9). But, to what extent do these trace a difference between somatic and germline gene editing and what are the moral implications of such a difference, if there is one?

10.2.2   Heritability

The fact that germline editing is hereditary is probably the difference between somatic and germline editing that has the most moral significance. At first glance, this seems to point to a more intrinsic feature of germline editing than those of risk or social costs, both of which point to potential consequences that may be avoidable. The fact that germline edits are heritable seems to be an unalienable fact of the kind of intervention it is. How accurate is this notion that what sets germline editing apart is the fact that such edits are heritable? And what is the moral significance of this exactly?

First, is it true that germline editing is heritable in a way that somatic gene editing is not? Is it true that heritability singles out germline editing as a class in some relevant way? On the face of it, this seems to be true, and it is often repeated. In fact, the line between germline gene editing and somatic gene editing is often described as the line between heritable and non-heritable editing. However, as we saw in a previous chapter, this difference is not as categorical as one may think (see Sects. 2.2.1 and 2.3). If heritability alone set germline editing apart, then we would need to include epigenetic changes that could be passed on to our future offspring in the same category.

Second, is heritability morally significant and, if so, in what way and on what grounds? Although it is true that edits to the germline are heritable, if there is a subsequent generation, this seems to be only half of what the moral concerns about germline editing are about. Many of the categorical objections do not focus on the next generation(s), but on the very child and person developed from an edited embryo. Any harm to them would be equally significant, even if it was never passed on. Thus, heritability cannot be the only morally significant aspect about germline editing, nor the only relevant difference. The fact that we edit germ cells and thus determine the genetics of a person before they are born also seems to be morally significant and morally different from somatic gene therapy.

Presumably, the main moral significance of heritability is about risk and *the scope* for potential harm. Should anything go wrong in the case of somatic therapy, the harm is limited to the actual patient (and indirectly to their next of kin, etc.), whereas if we edit the germline, should anything go wrong, this could affect later generations as well as the first generation. In theory, we could harm numerous people instead of one. However, if the harm were obvious to the first generation before they had any offspring, then, presumably, they would elect not to pass on such a heritance. Furthermore, that a change is heritable does not necessarily imply that it would be irreversible, such that the generation after could not be protected by a re-edit. Whether such re-edits are at all possible, and would be safe and not introduce additional risks, is, of course, highly speculative at this point, but just because there is heritability does not mean that actual harm to additional generations is unavoidable. The matter becomes much more difficult if harm appears later in life, such that the person already would have procreated, or if it appears in the next generation for the first time, and so on. In any case, the moral problem with heritability seems to be one of scope. Furthermore, the actual scope differs greatly depending on assumptions about what we know and do not know about irreversibility. Heritability matters because of the number of individuals potentially put in harm's way.

In general, the heritability aspect seems to function as an *amplifier* of all the other kinds of risks, such as those from off-target effects and unwanted on-target effects. It could also suggest something even more troubling, such as the potential for dynamic effects, when we consider that edits are not only heritable across multiple generations but that each generation could potentially add new edits and seek to undo other edits. If the technology becomes popular and useful, it is likely that its utility will increase. At some point, we may reach a level of editing and re-editing where things become complicated and perhaps even strange. This concern hinges on germline editing being risky in the first place and comes with epistemic gaps. By contrast, should germline editing largely be safe and beneficial, such effects would also be amplified with heritability. In sum, heritability is not morally significant in itself, but largely serves as an *amplifier* of ignorance, risk, and benefits.

There are, however, two other aspects that are related to the heritability aspect, which have to do with the fact that any alterations to the germline will affect a person *before they are born* and, likewise, heritability would amplify this aspect as well. Typically, this aspect has been raised in relation to consent (or, rather, the lack thereof), and the power it gives those in a position to alter the genome of another before they are born. But there is also an *intrusiveness* and *pervasiveness* part to this, given how central our genome is to what we can be and do. More than just an amplifier of risk, the concept of heritability could thus be seen as an umbrella term for a number of related concerns that all have to do with the kinds of effects that editing germ cells would have that the editing of somatic cells would not.

The fact that germline editing is performed on the germ cells, or on embryos at a very early stage, has several implications that could all be morally relevant: the fact that such edits will affect all cells (if successful), and are thus *pervasive*; the fact that germline alterations will affect the genetic limits and prerequisites of a person, and are thus *intrusive*; the fact that such alterations are made before birth, and thus *cannot be consented to*; and that such changes will affect that person's offspring and entire lineage, and thus *could affect their reproductive liberties* and abilities. All these aspects distinguish germline editing from somatic gene editing.

These aspects seem to have less to do with heritability being intrinsically wrong, and more about autonomy-related concerns. Autonomy is not merely about making one's own decisions, but about making one's own decisions about what is rightfully one's own. Traditionally, natural rights theory has given us a right to life and property as well as a right to decide what happens to these without intervention from others without our consent. Now, one could argue that of all the things that rightfully belong to us that no one else has a right to willfully experiment with or alter, it would be our own DNA. This comes close to the ideas we mentioned earlier as the right to be born with an unaltered inheritance. There is a tricky landscape to navigate here, in order to propose a consistent argument that does not become entangled in all kinds of rights of unborn persons, or rights against natural consequences of events when in the womb, and women's rights over their bodies and their reproductive rights. The point here is merely to highlight that there may be an intrusiveness argument to be made: There are certain things one must never do to an unborn person if those things could drastically affect who that person would be and could be in a way that would run counter to what they could hypothetically accept or embrace. The idea is that there is a gene editing equivalence to a parent who dresses a boy in a dress or in clothes fit for a much younger person to suit their own desires, and that there is something particularly problematic if such changes were imposed on someone before they are born and cannot be undone. The potential exists to be born with genes that someone else has decided for you, which could be humiliating and demoralizing. Both consent and heritability have been widely discussed; however, it is quite possible that one of the most significant aspects of germline editing is this *pervasiveness* aspect and the power this could give another person to alter what is not rightfully theirs to alter.

10.2.3 Risk

The second potential morally relevant difference between germline editing and somatic gene editing is that of risk. Risks are by far the most dominant reason for why edits to the germline are not legal in most countries and the most dominant reason behind calls of moratoria or general halts at the germline. Thus, if there ever was a dominant reason to draw a moral line at the germline it seems to be based on risk.

The question is to what degree this marks out a stark difference between somatic and germline editing. If one limits risks to those attached to the technology itself, at least some of the risk concerns apply to somatic gene editing as well. Thus, the difference seems to be one of degree rather than a categorical difference. Of course, there are differences in terms of risk. Not the least of which are attached to the aspects mentioned in the previous section: the fact that edits will affect all cells (if successful) and that they are inheritable. It seems to be this particular dimension to the risk aspect that makes it morally problematic in a different sense than ordinary medical interventions. That is paired with the concerns, also mentioned above, that these risks cannot be consented to, could be pervasive and could affect reproduction, and many risks could be largely unknown. All these aspects seem to suggest both that germline editing is too risky to be morally responsible to perform and decidedly more risky than somatic gene editing for the above reasons.

However, none of the above aspects provide any convincing grounds to argue that there is a categorical difference. Rather, it implies a threshold for unacceptably high risk or unacceptably high stakes. Thus, there is nothing to suggest that germline editing could not in the future fall below that threshold. Furthermore, the degree and kind of risk differs greatly within the class of potential germline edits. Presumably, germline edits to erase a monogenetic disease that has been well studied are different from multiple or more experimental edits. The point is that if risk is what is morally relevant, it does not seem to single out the germline as the morally relevant class, but rather some notion of acceptable versus unacceptable risk. There is thus no germline boundary, but an unacceptable risk boundary.

10.2.4   Social Implications and Slippery Slopes

The third potentially morally relevant difference lies in the risk for catastrophic outcomes and risks of a more social, psychological, and existential nature. Somatic gene therapy can only treat or enhance single patients. It cannot with a single intervention alter a lineage, nor can it determine who will and who will not be born in the future. The concern about eugenics could thus explain a potential moral difference.

Germline editing may allow us to determine what traits future generations may or may not be born with. It thus has the potential to rewrite what genetic majorities and minorities will look like and also how large or small those majorities and minorities will be, and how wide the gap between the genetically most privileged and the genetically least privilege will be. Thus, some view this as the real difference and threat. This could affect how those born with disability are met and treated, and the kinds of lives they will be able to live in terms of justice and fairness; and fear for a permanent underclass and elite where any social mobility would require genetic interventions in terms of a different social climate, outlook on fellow man, and social pressure to chase perfection.

This is also a risk argument of sorts, but one of social, moral, and existential risks. It marks out a difference between somatic gene editing and germline gene editing that is hard not to be regarded as morally significant. Somatic gene therapy is less convincing as a first step towards redesigning humanity. However, these kinds of risks seem to be more related to enhancement than other kinds of germline edits. Not all cases of germline edits pose these kinds of risks, unless one makes significant slippery slope assumptions.

Additionally, germline edits to prevent disease and functional variations could alter society and the social conditions for those currently living with such conditions, and it could have systemic effects that could deepen the divide between rich and poor nations and classes. There are thus two kinds of risks: more immediate social costs in terms of intolerance and injustice and risks of more far-reaching social consequences and genuine existential losses.

10.3   Second Direction: Morally Significant Features of the Germline

We will now look at the germline from the other direction and ask whether there is something morally distinct about the germline or something that makes altering it particularly morally problematic. We have referred loosely to "moral theory." Of course, moral theory is not a single theory, or even a set of received theories backed by a consensus, it is a vast and complex field of ongoing research informed by a scholarly tradition stretching thousands of years back. For our current purposes, we cannot do much more than allude to a way to approach the matter and draw some very rough sketches. However, certain things can be said about this approach. Most current moral theory focuses on actions, the role of the moral agent, and the overall question about what to do in a morally contestable situation. In this way of framing morality, the focal points of what could be of moral relevance could be narrowed down to three: the potential outcomes of the actions contemplated and the available alternatives; the kinds of reasons, rationale and in particular their agreement with certain principles or agreement with others; and the moral character and intentions of the moral agent.

According to this very rough sketch, one can broadly say that if there is something morally distinct about germline editing as a moral action, our best bet would be to look at the potential consequences, especially compared to other actions, any relevant principles that may single it out as particularly problematic, and whether such actions would go against what a wise and morally mature person ought to do. This still does not tell us much, since there are multiple theories about what makes a consequence good or bad in a morally relevant way, multiple theories about what kinds of conditions or principles determine moral rightness and wrongness, and various accounts of what constitutes a good person and what this implies for moral rightness of action. Of these three, the first two are dominant when the moral action is the main focus rather than the character or the person.

In Chap. 5, we introduced three basic kinds of logic that run through much of moral theory and can be applied to assess and analyze potential moral actions. This gives us a point of departure. These three kinds of logic also focus on different aspects of moral actions. The first focuses *on consequences as states of affairs*, the second *on principles* that the act considered may or may not violate or abide by, and the third is about the kind of *ideal* that the action promotes or undermines. With these three broad focal points, we can have a rough idea of where to look for potentially morally significant aspects of germline editing, and in what way germline gene editing could morally differ from somatic gene editing or other kinds of medical interventions. Germline editing may lead to *significantly different kinds of outcomes* and thus to a different kind or level of harm or benefit. Germline editing may *violate moral principles* or, conversely, *be required by moral principles*. Germline editing may *contribute to important ideals or undermine such ideals* that may illustrate a very promising or very bleak future, or it may *drastically alter* what our ideal future looks like.

10.3.1 Morally Significant Consequences

According to the value maximization logic, there is typically no special significance attached to different kinds of outcomes, what matters is one and the same thing: whether, overall, things get better or whether they, overall, get worse on some measure of good or bad. If that is the case, the moral issues raised by germline editing are not different in kind to any other moral problem ever raised: it is all about whether the benefits are worth the risks, and if we can expect to make things better. What we need to assess is whether the risks would be outweighed by the benefits, compared to the alternatives.

However, we have tried to argue (Chap. 8) that it may be that not all negative outcomes can be outweighed by greater gains. Perhaps certain things must never be lost, because they are not replaceable or reparable. If such risks are attached to germline editing but not to somatic gene editing, then this would be morally significant.

Furthermore, it could be argued that some potential outcomes, down certain slippery slopes, are so fundamentally different to the world we currently have that they may not be comparable, and that there is something morally significant about this, even if there were no issues about compensability or replaceability. Perhaps we can say that one state of the world is overall much better than another one, yet the losses and the costs that it took to get there make it morally very problematic.

But, ultimately, the value maximizer would want to know if there would be more happiness in a world where germline editing is available to parents who desire to use it to prevent genetic disease and have genetically related children; where fewer people are born with certain genetic diseases; where some people have been genetically enhanced and others have not; and where all future generations have modified genes. Any answer to this is bound to be extremely speculative. We do not know. There are too many parameters to make any kind of guess, and one complicating factor is our ability as humans to adapt to the circumstances we are given.

10.3.2 Morally Significant Principles

On the permissibility logic, the focus falls on moral principles and what we may and may not do. There may be certain things that *we simply must never do* under any circumstance, some things that we are *morally obliged* to do, and others that we are *at liberty to do* regardless of whether it is good or bad. Some things are not required but would overall be a good thing to do. When it comes to things we must never do, this would normally be restricted by some rule that made it impermissible and some kind of "off-limits" status of what we intended to affect. Thus, there are certain things we must not do to others, given that some things belong to them, and them alone, for reasons of property rights or privacy, or is for them and them alone to decide for reasons of autonomy. There are certain things we must not do to others, because it would be humiliating and harmful, for reasons of respect for persons and/or their happiness. Similarly, there are things we ought to do for others, because they have a right to them, for reasons of human need and a right to rescue.

In Chap. 6, we saw various arguments that appeal either to a line of impermissibility and/or a protected zone that implies such impermissibility. Usually, these two aspects come together: here is the line, because beyond this line lies what must be protected from interference. The logic here is perhaps not very different from the notions of taboo and that which is sacred. We saw such an argument based on the notion of hubris or playing God, suggesting that it would venture beyond our legitimate remit of action. We saw other arguments to the effect that the human genome or human "nature" constitutes such protected zones with which we must not interfere. Is this then what is morally significant and different about the germline? That germline editing constitutes a case of hubris, playing God, or playing around with nature, that somatic gene therapy does not? This seems neither to pinpoint a notable difference, nor what is morally most relevant here.

In more secular moral philosophy, the area that needs protecting is typically the moral rights and status of another individual as a moral equal. Thus, we must not venture beyond what is compatible with respect for another person, and we must not violate or infringe upon their equal rights, including rights to autonomy, liberty, and privacy. Here, there is more of a case that there is something notably different between somatic and germline gene editing. In somatic gene therapy, the other person who could have relevant rights claims is the person undergoing the therapy. In germline gene therapy, it is the person not yet born whose embryo it is and any future descendants from that embryo who would inherit such edits, and any third person who might be affected by the resulting outcomes of such edits, and any long-term effects resulting from norms changes and bigger changes in society as a consequence of many such edits. Of course, this difference is the same, regardless of whether we presume that the rights preclude or require edits. The point is that if we look for a morally significant difference between somatic and germline gene editing, there is an obvious difference in who they affect and whose potential rights it would potentially satisfy, violate, or infringe upon. To future generations, we must also add the interests and rights of the prospective parents and, depending on the kinds of edits, anyone who currently lives with various conditions. In short, the scope of potential rights claimants is significantly different.

Furthermore, we can assume that there might be many more conflicting interests in the case of germline editing compared to somatic gene therapy. All individual rights may not align in the same way: some rights may require that we perform certain edits and others that we abstain. For instance, perhaps a certain couple would not have a child at all unless they could ensure that it was genetically theirs and did not suffer from the genetic disease that they would pass on to them. Then it could be argued that the parents have a right to explore all options and are at liberty to make their own decisions with the available options. It could also be argued that the individual embryo and the resulting person would have a right to be born without a debilitating condition, should this be an option.

Now let us assume that the technological intervention and knowledge about it develops over time. Let us further assume that the first generation of such edits would suffer significant but not intolerable side effects. In the case of this first generation, the edit might even be a condition for being born at all. Now, let us consider the potential interests and rights of the next generation. Here, we could imagine that biotechnology has progressed. Perhaps there are now very successful treatments. Perhaps there are more advanced kinds of edits without the side effects. In short, we could assume that there are alternatives that are better than the inherited edit. If so, being born with such edits inherited from a previous generation is not a condition for being born at all, and it is not in the direct interests of that person. Of course, had their parents not had the edits done and their birth was conditional on such edits, then, presumably, the next generation owes their existence to the first generation's edit.

Nevertheless, we must not assume that for inherited alterations to our genome that the interest of future generations is the same and will not change due to various circumstances. This is likely to be exacerbated the further the aim of the edit is from removing direct sources of suffering and pain and the closer it is to attempts at improving odds for various benefits that rely on social factors and norms. Thus, edits with the aim of ensuring a decent height for an offspring in a society that premiers tallness in a family of shorter stature may seem like providing an advantage. However, the value of tallness is relative to the social and natural environment. Even seemingly unquestionable goods may come at a cost. For instance, moderate increases to cognitive capacities, if they required a higher intake of calories, could become a contested liability in a future world of extreme food shortage.

In short, if we look at germline editing from the perspective of rights and interests (and needs that might warrant rights), it becomes clear that germline editing will affect individuals; particularly individuals who are not part of the decision to make such edits. Furthermore, beyond the more obvious cases of prevention of severe suffering, it is not clear what can be concluded about whether germline edits would be in the interest of the edited individual or not. It is very likely that some cases would be and some would not. In any case, it seems obvious that merely from a rights perspective, the moral issues of germline gene editing are much more complex and the sources for making moral mistakes are much greater, given that the full set of moral implications are much harder to predict.

10.3.3   Unforgivables and Revolutionary Outcomes

Here, we will highlight two other notions that may be helpful. Some actions alter the ways things are in such dramatic ways that it is hard not to consider this fact alone as morally significant, even if they do not necessarily lead to on the whole worse or better outcomes than before but simply very different. We could refer to these as *revolutionary outcomes*. Something along these lines were alluded to when CRISPR was described as a revolutionary technology and compared with the Ford Model T of biotechnology (Mariscal & Petropaganos, 2016, see Chap. 9). There is no doubt that many arguments in the debate, particularly about enhancement and transhumanism, approach the matter as if there are revolutionary outcomes to consider here. The titles of some of the books cited in this debate clearly imply such revolutionary outcomes. These include *Humanity's End* (Agar, 2010), *Is Human Nature Obsolete?* (Baillie & Casey, 2005), *Beyond Humanity* (Buchanan, 2011), *Altered Inheritance* (Baylis, 2019), *The Future of Human Nature* (Habermas, 2003), *Our Posthuman Future* (Fukuyama, 2003), and *Fabricated Man* (Ramsey, 1970). All of these indicate that something radical and dramatic could be set in motion by germline gene therapy and editing of the human genome. This need not be good or bad in itself, and some argue that this is a positive opportunity to embrace, while others believe that this is reason for great concern. Nevertheless, it seems plausible to assume that if it is the case that germline gene editing could lead to revolutionary outcomes in a way that somatic gene editing could not, then this is a morally significant difference. Dramatic changes raise the stakes: We will need to know that what we create is something we have good reason to create.

Some moral outcomes and some moral acts are worse than others, and some acts are *dramatically worse* than others. Not only in the recent CRISPR debate, but also in the broader bioethical debate on genetic alterations of the human germline that precedes it, we have seen a constant reference to various dystopian arguments and various worst-case scenarios, which we could refer to as "unforgivable" (see also Sect. 9.3 on "A Most Serious Kind of Risk").

An act could be "unforgivable" in this sense if it could not be forgiven by moral agents themselves in hindsight, and/or by those directly affected and harmed by it, and/or by those close to them and their descendants, and/or by society at large and posterity. Here, we could consider all kinds of monstrosities of the past, such as mass murder, genocide, natural exploitation, mass starvation, transatlantic slave trade, scientific experimentation on vulnerable groups, and the like. If we have reason to believe that an act that we are considering could be unforgiveable, then we would have strong reasons not to proceed, all else equal, and to prevent situations where such unforgivable acts cannot be avoided.

If we apply this notion of "unforgivable acts," are there any such potential acts that could be performed with help of CRISPR and germline editing? We need not be very imaginative. We could simply imagine a totalitarian dream that includes specific ideas about what a perfect human ought to be, or what a perfect slave ought to be, and a plan to design all future individuals according to such a plan. Most such acts can be considered wrong in reference to violations of human dignity, human rights, and the like, or more broadly, as a case of treating another person as a mere means for one's own ends. However, not all cases that violate dignity and rights or treat someone as mere means belong in the category of unforgivables. In fact, most moral day-to-day failings seem perfectly rectifiable and forgivable. It may have violated women's rights not to be allowed to vote, but in hindsight, we celebrate the fact that such a right was won, rather than hold remembrances of the violations that preceded that right. Contrast this with the holocaust; here, we do not celebrate the end to it as much as we remember the horror of it: there is nothing that could rectify that suffering. Some acts and their outcomes are simply not compensable and are so dramatic in their horror that even if they were, strictly speaking, permissible, or even if they were a necessary step to some better outcome for the masses, such outcomes and the actions that led to them are unforgiveable.

Thus, should we have reason to believe that germline editing, in contrast to somatic gene editing, could lead to unforgivables or poorly understood revolutionary outcomes, then this implies that there is a morally significant difference between the two. Furthermore, on the assumption that there are slippery slopes that cannot be dismissed, this could be the case. However, it is unclear what kinds of conclusions about germline editing this would imply. First, just because something is less likely to result from somatic gene editing than from germline gene editing does not mean that the distinction is as sharp as one may think, nor that the revolutionary or unforgivable outcome is more likely or cannot be prevented. However, should we have reason to believe that germline gene editing could lead to unforgiveable or revolutionary outcomes in a way that somatic gene editing could not, then this seems to provide good reason to think that there is a morally relevant difference between the two.

10.4 The Case for a Categorical Moral Boundary at the Germline

We will now turn to the question about the germline as a categorical boundary. Is there a categorical moral boundary at the germline? In the introduction to Chap. 6, we referred to a categorical claim against germline editing as the Categorically Wrong Claim. It read as follows:

Categorically Wrong Claim (CW): Every act of human germline editing is categorically morally wrong.

For there to be a categorical moral boundary at the germline, two conditions must be met. It must be the case that (a) all instances of germline editing are morally wrong (that CW above is true); and (b) that there is something morally significant occurring at the boundary between germline editing and somatic editing, such that "crossing the germline boundary" is morally significant.

It is worth noting that the Categorically Wrong Claim can be true without there being a particular boundary at the germline. This would be the case if, for instance, most somatic gene therapy was also impermissible. For there to be a categorical moral boundary at the germline, there must be something about the kinds of acts that germline editing involves or the somatic/germline distinctions that carry such moral weight that we must never cross that boundary.

There are essentially only two answers to the question of whether the germline marks out a categorical moral boundary: There is either a categorical moral boundary at the germline or there is not.

The Categorical Boundary Claim: There is a categorical moral boundary at the germline. Every act of human germline editing is morally wrong and every time such an edit is performed, a line of moral impermissibility is crossed.

The No Categorical Boundary Claim: There is no categorical moral boundary at the germline. Whether an act of human germline editing is morally wrong or not is not determined by the fact that the germline is crossed.

The Categorical Boundary Claim would be true if it were the case that something that applies to every case of germline editing makes such editing impermissible and there is some categorical moral principle that explains such impermissibility.

From the previous section, we now have some idea of what could justify a categorical moral boundary. There could be a case to the effect that *because germline editing is inheritable, risky, or could bring about social costs*, it is categorically impermissible to edit the germline. There could be a case to the effect that because germline edits constitute an act of hubris or playing God, or seeks to alter nature itself, it is categorically impermissible to edit the germline. There could be a case to the effect that because the moral consequences are too difficult to predict that we might violate individual rights or make life harder for some while making it better for others, it is categorically impermissible to edit the germline. Finally, there could be a case to the effect that there is considerable risk in editing the germline for bringing about an unforgivable outcome, and therefore it is categorically impermissible to edit the germline.

However, all of these arguments are centered on risk. They all point to potential outcomes or likely consequences in some cases but not in others. In short, none of them make a very convincing case for the first condition that must be met, namely "all acts of germline editing are morally wrong." In other words, that the CW claim is true, even if they make a plausible case that there is something morally significant going on at the boundary between germline editing and somatic editing. In sum, the case that there is something morally significant about germline editing is much more compelling than the case that this significance underscores categorical wrongness.

10.4.1 The General Case for a Categorical Boundary

Before we can dismiss any claims about germline editing being categorically wrong, it would be useful to revisit the general case of categorical boundaries. The general claim that there are certain things that we must simply never do, no matter the circumstances or consequences, does not ring obviously false or mistaken. Perhaps germline editing belongs to a broader category of actions that are never permissible; or rather, some acts of germline editing might belong to this category. If we already know where the firm moral boundaries are to be drawn and on what grounds, we could simply investigate whether such a boundary coincides with the germline, or whether some, or all, uses of germline editing are off-limits. This would provide us with a clear moral answer.

Not all moral theories support some notion of categorical boundaries, but some do: versions of rights-based accounts on the one hand and Kantian theories based on some version of the categorical imperative on the other.

According to rights theory, it could be argued that rights are such that they must never be violated and are essentially non-negotiable. Thus, if it is the case that a particular act violates the right of a person, then this would make such acts categorically impermissible. Applied to germline editing, this would imply that if there are some cases of germline editing that violate individual rights, then those would be categorically impermissible; and, if all cases of germline editing violate such rights, then germline editing is categorically impermissible.

However, this is not very helpful unless we know whose rights, and rights to what precisely, we are discussing. Furthermore, should germline editing affect the rights of many different individuals with very different interests, then these various rights may conflict with each other.

Rights could be understood as a kind of formalized and explicit version of what respecting others as equals requires based on the fact that we are all born equal with the same right to a decent life. One cannot make sense of rights without some notion of the fundamental needs or interests protected by those rights. The moral force of rights comes from the fact that we are born moral equals and thus have the right to the same kind of respect and the same kinds of needs met. Two things make applying the notion of rights to germline editing difficult. First, most of those who are likely to have their rights-based interests affected are future individuals who do not yet exist and who may or may not exist depending on the choices we make, including the very act of editing their germline. It is a matter of scholarly debate what weight we should give to the rights of future individuals compared to existing ones. Here, it becomes even more challenging in that it is not merely a matter of potentially conflicting interests between the current generation and the next, but also between the next and those after. Second, rights are normally assigned on the assumption that we acquire them at birth because we are all born equal. The whole point of rights is to indicate some aspect of the universe that has a greater moral claim than other things.

Rights-based ethics cannot assign rights to everything. We cannot both have a right to eat and food have a right not to be eaten. Typically, rights are thus reserved for humans; even though this has been expanded to other species in recent years, the latter is seldom as expansive as human rights. However, both of the premises could be undermined by germline editing itself: A person not born equal to others may not have the same rights as everyone else. Yet, such differentiation may also undermine the notion of human rights. Consider the transhumanist vision; let us presume that this transhuman is 1000 times our superior, but we all have rights. It is unlikely that the content of those rights would be the same, given that our needs and interests would not be the same. This could, again, imply that even though it would violate a human right to kill a human, perhaps this right, when all things are considered, weighs quite lightly compared to the transhuman right not to be killed. This might relativize our human rights, make them appear less categorical, and weaken our moral standing. Perhaps it only makes sense for the transhuman to respect other transhumans as their equals.

But even with future generations consisting of "perfectly human" humans, we may not know enough about their needs and interests to predict the content of their rights. In order to know what their rights are, we must know what their fundamental interests are. What constitutes human rights cannot be absolute, but will depend on what is possible, what is available, what could be provided by others and by nature, what could be avoided, and what could be respected. Thus, the challenge of predicting the future rights of future people across many generations in a radically changing world may be as epistemically challenging as it would be to predict consequences. Thus, even if we agreed that it is categorically wrong to edit the germline in each case when such edits violate the individual rights of that person, it is hard to know exactly what edits this would rule out, if any. It complicates the matter even further, if we also agree that it is categorically wrong not to edit the germline of a person who has a right to such edits. It seems that we would need much more information before we can reliably predict where any such lines would go.

Some acts are so obviously problematic that it seems safe to assume that they would violate human rights. For instance, it seems likely that it would be categorically impermissible to bring about children as part of some experiment that would not be in the child's best interest but as a means for some other purpose. One could, for instance, imagine that the child was edited for some military purpose or as part of a medical experiment. Here, it seems easy to make a case based on universal rights and fundamental interests of the person. But all cases of germline editing are not like those. Some germline edits clearly seem to be, if they could be assumed to be safe and socially accepted in the society the child would inhabit, in the child's best interest.

Perhaps, then, there is a categorical moral boundary against some germline edits based on rights and that we should seek to replace the idea of a categorical germline boundary with a categorical human-rights boundary. This would not support the germline as a categorical boundary, but it would support the idea of a categorical boundary that is applicable to the moral issues of germline editing. The problem is that there is something troubling about the notion of using rights to guide moral actions that may undermine the prerequisites upon which the moral concept of rights depend. If rights are assigned at birth, then it seems we could not have rights that concern what happened to us before our birth. Thus, we could not have any rights against the removal of the prerequisites for having such rights. This could be amended by either claims to what can be done to an embryo that could develop into a person or by assigning embryos rights.

Rights make the most sense when they are universal and equal. This can explain both how we can have rights (to things from others) and how we can have an obligation to meet the rights of others. However, if we add unborn children to the claimants and future generations, then the population of claimants could be very large. Perhaps then a mother could be required to give birth even at the cost of her life, given all the claim rights of future generations (from all her potential descendants, in fact). This does not seem right. This would allow for her to be used as a mere means for future generations. Conversely, to create new humans as a mere means to promote some other interests does not seem right either.

From Kantian ethics, at least from the categorical imperative in its formulation of humanity, this is the key moral aspect that determines impermissibility. We must never treat the humanity in a person as a mere means, but also simultaneously as an end in themselves. Such a duty could be fulfilled without leading to any obvious conflicting interests: we could simply refrain from using others, whomever they might be, as mere means for some purpose that is not in their own interest. This would suggest that we are categorically prohibited from editing a person solely for someone else's interest. This, again, would not exclude medically motivated interventions if these were clearly in the person's own interest. Where that line is to be drawn in terms of genetic disease and disability is, of course, difficult to determine, but the point is that the line must be drawn on the grounds of what would be in the person's interest.

It is quite plausible that, depending on what one emphasizes in the Kantian framework, different conclusions can be drawn. On the one hand, to "never treat the humanity in yourself or someone else as a mere means" suggests that we should not regard human nature as a means to an end, such as the ideal of a perfect posthuman. This could be read as making it impermissible to edit an embryo for any other reason than its own interest as a human being. Thus, it would be impermissible to use the humanity of the embryo as a mere means to achieve a perfect posthuman. On the other hand, if humanity resides in our autonomy and rationality, perhaps enhancing those capacities would be to enhance our humanity, and thus to treat our humanity as a means as well as an end in itself. If so, the categorical imperative, also non-negotiable, may neither draw a line at the germline nor at enhancement, but only against edits that would negatively affect the person's autonomy or rationality. This is not the place for a Kantian analysis (see Gunderson, 2007 for a few indicative ideas); the point is that the two most convincing cases for categorical boundaries in moral theory do not provide definitive support for a categorical boundary at either of the two established boundaries of the debate, against germline editing or enhancement, but suggest two other categorical boundaries based on rights and respect for persons.

Another categorical moral boundary could perhaps be based on moral responsibility, such that it is categorically impermissible to act in such a way that one cannot take full responsibility for the consequences. Such a principle would prohibit edits to future generations that we could neither fully predict nor repair or compensate for, should anything go wrong. However, such a moral category of wrongs would go beyond germline editing and could potentially exclude all kinds of actions that we normally take as perfectly acceptable. Indeed, one cannot take full responsibility for all the consequences of bringing new persons into the world in the first place. But maybe there are limited variations to such a principle, such that potential harms and wrongs above a certain threshold or of a certain magnitude that were in principle irreversible and irreparable would be morally impermissible. If so, then perhaps what is of relevance is the fact that germline editing is, for now at least, irreversible and could potentially harm someone of moral importance. This would mean, however, that, should we be able to reverse-engineer any edits, it would no longer be impermissible in the same way.

10.4.2 Categorically Impermissible for Contingent Reasons

Germline editing could also, for more contingent reasons, be categorically impermissible. Perhaps all acts of germline editing are morally impermissible, not because they constitute an act of germline editing, but for some other reasons that make it so. For instance, it may be the case that germline editing is not morally permissible because animal experiments are categorically impermissible; therefore, any science that depends on animal experiments is impermissible.

We could even find grounds for a categorical line based on consequences, but these are weaker. It could be that certain outcomes are so bad that we must never risk bringing them about (Sects. 6.3 and 9.3). However, such worst-cases or high-stake risks, would more likely imply that such risks are impermissible, not the act of germline editing itself. Thus, the obligation would be to seek to lower or avoid the risk or mitigate or circumvent the outcome. A general right against risk of harm is problematic in that it could lead to paralysis (see, e.g., Hayenhjelm & Wolf, 2012).

A strict consequentialist could argue that we have a categorical moral obligation to maximize the value of the outcomes; thus, we must select the best possible child, edit a child so that they had the best possible genes—or on a larger scale, edit the wider population and the human gene pool. On such an account, it would be wrong not only to neglect to edit a single child who would experience greater well-being had we done so, but also to neglect to maximize their capacities and faculties should this increase their potential for well-being even further. Thus, if morality requires us to maximize value, then this would suggest a moral imperative to pursue this end, and if the maximum value could only be achieved by means of germline editing, then this would be non-optional. It is for these reasons that it has been suggested that we ought to edit the germline or even ought to engage in enhancement (Sects. 7.2 and 8.5). However, any such calculus depends on a long list of assumptions, many of which are little more than conjectures. According to the value maximization logic, what we must maximize is not the genetic capacities as such, but the total well-being, or something similar. Thus, should it be the case that the world would be much happier if we completely forgot the possibility of germline editing and simply accepted life as it is, then this is what we must do and all else would be morally wrong. Should it be the case that editing a fifth of humanity so that they looked ridiculous, but would create so much amusement for the rest of the population that there was no possible way to achieve greater sums of happiness, then this would be what we must categorically do. In short, maximizing value depends entirely on what the actual numbers would be when taking all consequences into account.

The strongest case for a categorical boundary would then be if there was a substantial and unavoidable risk for potentially unforgiveable outcomes that are also irreversible and irreparable.

10.5 Beyond a Categorical Boundary at the Germline

From the previous sections, we can conclude two things: The case for a categorical boundary at the germline is weak, and there are some serious concerns about germline editing that may imply a serious risk, at least in some instances. Now, if it is the case that some acts of germline editing ought never to be performed, whereas some could be highly beneficial and not obviously morally wrong, then perhaps we have looked for a categorical boundary in the wrong place. We will now turn to the next set of questions. Have we been looking at the wrong categorical boundary? Is there another moral boundary that better demarcates what we must never do when it comes to human gene editing? Or is there a moral boundary at the germline, only not a categorical one but a conditional one, such that germline editing would be morally permissible in some cases, should the conditions be met, but otherwise not? Both of these boundaries suggest that some germline edits may be permissible but not all of them. The first because there is a distinct subgroup of germline edits that are categorically impermissible. The second because there are criteria that need to be met for germline editing to be permissible.

Here, we will take a brief look at two alternatives to the germline as a categorical boundary. First, moving the categorical boundary forward so that it aligns not with the somatic/germline boundary but with *the therapy/enhancement boundary*. Second, listing the moral conditions that need to be satisfied for germline editing to be permissible, thus replacing a categorical boundary with *a conditional one*.

10.5.1 A Categorical Moral Boundary Against Enhancement

Almost all the worst-case scenarios that motivate the categorical objections to germline editing seem to be about the long-term effects of enhancement or non-therapeutic interventions. The exception to this is the concerns raised by the disability community for fear of increased intolerance and discrimination that may also result from therapeutic edits, at least if interpreted broadly (Garland-Thompson, 2020). However, even when taking such concerns into account, there may be cases of genetic disease that we would not wish upon anyone and that could be edited for the benefit of all in a way that adding properties or reinforcing some favored norm would not be. Furthermore, there may be diseases so severe that parents would never knowingly seek to give birth to a child that would inherit such a disease, and thus germline editing would enable them to have a child who would otherwise never have been born. Thus, there are reasons to think that the enhancement boundary captures the dominant moral concerns of the debate more closely than the somatic/germline editing does.

If what we are really concerned about is enhancement rather than germline editing per se, then perhaps the moral line should be drawn between therapy and enhancement. This has been a prominent position and the somatic/germline and therapy/enhancement boundaries are both widely referred to as moral boundaries that prevent impermissible edits (see Evans, 2020). We discussed this notion in a previous chapter (Sect. 2.2.2). Perhaps it is time to revisit it.

We would, then, end up with one claim about what is categorically wrong and a slightly different claim about where to draw a possible categorical line:

Categorically Wrong Claim (Enhancement): Every act of human germline editing for enhancement purposes is categorically morally wrong.

The Categorical Boundary Claim (Enhancement): There is a categorical moral boundary of using germline editing for enhancement; every act of human germline editing
for enhancement purposes is morally wrong and morally impermissible.

However, as we have seen earlier, the distinction between therapy and enhancement is porous (Sects. 2.2.3 and 2.3). This means that even if it does trace the
actual moral concerns about germline editing better than the germline boundary,
it would not be a very strong barrier against any slippery slopes towards such
enhancements. Even if we begin with definitive cases of therapeutic germline
editing, there are cases of germline editing that are not strictly speaking therapeutic but "therapeutic enough" not to set off moral alarm bells, and slightly
more non-therapeutic interventions that seem similar enough to those cases not
to set off any alarm bells, and so on.

In contrast to the line between somatic and germline editing that, as a distinction, makes some descriptive sense, such that we would know when we edit the
one rather than the other, it is much harder to point to what constitutes therapy
and what constitutes enhancement. In the end, this depends on how one defines
what is normal, healthy, unhealthy, and so on. Furthermore, the very notion of
"therapy" may not strictly apply to germline edits in that it aims to prevent a
disease rather than treat it. Thus, we could refer to such prevention as a form of
enhancement, as well as improvements of the immune system, removal of genes
that merely increase the probability of a disease that one may or may not have
developed, and so on.

More worryingly, even though nearly all of the worst-case scenarios discussed are premised on the practice of germline enhancement, not all cases of
enhancement seem equally morally problematic. Some cases of non-therapeutic
interventions are not obviously more controversial than other kinds of germline
editing. There is no obvious reason why, for instance, correcting for shortness or
improving the immune system morally belong together with fluorescent fish and
transhuman cognitive powers. If anything, they seem to remove a potential genetic
disadvantage rather than adding to or expanding upon our genetic heritage.

Cwik (2020b, p. 8) has argued that germline editing is not a unified category,
but instead "a short-hand for a heterogenous category of translational projects
and possible future applications." According to him, the therapy/enhancement
distinction is too crude. Instead, he suggests that we replace that twofold division
with three other morally relevant categories: "revising," "correcting," and "transferring" genes at the germline (Cwik, 2020b, p. 8). Gene correction refers to
"correcting pathogenic mutations" and the "goal of the editing is to remove the
pathogenic mutation and alter the gene to match a nonpathogenic allele prevalent

in the (healthy) population" (p. 13). Gene revision would be to "revise an otherwise healthy genotype in line with a judgement about what, in respect to this
gene, would be most valuable for an individual" (p. 14). Genetic transferal refers
to cases where new genetic material is transferred. (Interestingly, Cwik reminds
us that mitochondrial DNA transfers belong to this category.) Cwik is careful to
point out that these categories are descriptive, and although they raise different
kinds of moral questions, he does not assume that they trace permissibility (p. 14)
or that the three categories overlap with the degree of moral controversy:

> The point here is not that we can answer ethical questions merely by pointing to
> whether a procedure is revision, correction, or transferring, as has been assumed about
> whether something is a "therapy" or an "enhancement." The point is that by making
> these distinctions and getting a more precise categorization schema, we can get a bet-
> ter overall map of the ethical terrain here, one which will have multiple benefits in
> sorting through the ethics of gene editing. (Cwik, 2020b, p. 14)

Nevertheless, it could help us to differentiate between, for instance, removing a
genetic disposition to develop blindness ("correct") on the one hand, and adding
night vision through recombining DNA ("transfer") on the other. Or, between
removing the genetic disposition to develop Alzheimer's disease ("correct") and
boosting memory function ("revise") and adding genes to develop supercognitive
functions ("transfer"). However, if what we seek is a way to draw categorical
moral lines, these three do not seem to be any more helpful than enhancement.
As Cwik pointed out, mitochondrial DNA transfer is a case of transfer; thus, one
of the least controversial examples belongs to the potentially most controversial
category of the three. Furthermore, what counts as "revising" and what counts
as "correcting" are not necessarily much more definitive than what counts as
"therapy" and what counts as "enhancement." Nevertheless, mitochondrial DNA
aside, once we add the possibilities of DNA transferred and not just edited, we do
seem to cross a different kind of line, given that this could drastically expand the
possibilities for what could be done if such transfers include recombinant DNA
from other species.

Perhaps, then, the relevant moral categories are, in fact, something like the following: therapeutic germline intervention, moderate enhancement (up to normal
species functioning), and radical enhancement (beyond normal species functioning), with the potential categorical boundary to be drawn between moderate
and *radical* enhancement. This seems to be Agar's position, who has defended
more moderate kinds of enhancement, but has also been very critical of radical
enhancement (2010, 2013). However, it is far from clear where such a line should
be drawn and whether such a line would be any more robust than the one between

therapy and enhancement. Such a line would need to depend on some notion of what normal species function amounts to, while what is and is not normal would not remain fixed, but change with the very introduction of such edits.

Furthermore, moderate enhancement seems perfectly sufficient to bring about injustice and decreased tolerance for difference and increased discrimination. Additionally, moderate enhancement could decrease diversity in the population in ways that could affect both norms for normality and bring about dramatic differences in genetic health between different groups in society or rich and poor nations. (If those differences are influential enough and also sufficient for various kinds of illegal or amateur germline editing services to emerge to meet the demand for low-cost alternatives, this could add additional risk and justice concerns). It is not very likely, from a global perspective, that access to expensive prenatal technologies would be evenly accessed; thus, we would end up with a very real concern about justice.

As a moral boundary, drawing the line at radical enhancement only address one kind of concern: jeopardizing and altering the meaning of being human and threats of transhumanism. It does not address the older concerns about eugenics, desirable and undesirable genetic properties, and injustice. A line drawn at the normal human perfections could still become a society of intolerance and injustice. This does not exclude the fears of a genetic class society where social mobility must become genetic mobility. This could also open the door to various totalitarian temptations, such as programs to breed future sports talents or complacent and hardy workers and soldiers well within what is normal species functioning. The old concern about eugenics was not one about capacities beyond what is considered normal, but rather one about a society that regards some as wanted and others as unwanted—where a dignified life is a privilege reserved only for some. For the ideal of human equality to hold, there must be something that is shared among all humans on some level, and merely remaining on one side of the moderate/radical boundary may not be sufficient for this.

To conclude, it may seem like a good thing, at least from a more bioliberal perspective, to replace the germline boundary with an enhancement boundary. Predominantly, the gain would be to include a bit more in the category of potentially morally permissible gene edits. This would allow for all therapeutically motivated germline edits. Furthermore, if one considers removing the genetic propensity for developing certain genetic diseases, then perhaps increasing lifespan would also be a good thing, and thus replacing the enhancement boundary with "radical" enhancement would seem like the best move. One would think that most bioliberals would thus seek to make as strong a case as possible for the enhancement boundary over the germline boundary. Interestingly, this does not seem to be the case. Rather, it seems common to point out that there is no intuitive boundary between therapy and enhancement, but that therapy is enhancement, and enhancement is everything we do to boost capacity, including education, wearing glasses, and so on. Thus, this undermines the case for the enhancement boundary, since one of its primary roles (just as the germline boundary) has been to prevent a slippery slope of radical changes to our nature, relations, and society that may prove detrimental.

For all the weakness of the moral distinction between somatic and germline editing, including the possibility that it is too restrictive, the distinction between therapy and enhancement seems even less helpful. First, it is conceptually vague. Second, it is hard to draw a clear line in practice, thus it is not very action-guiding. Third, it is not clear that it makes any crucial moral demarcation.

10.5.2 A Conditional Boundary at the Germline

If there is no convincing case for a categorical boundary at the germline, or even at enhancement, what about a conditional boundary? A conditional boundary would not make all cases of germline editing morally impermissible, only those that fail to meet certain specified and morally necessary conditions. Such a conditional boundary would address the concerns that motivated a call for a categorical boundary, while recognizing that these concerns need not apply to all cases under all conditions and allowing germline editing when the right criteria are fulfilled.

> The germline as a conditional boundary: Germline gene editing is only morally per-missible when a number of specified and explicit moral conditions are fulfilled and impermissible when they are not.

This may seem like the most plausible and morally accurate version of a germline boundary. However, the exact meaning and implication of the principle depends entirely on what those specified conditions are and how accurate and equally exhausting they are. Should a single, necessary condition be missed from those listed, it would not block impermissible acts. Should a condition that is not necessary be added, then acts may be unnecessarily blocked. The notion of a conditional boundary is somewhat useless unless we specify what the conditions are. Basically, any of the moral concerns that we have raised throughout this book could provide grounds for a condition of some sort: injustice, playing God, meta-physical risks, dignity, rights, well-being, safety, and so on. Thus, it seems that we would need to have the moral question answered before we can specify the actual boundary. That is, we need to bridge the gap of moral uncertainty in order to know what the right moral conditions are, whether they make permissibility conditional on maximizing well-being or not violating individual rights; on not imposing metaphysical risks or not contributing to injustice, or some combination of these. Depending on how many of these conditions are thought to apply, a conditional boundary could be very restrictive or very permissible, or anything in between. It would be very permissible if only a few and relatively rare conditions were to apply. It would be very restrictive if so many conditions apply that they covered most cases. Either way, we would first need to know what makes it permissible and impermissible before we can flesh out the principle.

A promising version of this kind of boundary can be found in the two principles that the Nuffield Council proposed in their second report on germline editing (Nuffield Council, 2018):

Principle 1: The welfare of the future person

Gametes or embryos that have been subject to genome editing procedures (or that are derived from cells that have been subject to such procedures) should be used only where the procedure is carried out in a manner and for a purpose that is intended to secure the welfare of and is consistent with the welfare of a person who may be born as a consequence of treatment using those cells.

Principle 2: Social justice and solidarity

The use of gametes or embryos that have been subject to genome editing procedures (or that are derived from cells that have been subject to such procedures) should be permitted only in circumstances in which it cannot reasonably be expected to produce or exacerbate social division or the unmitigated marginalisation or disadvantage of groups within society.

These proposed principles are interesting and ambitious in that they seem to single out two of the most dominant concerns about germline editing, besides safety, and in a very elegant way. Both principles thus block uses and outcomes that have given rise to some of the most serious objections. It is worth considering in some detail what these two principles allow and what they prohibit, as stated.

The first principle only allows for germline edits that are motivated by, and consistent with, the welfare of the person born with those edits. This principle effectively blocks all uses of germline editing that treats the developing person to be edited only instrumentally for some purpose that would not be in their own interest. We can compare this with Kant's categorical imperative in the formulation of humanity, which prohibits using the person of another as a mere means.

Thus, we would not be allowed to breed children for a grand program, whether nationalistic, aesthetic, or experimental, and so on: it is only justified if it is expected to be in the person's interest. This could, however, include all kinds of editing if it would promote their welfare; hence, it would not be limited to addressing genetic disease. But if one could prolong life expectancy and improve hearing, memory, immune system, cognitive abilities, and so on, this could presumably all be in the person's interest. In other words, this first principle does not prevent enhancement but rather exploitation and violations of human rights and dignity; and it would most likely need to be free from any individual, social or psychological cost. Furthermore, it would presumably also prevent ambitious parents from designing their offspring to fit their own aspirations if such edits would infringe on the person's right to an open future.

This interest in welfare, at least in some sense, seems limited to the first generation born with those edits, since the subsequent generations would, presumably, not be born "as a consequence of treatment using those cells." Thus, the first principle essentially states that, unless human individual rights are respected, it is not permissible to bring about a child from an edited embryo or germ cells. This takes care of several concerns that motivated a categorical boundary, especially the deontological objections. It also makes it clear that the welfare must outweigh the risks; thus, implicitly ruling out risky interventions that would not be conducive to the person's welfare.

The second principle only allows for germline edits that do not threaten to bring about injustice. This principle thus effectively prevents all the worst-case scenarios in the form of totalitarian eugenics programs, genetically divided societies, increased intolerance and discrimination, and outright genocide and conflict resulting from a genetic divide. In short, it prevents all "Gattaca" concerns. This principle thus prevents all the concerns about worst-case scenarios, societal risk, as well as the objections from the disability community.

Together, they do not categorically rule out germline editing for medical or enhancement purposes, but only on the condition that injustice does not result and that it is conducive to the welfare of the person. Of course, even if we strictly apply these principles, there is no guarantee that we will not make epistemic mistakes, and something that was both motivated by and believed to be in the best interest of the future person, in fact, is not, or what was believed to not promote injustice, in fact, did. What is interesting here is that, those epistemic reservations aside, these two principles seem to sum up all the main objections. The only two kinds of concerns from the debate they do not address are those based on the notion that there is something intrinsically wrong with editing the human germline (Sect. 6.1) and slippery slope arguments. In any case, any arguments to the effect that germline editing is intrinsically wrong would presumably imply a categorical rule against such editing, not a conditional one.

The slippery slope concerns are, however, not likely to disappear anytime soon, for two reasons. First, technology, especially when paired with market interests, has a tendency to push forward fast and deliver new versions and solutions replacing the previous ones. It is therefore unlikely that the development would stop at any particular point rather than continue. Second, small steps paired with immediate benefits do not seem that significant, even if they push the boundary forward slightly. Third, the matter of germline editing is multigenerational and does not expire. Thus, we cannot think of the full consequences of germline editing, while only considering how it will affect our current generation and the next. Nor can we assume that regulations, values, laws, leaders, ideologies, or governments will be the same over the technologies' entire lifespan. In the end, there is a challenge of responsibility here: How far does our responsibility reach, should we set things in motion that would not otherwise have occurred? This goes both ways; we cannot currently rule out that, in future, germline editing could become essential to the survival of humanity.

To return to the matter of conditional boundaries: Unless we have all the right criteria, we cannot know that following such a principle would lead to the right kind of decisions.

10.6 The Germline as a Line of Precaution

All the previous positions on the germline as a boundary require sufficiently reliable moral knowledge that enables us to determine right from wrong in the case of human germline gene editing. But what if we do not have such reliable knowledge? This brings us to the fourth and final step in our inquiry of the germline as a boundary for what we morally ought to do when the previous steps have failed in yielding a reliable answer. In fact, it seems that we cannot safely conclude that there is a categorical moral boundary at the germline. Nor can we safely conclude that there is a categorical moral boundary at the point of enhancement. Furthermore, we do not seem to be in a position where we could replace a categorical boundary with a reliable conditional boundary for reasons of epistemic and moral uncertainty. What then? Must we conclude that there is no case for a boundary at all? That somatic and germline gene editing are on a par? Or, that germline editing is not morally different to any other kind of medical or public health intervention?

There is a third option that we have not discussed yet, a somewhat more pragmatic moral answer: perhaps the germline could serve as *a kind of precautionary boundary*. In this way, it would still serve as a red line, but not because germline edits are categorically wrong, but because, overall, *it is riskier* to proceed with germline gene editing than it is not to—and those risks are significant.

> The Moral Precautionary Claim: Every act of human germline editing violates, all else equal, a moral boundary of precaution.

There are two ways to understand the germline as a precautionary boundary. We could view the germline as a *moral threshold*. Such a threshold would require a different kind of rationale to be in place in order for germline editing to be justified. It would not be that germline editing is categorically impermissible, only that it is permissible in rare and exceptional circumstances. However, this threshold alternative would not really solve the challenges faced by germline editing as a conditional principle. It would still need to specify the conditions that could justify an exception to an overall rule of caution against germline editing. It is thus a version of the conditional principle; and should it miss specifying any crucial criterion, then it may fail to be properly cautious.

Alternatively, we could view the germline as a categorical boundary, but on precautionary grounds against risking moral wrongdoing, rather than on grounds of moral wrongness. Such a moral precautionary line would not necessarily indicate an underlying categorical principle, but would serve *as a placeholder* for a future moral principle (categorical or conditional) that would be more accurate and precise. Such a principle would, on precautionary grounds, draw a categorical line at the germline, not because it is assumed that it is categorically wrong to edit the germline, but because it is morally too risky. We will refer to such a placeholder principle as a *locum tenens* principle. It should not be confused with a *pro tanto* or *prima facie* principle: it is not about potential waivers or partial and competing moral truths, but about minimal moral advice when we do not have access to the right answer. Just as in the ordinary case of the precautionary principle, it only makes sense to appeal to such a principle in special circumstances: When the stakes are high, especially when it comes to potential harm or losses for proceeding, and we are epistemically in an impoverished situation. This means that the principle would have no moral validity once the epistemic situation changes such that we have reliable moral knowledge.

A boundary drawn at the germline based on such a precautionary *locum tenens* principle would acknowledge the lack of moral certainty, while simultaneously also acknowledging that some classes of actions are much riskier than others, morally speaking. As long as we know that one class of action is considerably morally riskier than the other, and that those risks are such that we would not want them to materialize, we would know what to do.

There are two main reasons that could speak in favor of a precautionary boundary at the germline. The first is *an epistemic argument*. A precautionary boundary does not require the same degree of moral knowledge to be action-guiding as laying down a categorical moral boundary or specifying the exact moral conditions would; nor does it need to draw the right moral line of permissibility in the exact right place, nor identify all the necessary conditions for making germline editing permissible. All we need to know is whether, *overall, it is safer not to edit the germline*. This also means that the principle is replaceable with a more accurate and precise principle at any point, should moral certainty improve.

The second reason is that it *would prevent all the serious worst-case scenarios*. It would block the more hypothetical worst-case scenarios at the end of potential slippery slopes as well as more immediate risks of harm without making moral postulates about categorical boundaries, and the like. It would thus provide a red line of sorts against all the outcomes that we are concerned about. The challenge, here, is to demonstrate that such a red line is warranted and does not unnecessarily halt promising progress.

This position on the germline would thus have all the preventive advantages of a categorical position without making the same morally questionable assumptions and requiring the same degree of moral knowledge. It would only hold the positions until we find a more accurate principle, but, in the meantime, ensure that we do not risk what could not possibly be rectified.

10.6.1 Erring on the Side of Caution

Would a boundary at the germline err on the side of caution? According to Koplin et al. (2019), it is an open question whether the precautionary principle would support or oppose germline editing, as both options carry risks:

> … we want to draw attention to a general difficulty associated with applying the precautionary principle in the context of GGE [*germline gene editing*]. It might seem that insofar as GGE carries plausible and significant risks to future generations, most plausible versions of the precautionary principle would weigh against pursuing GGE. This is not necessarily the case, as failing to pursue GGE may also carry plausible and significant risks to future generations. (Koplin et al., 2019, p. 58)

Harris (2009, 2010) makes a similar point. He argues that in order to determine which option is safer, we need to be able to compare two alternative trajectories— abstaining from germline gene editing and pursuing it:

> Unless we can compare the future progress of evolution uncontaminated by manipulation of the human genome with its progress influenced by any proposed genetic manipulations, we cannot know which would be best and hence where precaution lies. (Harris, 2009, p. 133)

Before we can make any case for a precautionary line at the germline, we need to take a closer look at these challenges. We have discussed the risks of germline gene editing at length, but what are the risks of *not* editing?

It may seem counterintuitive that *not* using a new technology could be viewed as a risk. The basic idea, here, is that we must compare two different kinds of futures. The first future is one where we do not use germline gene editing to correct for genetic disease (or more), but allow our gene pool to deteriorate and ultimately, over time and generations, bring about a future with poor genetic health, great medical costs, and a heavy reliance on medical and other support for a decent life. The second future is one where we use germline editing with the possible risk of harm, but also embrace all the benefits, not just for the first generation, but all the generations after, with increased genetic health and less need for medical treatment and support. Thus, unless we know for certain that there will be more harm in the latter scenario, we cannot safely conclude advise against germline editing. The implicit assumption seems to be that the risks of proceeding can roughly be expected to be manageable and acceptable, and that the benefits of proceeding will roughly be as hoped for multiplied over many generations, and no later innovation or turn of events would drastically alter that rough estimate. The force of this assumption depends on how realistic and broad the notion of risk is and to what extent epistemic and moral risk are not underestimated. It also depends on the extent to which the harms, losses and wrongs that could result from potential risks are, in principle or realistically, compensable, and possibly outweighed by benefits. Should there, for instance, be risks that could not even in principle be outweighed by benefits, this kind of calculation cannot really be done.

Furthermore, the comparative trajectory is based on a categorical position where all benefits and harms follow from categorically *never* using germline editing. If we replace the categorical position with a *locum tenens* principle, this will not exclude the possibility of using some eventual safer version of germline technology, should we later learn that this would be morally permissible in general or in cases of emergency or other exceptional circumstances. What we may and may not do will depend on the moral principle that replaces the *locum tenens* principle later, should moral knowledge improve. The comparison should perhaps not be one between saying "yes" or "no" to germline editing, but rather between "soon" or "definitely not now." New and largely untested technology will likely improve over time and therefore too much reliance on the first versions may prove irresponsible. It therefore seems that these "open question" arguments are less convincing when posed against a precautionary line than a strictly categorical line.

There are two main hypotheses here: either (a) we can safely assume that one of the two sides to the germline boundary is overall much safer than the other; or (b) it is an open question and could equally be either one of those two. If the former is true, then there are grounds for a precautionary approach (Hayenhjelm, 2024). If the latter is true, then there is not. The open question argument, as we have seen, posits that there are comparable risks on both sides; therefore, there is no obvious route of precaution.

The open question argument somewhat downplays the reasons and concerns that underpin the categorical objections. Even if germline editing is not categorically wrong, and even if it is not problematic because it violates human nature or the individual rights of an unaltered genome, among other things, there is potential for serious wrong and harm that cannot be dismissed entirely, and that may not be outweighed by benefits. The main line of argument, here, seems to be whether the slippery slope concerns can be ignored or must be taken seriously, whether the concerns about changed norms and society are serious moral concerns, and whether a fundamental loss to what it means to be human is morally significant.

10.6.2 Precaution as Protection Against Risk

What is and what is not precautionary depends on which risks we consider (Braun & Dabrock, 2018). Precaution only makes sense if there is a risk that we seek to avoid. There could be many reasons for caution and "caution" could refer to different kinds of risks or concerns that one would need to avoid, if possible.

The risk–benefit balance will look very different if we employ only a narrow notion of risk that merely covers anticipated technical risks and anticipated medical and health benefits compared to a calculus of a much broader notion of risk that includes potential social costs, potential existential costs, and so on. It also matters to what extent the epistemic dimension is taken into consideration, particularly to what extent we can expect unpredicted risk of harm and to what extent such effects might be systemic and irreversible. It will also matter whether moral uncertainty is taken into account. It also matters to what degree one takes all negative outcomes, such as harms, losses, and wrongs to possibly outweigh benefits or whether some kinds of harm, losses, or wrongs could never be rectified.

We have previously discussed three dimensions of risk: outcome risk (or risk of harm and/or losses), epistemic risk, and moral uncertainty and the risk of wrongdoing. The very notion and concept of moral precaution could be used as a preventive measure along all three of those dimensions: to avoid outcome risk of harm, moral risks of wrongdoing, and acting under ignorance, when such ignorance could obscure the true severity of outcome risk or moral risk, or make it difficult to prepare for such eventualities, given that they are largely unknown.

Most of the time when we discuss precaution, we are referring to measures to prevent *outcome risk*: we want to prevent certain outcomes. Such outcome risks span across distinct outcomes: from direct harm because of safety risks (Sects. 7.1 and 9.1.1), to societal and psychological outcomes (Sect. 9.1.2), and more fundamental losses due to metaphysical and existential risks (Sects. 9.1.3 and 9.3). Some of these concerns may seem unlikely and fanciful, while the expected benefits may seem tangible and immediate. In any case, there is potentially much to lose if things go seriously wrong.

Precaution could be a measure against *epistemic risk or risks resulting from ignorance*: We want to avoid actions of which we do not fully understand the consequences (Sect. 9.4). In the case of germline edits, the "ignorance about long-term consequences" (Juengst, 2017, p. 18) is substantial in terms of what we do not know and cannot reliably predict, not the least because the possible futures are many and complex and because they depend on many other circumstances than those that result directly from germline editing. Furthermore, given that some of the alterations may affect what we currently take as fundamental in various ways, the potential consequences are even harder to predict. We need to consider the moral matter as one that spans across multiple generations. Thus, the moral matter does not end with the edits that we could perform on the next generation, but also the kinds of decisions that the next generation may perform on the one after them, and so on. If the nature and preferences of some such future generation will be very different to ours, then so will their imagined ends and uses for the technology.

Additionally, precaution could also be a measure to avoid doing what is morally wrong under moral uncertainty. Moral uncertainty makes it difficult to know what one ought to do. This problem becomes accentuated in cases that affect not-yet-existing generations and where we cannot take full responsibility of the consequences in the sense of repairing them. If we do not know what is right or wrong on a small scale, we may do what we later realize is morally wrong. In such cases, we have access to the whole repertoire of reparation: apology, compensation, regret, repair, atonement, and so on. When it comes to future generations, this is no longer the case. Thus, there is strong reason to err on the side of safety; also when it comes to what would most likely not turn out to be morally wrong, if there is such a thing, rather than place our bet on a controversial moral theory being right.

All of these three parameters are relevant in the case of germline editing. First, there are serious outcome risks, some of which point to possibly the most serious kinds of risks. Second, there are substantial epistemic risks in that the actual consequences for future generations are not fully known or even fully predictable. Thus, it is impossible to rule out even greater harms or losses, including genuine losses we have not yet imagined. (This goes for gains as well, but the anticipated harms and gains are not symmetrical, and a gain postponed can still materialize later, but an avoidable harm could cause irreversible damage). Third, there is considerable risk that we might do what, in fact, turns out to be morally wrong. (This is not only increased by the fact that we are entering new territory, but are also affecting future beings who will live in a different world and perhaps have different needs and desires than us).

All three seem to add a layer to the stakes that come with the intrusiveness and pervasiveness of the technological intervention: If we alter the genome of a person, it better be safe, we better know what we are doing, and we better know that it is the morally right thing to do. The same goes for the collective and societal case: If we alter the genome of humanity and society in fundamental ways, it better be safe, we better know what we are doing, and we better know that it is the morally right thing to do.

All of this together means that we ought to act in a way that is precautionary on all three accounts, and we ought not to act on the presumption that it is safer than it is, that we know more than we do, or that we know more about what morality demands from us than we do. If there is some option or principle that in some sense diminishes the safety, epistemic, and moral risk, then we ought to opt for that. There are good reasons to think that human germline gene editing scores high in outcome risk and epistemic risk, and moral uncertainty makes it difficult to draw any definitive conclusions. This suggests that precaution is not neutral between editing and not editing but leans heavily towards not editing.

However, *to avoid all kinds of risks* would lead to stagnation. The precautionary principle itself has often been critiqued for being too conservative. Thus, to apply it, there would need to be sufficient risk to warrant such a precautionary approach. There needs to be sufficient epistemic challenges and/or sufficient stakes that could warrant a precautionary approach. In this case, we have argued for both of these points (see Chap. 9).

What, then, are the precise gains of a moral perspective opting for precaution? There are two moral reasons for precaution in order to avoid serious risk of harm. The first reason is a *consequence-based one*: If there are potential harms or losses at stake of such a magnitude that they could not possibly be repaired or compensated for, then it would be reason for precaution. Or, more generally, if certain harms or losses are such that they could never be outweighed by additional benefits, then we have precautionary reasons to avoid such outcomes.

The other reason is based on the requirements of *responsible action*. If potential consequences of risky influential actions are such that we would not be able to control them, then we would have precautionary reason to avoid such outcomes. Additionally, if the outcomes of risky influential actions are both so potentially dangerous and to such a large extent unknown that sufficient mitigation or preparatory steps cannot be taken, then this would give us reason for precaution.

If we translate the above to the context of human germline gene editing, we will arrive at something like the following claims:

1. Precaution requires us to avoid imposing risks of harm, loss, or wrongdoing, such that they could never be positively compensated for, repaired, or forgiven.
2. Precaution would require us not to impose such risks that we could not take responsibility or sufficiently prepare for.

The first claim is that if certain risks could lead to outcomes that both constitute severe negative states that could not be restored, we have reason to prevent them. The second claim is that if certain risks are such that we would lose control over them and could not take responsibility for their outcomes and implications, then we have reason to prevent them. The first appeals to harms that would leave the world a worse place in some respect, and the second to irresponsible actions, where unforeseeable consequences may not only make the world a worse place in some respect, but they would also be such that those who caused it cannot take responsibility for it.

The gain would then be moral: We would not risk bringing about a state of the world that we would have strong reason to regret and could not repair, and we would not risk bringing about a state of the world that may causally spiral away in a way that we lose control over it. Are there such risks attached to germline editing that those kinds of gains seem plausible? Most obviously, the multigenerational and hereditary aspect of germline editing combined with the epistemic gaps make it difficult to assure compensation and responsibility for any individuals that come to harm. The most troubling aspect being that we cannot safely exclude the possibility of imposing very serious risks, and we may not fully understand the full nature or scope of their implications.

10.6.3 The Germline as a Locum Tenens Moral Boundary

We are now in the following situation: There are strong reasons to be cautious, but we have no firm moral boundary to rely on, and there is still need for action-guidance.

The categorical case against germline editing is weak. We could always imagine situations where our only hope for human survival depends upon germline editing. It does not seem plausible that we should not be morally permitted to use germline editing in such circumstances, and if so, germline editing cannot be categorically impermissible. The trouble is that we do not know enough to specify the exact conditions that could be relied upon to separate the permissible from the impermissible, and there are a number of most serious outcomes that we have very good reason to avoid as best as we can.

For these reasons, there might be a case for treating the germline boundary as what we have referred to as a *locum tenens* moral boundary. A moral principle is a *locum tenens* principle in this sense only if it is a principle that advises moral actions in want of moral knowledge of a proper moral principle. Here, we could use the somatic/germline distinction that already has an established meaning and is fairly definitive in terms of action-guidance. If it is the case that that boundary could fulfill both precautionary reasons; that is, it would prevent all the incompensable harms, losses, and wrongs, and it would prevent imposing risks that we would not be able to control, then this could suggest that the germline could serve as such a *locum tenens* principle. It is important to see what such a principle can and cannot do in this case. It is not a proper moral principle in the way that it can accurately determine what is and is not morally permissible actions in a precise way. What it can provide is an action-guiding principle *in want* of such a moral principle on the basis that we know enough to conclude which of the two sides of the germline is the "safer one" and *on the assumption that the risks on the less safe side are severe enough* to warrant precaution (rather than attempts at value maximization), or that we have *too little knowledge to preclude* that there could be such severe risks. In such cases, we ought to regard the germline as a *locum tenens* moral principle. It will thus serve as a kind of precautionary moral principle. This means that it will err on the side of caution, and it will be biased towards conservatism.

> The germline boundary as stand-in moral barrier based on a *locum tenens* moral principle. The human germline could serve as a moral boundary on the grounds of a *locum tenens* principle that would make it impermissible to edit the germline as a moral precaution (in the absence of a more precise moral principle). The principle, and hence its support for the germline boundary, would only apply under moral and epistemic uncertainty in want of a more precise moral principle and under condition that it can be presumed to err on the side of moral caution.

There are two reasons for why this would be a sound principle. The first has to do with the stakes involved, what we stand to lose, and the fact that some such losses may be genuinely irreparable. The second reason has to do with the moral implications of responsibility. Imposing risks that could lead to harmful outcomes exceeding what we could possibly repair or resolve does not seem to be compatible with acting responsibly.

It does not mean that the germline boundary is a proper moral principle, not even a *pro tanto* or *prima facie* principle; it is not one of many possibly relevant moral principles that could be overturned by another, but a placeholder for a proper moral principle. This means that should the epistemic situation change with regard to the moral knowledge and we have a better principle to replace it with, then it would have served its purpose. It also means that the fact that in some cases it would give the wrong advice need not be an objection to its relevance and soundness, as long as it avoids all the incompensable and most serious kinds of harms, wrongs, and losses. Such a principle does not determine what is and is not morally permissible, only what is and is not morally responsible when acting under moral uncertainty; it could at any point be replaced with a more accurate and less precautious principle once moral certainty improves.

How would such a principle compare to the other ones we have discussed in this book? First, as a *locum tenens* principle, it would be less epistemically demanding than a categorical or conditional principle. Second, it would, as stated above, prevent the worst-case scenarios and serious risks, including the technological risks and risks from increased intolerance for genetic variations. In this respect, it would have advantages over drawing such a precautionary line else-where, such as at the point of enhancement that would not prevent risks from the technology itself or from social costs attached to therapeutic interventions. Third, also in contrast to drawing such a precautionary line at enhancement, it is, as has been argued earlier, fairly definitive and easy to abide by in practice. There are, with the exception of mitochondrial DNA, relatively few gray areas—at least when compared to the therapy/enhancement distinction. Fourth, as a stand-in for moral principles while we look for a true moral principle, it is also perfectly replaceable with a different principle once our knowledge improves. It is a pre-cautionary principle of sorts, but one of moral precaution. The basic idea could translate into something like "hold off until we have better moral knowledge that can give us more precise advice."

This position on the human germline would afford it the status of the next-best thing to a more morally accurate boundary. There seems to be at least some cases of germline editing that are definitely morally impermissible and some risks that we cannot fully rule out. Even if there are, in addition to this, cases of perfectly permissible germline edits, few of those are likely to be obligatory. Thus, even if a strict boundary at the germline is too crude, morally speaking, the epistemic gaps are too significant to allow for any reliable conditional principle that successfully excludes all the unwanted outcomes. Perhaps it would be wise to stick with the germline boundary. Not only until it is safe and efficient enough, as the Technical View suggests, not only until there is public consensus and trust, as the Democratic View suggests, but until we know more about what is and is not the right thing to do in this context. What complicates the picture is not merely factual uncertainty but moral uncertainty. Thus, we must not overlook things that may morally matter in the long run.

The germline as a *locum tenens* moral principle is in a sense both a pragmatic and precautionary position, but on *moral* grounds rather than on safety grounds in a technical sense.[2] The idea is that the epistemic gaps, including moral uncer-tainty, make it difficult to replace the boundary with a stronger boundary that only excludes those cases that need to be so and allowing all others, all while the

---

[2] There may also be independent reasons to draw the boundary at the germline on the basis of the reparability principle that would advise us never to impose risks that could cause the loss of a kind qua kind (here, the loss of humanity); and, furthermore, never to impose risk for incompensable losses greater than that we know we can reverse or repair (see Hayenhjelm, 2018). If so, even if we could dismiss or control for the risks of loss of humanity, we could still not impose risks of harm that we may not be able to repair. Thus, until it is sufficiently safe in that sense, we ought not to cross the germline.

germline itself is both identifiable as a boundary (and thus action-guiding) and precautionary.

Given the epistemic gaps and uncertainties, there is merit for the germline as a moral *locum tenens* principle. However, a *locum tenens* principle is still not the "real deal" morally speaking, but a temporary solution in want of the real deal. At some point, we would want to replace it with a more precise moral principle that is both practically applicable and sufficiently safe (prevents all the morally concerning consequences), while allowing those applications that would benefit mankind (should it be safe to do so). Ideally, we would want a boundary that rests on firm moral foundations and that is also action-guiding and would in practice avoid the outcomes we are most concerned about.

However, even if a "real deal" moral principle is the ideal, we may never find such a principle, or even if we did find it, such a principle may not be sufficiently action-guiding. If so, a *locum tenens* moral principle could be the best that we could do. Such a principle could at least provide the minimum for sound moral guidance if it were to get things somewhat right; in other words, morally block the most concerning outcomes and be action-guiding.

10.6.4 Objections to the Idea

Does the idea of the germline as a *locum tenens* principle, or a moral line of precaution, add anything to the moral matter of the germline? Is it not, for instance, merely the call of a moratorium restated in a more complicated way? Is it not too conservative? Why opt for this alternative when we could, say, employ Nuffield's dual principles instead, which seem to avoid all the worst outcomes equally well, while still holding the door open to responsible germline gene editing? This will be discussed in the following.

10.6.4.1 The Moratorium in New Clothes?
Now, if the above idea of the germline as a *locum tenens* principle is nothing but a temporary halt to germline editing until it is sufficiently safe and we have found a moral resolution, is it not just the same idea as the idea of a moratorium?

The moratorium and our idea of the germline as a *locum tenens* principle against germline editing answer different kinds of questions. The moratorium is a decision or stance answering to the need for a policy or a professional stance. However, such a stance would ideally come with some kind of moral justification as part of its rationale. The germline as a moral precaution is a response to the underlying moral question about what is and is not the morally right thing to do. Thus, whereas the first is a response to the need for responsible policy decisions and boundaries in professional ethics, the latter is a response to the more abstract question about what morality requires from us. That said, the germline boundary as a case of moral precaution could support a moratorium (as would the categorical arguments or various safety-based risk arguments).

However, when we look at the specific calls for a moratorium, these are thought to be temporary measures until the technology is sufficiently safe and there is societal consensus. Of course, if there is no consensus, or if the right level of safety cannot be reached, then it may become a somewhat permanent ban. But, from the perspective of morality and the germline as a *locum tenens*, the boundary is not merely a temporary measure until safety and consensus is assured. It is a placeholder until we are in an epistemically better place, not just in general, but in terms of moral knowledge. A consensus would suggest wide agreement and less controversy, but would not normally hold as a reliable indication of moral truth. Safety, as we have seen, is only part of the moral concern.

Furthermore, even if the germline boundary as a precautionary moral boundary can support a moratorium, in that the rationale and the conditions are different, it is not obvious that that is the only policy implication. It could also support a ban. It is quite possible that cases that are very far from any slippery slopes could be permitted if specified clearly enough (such as mitochondrial DNA transfer). What it would not support is a case-by-case approach that would undermine any red lines.

10.6.4.2 Too Conservative?

The second objection worth addressing is the concern that the position above is simply too conservative. We can look at germline editing in a slightly more "local" way. We could limit our moral perspective to the benefits and risks of the technology's most immediate applications. We could assess the risks, limited to off-target risks, unwanted mutations, and mosaicism, and compare these with the prospective benefits, limited to the interests of those parents who it would enable to have biological children, along with additional benefits for the overall gene pool and reduction of the burden of disease. From this perspective, there are obvious concerns about the technical safety, and there may be some issues about accessibility, but on the whole, it seems like a beneficial project. Furthermore, any concerns about genocide, the end of humanity, and fears about a deep divide between a genetically improved upper class versus an unmodified underclass, such that conflict will arise, may seem very farfetched, perhaps so farfetched as to not deserve any serious consideration.

We could also look at it from a more "universal" perspective. Here, we know that there are certain things that could not be done unless germline editing makes this possible. We also know that once a technology is introduced, it does not remain under democratic rule or loyal to geographical boundaries. It will be as accessible to the totalitarian regime as the democratic one, and to both private and public enterprises. We also know that scarcity affects the kinds of chances people are willing to take. There are many future scenarios where people, out of desperation, may try anything to ensure a decent life for their future offspring. In a free market, this could easily be exploited. The point is that whatever the limits are for reigning in human germline gene editing in our current political and societal climate, we cannot be certain that that climate will remain for the length of the technology's availability.

The underlying rationale for the principle is this: There are certain things that are never worth risking and it is likely that these apply to some cases of germline editing. Given the amount of convincing slippery slope concerns, we cannot know for certain where those risks begin to draw a closer line; any alternative non-categorical line would increase the likelihood of slippery slopes or drawing the line in a place where some unacceptable risks are not excluded.

Would this be overstating the risks and understating the gains? Possibly. But as has been argued, interventions in the human germline are not just any kind of venture. Thus, the safety argument is strong. Secondly, as with all new technology, what we know about risks and benefits is likely to be asymmetrical; we are likely to know much more about the anticipated benefits, as these will be the very purpose of the technology, whereas the risks may only be discovered after they have materialized. In particular, with technological leaps that could have a systemic and revolutionary impact, the full scope of consequences may be very hard to assess *ex ante*. A simple rule of thumb in such cases could be to look at what we are likely to be able to repair, heal, or reverse (Hayenhjelm, 2018). Far-reaching experiments with human DNA before birth does not obviously belong to the category of things that we could repair, should things go wrong.

It could be argued that this would not be our responsibility, but unless *we are sure* that this it is not, we are taking a moral risk and we may do what is wrong, and that wrong could be irreparable or irreversible. There are thus reasons to be cautious, but, that said, ultimately, the weight one attaches to the need for caution will depend on how convincing the slippery slope arguments are and how serious the epistemic gaps are considered to be, including the moral ones.

10.6.4.3 The Nuffield Council's Two Principles

If there is reason to think that the most accurate moral principle will not draw a moral line at the germline, then why draw a categorical line there if we can simply exclude the exact worst-case scenarios that we are actually morally concerned about? This would allow for the "benign" uses and exclude those that can be expected to lead to harm. The Nuffield Council's two principles would clearly exclude any kind of exploitation or intervention that was not directly in the best interest of the person whose genome was edited, and it would clearly exclude any kind of intervention that would be contrary to justice. If that sums up all our moral concerns about outcome risks, while also opening the door to germline edits that do not strike us as obviously morally problematic, then why advocate anything as conservative as a moral boundary at the germline based on a *locum tenens* principle of moral precaution? Is this not simply too risk averse a position to be rational?

The Nuffield Council's principles elegantly draw the lines. There are two main differences. First, as we have argued, the Nuffield Council's principles presume that all of the most pressing moral concerns have already been articulated. This may, according to us, be overly optimistic from an epistemic perspective. We may have good reason to believe that we do not yet know what all the major concerns are, because we do not know the full scope of its impact, possible uses and misuses, all the settings where it may be applied, and so on. Nor do we know what all the future worlds where that technology could be used may look like, which could pressurize development in various directions. There are two general points here. First, again, it seems safe to assume that we will always know more about the benefits of a new and potentially revolutionary technology than about its side effects and negative impact, especially if those are systemic. Second, any precautionary line will always be more risk averse than weighing known risks against known benefits would suggest was optimal.

In other words, the Nuffield Council's principles are epistemically more optimistic and thus more vulnerable to new knowledge. If the two concerns that underpin the two principles overlook a third, even more serious, concern, then its moral advice is simply wrong. Furthermore, we would not be able to say that we had erred on the side of caution.

Third, as moral advice that could provide clear guidance, it is more open to interpretation in practice. How, for instance, will we determine whether a particular germline gene intervention will or will not be compatible with justice in the long run? Or, what will or will not be in the long-term interest of a child born with such edits? The germline as a boundary of moral precaution is definitive and thus unambiguous in its moral advice. This means that it could provide a clear idea of what precaution in the context of germline gene editing would look like and any deviation from that would also be understood as moral risk in some sense. Such risks may sometimes be warranted, but at least the line for where precaution goes would be clear.

Ultimately, we cannot get around these two points: We are editing our own DNA and the moral conclusions will depend on what weight one attaches to the epistemic gaps and slippery slopes on the one hand, and the scope for moral responsibility on the other. Here, it is argued that the epistemic gaps are considerable, the slippery slopes cannot be ignored, and several of the outcomes could prove to be incompensable in terms of their harm or impact, or otherwise unforgiveable, and that moral responsibility is partly about what remains within our control and what we could rectify, should things go wrong. Heritable changes to the human genome are imposing risks for which we may not be able to take responsibility.

10.7   Concluding Words

If we review what we have argued for in the present book, a number of conclusions can be drawn. First, the safety concerns will not disappear. Second, beyond safety concerns, there is something more problematic about germline editing than many (or even most) kinds of moral actions—not just because of the epistemic and safety risks (of actual harm), the long-term risks of injustice and a change in culture, but also because of the subject matter itself— the very act of meddling with our own DNA in ways that could alter humans in fundamental ways. There is a scope of power in the tool that could be used, abused, and cause unknown side effects that we cannot currently predict. In short, it is, if nothing else, a very risky endeavor. Additionally, all institutional, conventional, and political solutions will only apply as long as those institutions, conventions, and political majorities last. For heritable practices, the moral perspective must be able to survive the changes in trends, ideologies, and institutions. When it comes to democracy and political rights, these are protected by a constitution to disallow a majority at any one point in time to limit or remove such rights. However, when it comes to our own DNA, if we would only be protected by societal consensus, this would not protect us from ideologically motivated genetic alterations.

The concerns about risk and safety will not disappear any time soon, if we take risks to include not only technical risks, but also societal risks and risks for moral wrongdoing, including the risks for irreparable consequences ("unforgivables") and apply the notion of epistemic risk to all three of those dimensions. We do not know enough to conclude that germline gene editing will be technically safe, we do not know enough to conclude that it will promote a society that we would want to live in and pass on to future generations, and we do not know whether it would be the morally right thing to do. Thus, the relevant notion of precaution ought to match all of those dimensions of risk.

This means that the precautionary concerns are of at least three different kinds: (i) to *avoid or minimize direct technical risks and side effects*, (ii) to *avoid or minimize psychological and societal consequences*, such as discrimination and injustice, and to *avoid or minimize moral risks of wrongdoing* and paving the way for a future we could neither reverse nor stand for. Should germline editing cause off-target or on-target side effects, this could be rectified in a sense: the technology could be improved and harms to one generation need not affect later ones, and so on. Harms to individuals would not be avoided, but it could be rectified before a whole generation or humanity as a whole was harmed. There is a difference between what is not safe—that we cannot guarantee that individuals will not come to harm—and vast changes to humanity or the world that we cannot reverse. Likewise, should germline editing come to cause social injustice, this could in principle be rectified with compensatory public policy and compensation over a few generations.

The risk of moral wrongdoing arises from the problem of moral uncertainty: all things considered, we do not know for certain what the right thing to do is. What may seem rational at one point may turn out to be morally unforgiveable by a later generation. Moral uncertainty here refers to a particular kind of uncertainty or lack of knowledge: not about descriptive facts but about morality as such, including which moral theory, if any is accurate. We introduced three kinds of moral logic in Chap. 5 that provide three different kinds of perspectives on the dimensions of moral risk. The first risk is that what was meant to improve the world, in fact, made it worse, and caused more harm than benefit. Such outcomes may be unfortunate, but as long as enough resources have been set aside, they could be compensated for. Unless they are in principle incompensable. The second kind of risk is that what we thought was permissible, in fact, turned out to be impermissible. Such risks could be forgivable, if motivated by the appropriate reasons and, hence, something we could be answerable for—unless it is something we could not possibly stand for. The third kind of risk is that what we thought would lead us to a better society ultimately led to a society we could not possibly stand for, or could not live with having created. It need not be that any particular person comes to harm or that we did something objectively impermissible, but that we have brought about some turn of events that we could not possibly support. For instance, should all of humanity come to an end, then there would be no future claimants to complain about harm or loss, nor may the universe or our planet suffer any direct harm or loss. Alternatively, our actions could pave the way for a dystopian future that was our fault. In this way, all the calls for consensus and broad debates make sense in that the moral question is not only about what is and is not permissible, but also about what kind of visions we have for the future, which seems to be more of a democratic matter for all of us than a matter that has any one particular answer.

In any case, moral precaution would advise us not to yield outcomes that could ultimately lead to great harm and suffering, not risk violating fundamental moral norms, and not limit our future to specific trajectories that we could not possibly endorse. Responsible agency implies taking responsibility not only for one's most favored outcome, but also for all future societies that could come to pass when such attempts fail or lead to unexpected outcomes. Here, what can be compensated for, reversed, and forgiven is key. Many moral actions can be repaired one way or another, and thus could be risked as long as there were sufficient means, skills, and will for such reparations. Some moral actions, by contrast, are such that they could not even in principle be repaired—these we must avoid. Wrecking the human genetic code by mistake would be such an act. Undermining humanity as a shared community may be another. This latter point is more abstract and thus perhaps easier to dismiss without consideration. But, in contrast to the other more serious concerns, it points to a kind of harm that cannot even in principle be repaired or compensated.

Careful alterations and improvements may ultimately be morally called for, but given the stakes, this can only be done with full awareness of the epistemic risks and immediate outcome risks—whether biological, psychological, social, or political—as well as the moral risks. What makes the ethical issues raised by the germline interesting is that it brings the importance of all three kinds of moral logic in view. Most moral questions only call upon the first two: "Is it impermissible?" and if so, "Would it be advisable, given the risks, costs, and expected benefits"? Here, we cannot fully address the moral question about the germline by only examining risks (such as mosaicism, off-target risks, or even social and psychological risks) nor by considering whether there are matters that pertain to rights, obligations, and duties. Nor by weighing the expected gains against the risks. It seems that we cannot get very far without considering more fundamental moral questions, such as what kind of society it is that we want to promote, and ultimately, what matters to us, what kind of world we want to live in, and what kinds of beings we wish to be. In this, at least, the democratic voices are right about the kinds of questions that we need to ask, and the transhumanists and theologians are right in raising concerns about ideals and core values. The right kind of moral precaution would need to address all of these moral aspects: risks, benefits, obligations, and visions for the future and the underlying values they make possible or impossible to realize.

If this is right, the question about impermissibility does not merely cover the potential violation of rights or harm to others, but also various kinds of possible and impossible futures. One particular future we need to include in the possibilities is one where we do not exist, or where our values do not make sense, and where unforgiveable outcomes cannot be dismissed. If this is true, then it would seem that a precautionary approach that merely applies a precautionary halt to technical risks is insufficient; we need to also recognize the full scope of epistemic risks and moral uncertainty. We have argued that this supports the case for the germline as a *locum tenens* moral boundary. This would mean that unless we know differently, we ought to, for now, treat the germline as a categorical boundary of impermissibility. Not because it would be morally impermissible to cross it in an objective sense, but because we do not know where to draw an exact line and because it would be both action-guiding and steer away from the worst-case outcomes in a moral sense. Perhaps this is overly cautious; however, it is revisable in light of new technical, social, and moral knowledge.

The strongest case for the germline boundary would be if it overlapped and was supported by a moral principle that drew a categorical moral line of permissibility in the same location. There would then be a moral principle that stated that any action of germline gene editing is impermissible, because it is morally wrong, and this would be the final word on the matter. We have argued for a weaker position on the grounds of moral uncertainty: The germline boundary can be supported as a moral *locum tenens* barrier that, in want of a more definite moral boundary, draws the line at the germline. This principle says that we should not edit the germline, not because we know it to be morally wrong, but because we do not know which acts are permissible and impermissible and because it would be best to err on the side of caution—also in a moral sense. Given that the germline boundary is (a) well-established; (b) sufficiently conceptually clear to avoid slippery slopes and to be action-guiding; (c) that we have good grounds to presume that it errs on the side of caution in that it avoids the relevant worst-case scenarios; and (d) some of the worst-outcomes may in principle be irreparable, then the best we can do for now is to treat the germline as a *locum tenens* moral barrier.

References

The Academy of Sciences of Hong Kong, the U.S. National Academy of Sciences, the U.S. National Academy of Medicine, & the Royal Society. (2018). *On Human Genome Editing II: Statement by the Organizing Committee of the Second International Summit on Human Genome Editing, November 29, 2018*. Retrieved September 30, 2024, from https://royalsociety.org/-/media/news/2018/human-genome-editing-statement-29-11-2018.pdf.

Act for Protection of Embryos (The Embryo Protection Act) [Embryonenschutzgesetz – ESchG]. (1990, December 13). *Federal Law Gazette, Part I, No. 69, Bonn, 19th December 1990*. Retrieved September 28, 2024, from https://www.rki.de/SharedDocs/Gesetzexte/Embryonenschutzgesetz_englisch.pdf?__blob=publicationFile.

Adler, M. D., & Posner, E. A. (2001). *Cost-Benefit Analysis: Legal, Economic, and Philosophical Perspectives*. University of Chicago Press.

Agar, N. (1998). Liberal eugenics. *Public Affairs Quarterly, 12*(2), 137–155.

Agar, N. (2004). *Liberal Eugenics: In Defense of Human Enhancement*. Blackwell-Wiley.

Agar, N. (2010). *Humanity's End: Why We Should Reject Radical Enhancement*. MIT Press.

Agar, N. (2013). *Truly Human Enhancement: A Philosophical Defense of Limits*. MIT Press.

Angrist, M., Barrangou, R., Baylis, F., Brokowski, C., Burgio, G., Caplan, A., Riley Chapman, C., Church, G. M., Cook-Deegan, R., Cwik, B., Doudna, J. A., Evans, J. H., Greely, H. T., Hercher, L., Hurlbut, J. B., Hynes, R. O., Ishii, T., Kiani, S., Hoskins Lee, L. T., … Davies, K. (2020). Reactions to the national academies/royal society report on *heritable human genome editing. The CRISPR Journal, 3*(5), 333–349. https://doi.org/10.1089/crispr.2020.29106.man.

Annas, G. J. (2000). The man on the moon, immortality, and other millennial myths: The prospects and perils of human genetic engineering. *Emory Law Journal, 49*(3), 753–782.

Annas, G. J. (2010). *Worst Case Bioethics: Death, Disaster, and Public Health*. Oxford University Press.

Annas, G. J., Andrews, L. B., & Isasi, R. M. (2002). Protecting the endangered human: Toward an international treaty prohibiting cloning and inheritable alterations. *American Journal of Law & Medicine, 28*(2–3), 151–178. https://doi.org/10.1017/S00988588000 1162X.

Anscombe, G. E. M. (1958). Modern moral philosophy. *Philosophy, 33*(124), 1–19. Retrieved October 15, 2024, from http://www.jstor.org/stable/3749051.

© The Editor(s) (if applicable) and The Author(s) 2025
M. Hayenhjelm and C. Nordlund, *The Risks and Ethics of Human Gene Editing*,
Technikzukünfte, Wissenschaft und Gesellschaft / Futures of Technology, Science
and Society, https://doi.org/10.1007/978-3-658-46979-5

Ashford, E. (2003). The Demandingness of Scanlon's Contractualism. *Ethics, 113*(2), 273–302. 10.1086/342853.

Ashford, E., & Mulgan, T. (2018). Contractualism. In E. N. Zalta (Ed.), *The Stanford Encyclopedia of Philosophy* (Summer 2018 ed.). Retrieved September 28, 2024, from https://plato.stanford.edu/archives/sum2018/entries/contractualism.

Aydin, C. (2017). The posthuman as hollow idol: A Nietzschean critique of human enhancement. *The Journal of Medicine and Philosophy: A Forum for Bioethics and Philosophy of Medicine, 42*(3), 304–327. https://doi.org/10.1093/jmp/jhx002.

Baillie, H. W., & Casey, T. K. (Eds.). (2005). *Is Human Nature Obsolete? Genetics, Bioengineering, and the Future of the Human Condition.* MIT Press. https://doi.org/10.7551/mitpress/3977.001.0001.

Baltimore, D., Berg, P., Botchan, M., Carroll, D., Charo, R. A., Church, G., Corn, J. E., Daley, G. Q., Doudna, J. A., Fenner, M., Greely, H. T., Jinek, M., Martin, G. S., Penhoet, E., Puck, J., Sternberg, S. H., Weissman, J. S., & Yamamoto, K. R. (2015). A prudent path forward for genomic engineering and germline gene modification. *Science, 348*(6230), 36–38. https://www.science.org/doi/10.1126/science.aab1028.

Baltimore, D., Charo, A., Daley, G. Q., Doudna, J. A., Kato, K., Kim, J-S., Lovell-Badge, R., Merchant, J., Nath, I., Pei, D., Porteus, M., Skehel, J., Tam, P., & Zhai, X. (2018). *Statement by the Organizing Committee of the Second International Summit on Human Genome Editing.* The National Academies of Sciences, Engineering and Medicine. Retrieved, September 28, 2024, from https://www.nationalacademies.org/news/2018/11/statement-by-the-organizing-committee-of-the-second-international-summit-on-human-genome-editing.

Baruch, S., Pritchard, D., Javitt, G., Scott, J., Borchelt, R., Kalfoglou, A., & Hudson, K. (2005). *Human Germline Genetic Modification: Issues and Options for Policymakers.* Genetics and Public Policy Center. Retrieved, September 28, 2024, from https://jscholarship.library.jhu.edu/server/api/core/bitstreams/a4e4958a-df37-41be-8d38-d8a6b8e03d49/content.

Baumann, M. (2016). CRISPR/Cas9 genome editing—New and old ethical issues arising from a revolutionary technology. *NanoEthics, 10*(2), 139–159. https://doi.org/10.1007/s11569-016-0259-0.

Baylis, F. (2019). *Altered Inheritance: CRISPR and the Ethics of Human Genome Editing.* Harvard University Press.

Baylis, F., & Robert, J. S. (2004). The inevitability of genetic enhancement technologies. *Bioethics, 18*(1), 1–26. https://doi.org/10.1111/j.1467-8519.2004.00376.x.

BBC News (2018, July 17). *Editing human embryos 'morally permissible'.* https://www.bbc.com/news/health-44849034.

Beauchamp, T. (2019). The principle of beneficence in applied ethics. In E. N. Zalta (Ed.), *The Stanford Encyclopedia of Philosophy* (Spring 2019 ed.). Retrieved September 28, 2024, from https://plato.stanford.edu/archives/spr2019/entries/principle-beneficence/.

Beauchamp, T. L., & Childress, J. F. (2019). *Principles of Biomedical Ethics* (8th ed.). Oxford University Press. (Original work published 1979).

Beccalossi, C. (2020). Optimizing and normalizing the population through hormone therapies in Italian science, c. 1926–1950. *The British Journal for the History of Science, 53*(1), 67–88. https://doi.org/10.1017/S0007087419000906.

Bentham, J. (2011). *An Introduction to the Principles of Morals and Legislation.* Bottom of the Hill Publishing. (Original work published 1789).

Birnbacher, D. (2018). Prospects of human germline modification by CRISPR-cas9–an ethicist's view. In M. Braun, H. Schickl, & P. Dabrock (Eds.), *Between Moral Hazard and Legal Uncertainty: Ethical, Legal and Societal Challenges of Human Genome Editing* (pp. 53–66). Springer VS. 10.1007/978-3-658-22660-2_4.

Boggio, A., Romano, C. P., & Almqvist, J. (2019). The regulation of Human Germline Genome Modification (HGGM) at the national level: A call for comprehensive legal reform. *Loyola of Los Angeles International and Comparative Law Review, 43*(3), 201–226. https://digitalcommons.lmu.edu/cgi/viewcontent.cgi?article=1805&context=ilr.

Bosley, K. S., Botchan, M., Bredenoord, A. L., Carroll, D., Charo, R. A., Charpentier, E., Cohen, R., Corn, J., Doudna, J., Feng, G., Greely, H. T., Isasi, R., Ji, W., Kim, J.-S., Knoppers, B., Lanphier, E., Li, J., Lovell-Badge, R., Martin, G. S., … Zhou, Q. (2015). CRISPR germline engineering—The community speaks. *Nature Biotechnology, 33*(5), 478–486. https://doi.org/10.1038/nbt.3227.

Bostrom, N. (2003). Human genetic enhancement: A transhumanist perspective. *Journal of Value Inquiry, 37*(4), 493–506. https://doi.org/10.1023/B:INQU.0000019037.67783.d5.

Bostrom, N. (2005). Transhumanist values. *Journal of Philosophical Research, 30*(Supplement), 3–14. https://doi.org/10.5840/jpr_2005_26.

Bostrom, N. (2008a). Dignity and enhancement. In A. Schulman, & T. M. Merrill (Eds.), *Human Dignity and Bioethics: Essays Commissioned by the President's Council on Bioethics* (pp. 173–207). U.S. Independent Agencies and Commissions. http://hdl.handle.net/10822/559351.

Bostrom, N. (2008b). *Letter from Utopia.* Retrieved September 28, 2024, from https://www.nickbostrom.com/utopia.html.

Bostrom, N. (2008c). Why I want to be a posthuman when I grow up. In B. Gordijn & R. Chadwick (Eds.), *Medical Enhancement and Posthumanity* (pp. 107–136). Springer Science & Business Media.

Bostrom, N., & Ord, T. (2006). The reversal test: Eliminating status quo bias in applied ethics. *Ethics, 116*(4), 656–679. 10.1086/505233.

Bostrom, N., & Sandberg, A. (2009). The wisdom of nature: An evolutionary heuristic for human enhancement. In J. Savulescu, & N. Bostrom (Eds.), *Human Enhancement* (pp. 375–416). Oxford University Press. https://doi.org/10.1093/oso/9780199299720.003.0019.

Braun, K. (2005). Not just for experts: The public debate about reprogenetics in Germany. *The Hastings Center Report, 35*(3), 42–49. https://doi.org/10.1353/hcr.2005.0054.

Braun, M., & Dabrock, P. (2018) Mind the gaps! Towards an ethical framework for genome editing. *EMBO Reports, 19*(2), 197–200. https://doi.org/10.15252/embr.201745542.

Braun, M., Schickl, H., & Dabrock, P. (2018). Between moral hazard and legal uncertainty: An introduction. In M. Braun, H. Schickl, & P. Dabrock (Eds.), *Between Moral Hazard and Legal Uncertainty: Ethical, Legal and Societal Challenges of Human Genome Editing* (pp. 1–14). Springer VS. 10.1007/978-3-658-22660-2_1.

Brokowski, C. (2018). Do CRISPR germline ethics statements cut it? *The CRISPR Journal, 1*(2), 115–125. https://doi.org/10.1089/crispr.2017.0024.

Brokowski, C., & Adli, M. (2019). CRISPR ethics: Moral considerations for applications of a powerful tool. *Journal of Molecular Biology, 431*(1), 88–101. https://doi.org/10.1016/j.jmb.2018.05.044.

Broome J. (2002). Modern utilitarianism. In P. Newman (Ed.), *The New Palgrave Dictionary of Economics and the Law* (pp. 1309–1314). Palgrave Macmillan. 10.1007/978-1-349-74173-1_248.

Broome, J. (2004). Weighing lives. *Oxford University Press.* https://doi.org/10.1093/019924376X.001.0001.

Buchanan, A. (2011). *Beyond Humanity?* Oxford University Press. https://doi.org/10.1093/acprof:oso/9780199587810.001.0001.

Byron, M. (Ed.). (2004). *Satisficing and Maximizing: Moral Theorists on Practical Reason.* Cambridge University Press. https://doi.org/10.1017/CBO9780511617058.

Caplan, A. L. (2009). Good, better, or best? In J. Savulescu, & N. Bostrom (Eds.), *Human Enhancement* (pp. 199–209). Oxford University Press. https://doi.org/10.1093/oso/9780199299720.003.0010.

Cavaliere, G. (2019, March 18–19). Background paper: The ethics of human genome editing. Commissioned ethics paper for WHO Expert Advisory Committee on Developing Global Standards for Governance and Oversight of Human Genome Editing.

Chan, S., & Harris, J. (2007). In support of human enhancement. *Studies in Ethics, Law, and Technology, 1*(1), 1–3. Retrieved September 28, 2024, from https://summerschool.globalbioethics.org/wp-content/uploads/2015/11/ChanHarris.2007.pdf.

Charo, R. A. (2020). Who's afraid of the big bad (Germline editing) wolf? *Perspectives in Biology and Medicine, 63*(1), 93–100. https://doi.org/10.1353/pbm.2020.0007.

Coady, C. A. J. (2009). Playing God. In J. Savulescu & N. Bostrom (Eds.), *Human Enhancement* (pp. 155–180). Oxford University Press. https://doi.org/10.1093/oso/9780199299720.003.0008.

Cohen, G. A. (2011). Rescuing conservatism: A defense of existing value. In R. Jay, Wallace, R. Kumar, & S. Freeman (Eds.), *Reasons and Recognition: Essays on the Philosophy of T.M. Scanlon* (pp. 203–230). Oxford University Press. https://doi.org/10.1093/acprof:oso/9780199753673.003.0009.

Collins, F. S. (2015, April 28). *Statement on NIH funding of research using gene-editing technologies in human embryos.* Retrieved September 28, 2024, from https://www.nih.gov/about-nih/who-we-are/nih-director/statements/statement-nih-funding-research-using-gene-editing-technologies-human-embryos.

Comfort, N. (2012). *The Science of Human Perfection: How Genes Became the Heart of American Medicine.* Yale University Press.

Comfort, N. (2015, July 16). Can we cure genetic diseases without slipping into eugenics? *The Nation.* Retrieved September 28, 2024, from https://www.thenation.com/article/archive/can-we-cure-genetic-diseases-without-slipping-into-eugenics/.

Condit, C. M. (1999). *The Meanings of the Gene: Public Debates about Human Heredity.* University of Wisconsin Press.

Cong, L., Ran, F. A., Cox, D., Lin, S., Barretto, R., Habib, N., Hsu, P. D., Wu, X., Jiang, W., Marraffini, L. A., & Zhang, F. (2013). Multiplex genome engineering using CRISPR/Cas systems. *Science, 339*(6121), 819–823. https://doi.org/10.1126/science.1231143.

Council of Europe. (1997). European Treatise Series No. 164. Convention for the Protection of Human Rights and Dignity of the Human Being with regard to the Application of

Biology and Medicine: Convention on Human Rights and Biomedicine. European Treaty Series No. 164, Oviedo, 4.IV.1997. Retrieved September 28, 2024, from https://www.coe.int/en/web/bioethics/oviedo-convention.

Crisp, R. (2021). Well-being. In: E. N. Zalta (Ed.), *The Stanford Encyclopedia of Philosophy* (Winter 2021 ed.). Retrieved September 28, 2024, from https://plato.stanford.edu/archives/win2021/entries/well-being.

Cwik, B. (2019). Moving beyond 'therapy' and 'enhancement' in the ethics of gene editing. *Cambridge Quarterly of Healthcare Ethics, 28*(4), 695–707. https://doi.org/10.1017/S0963180119000641.

Cwik, B. (2020a). Responsible translational pathways for Germline gene editing? *Current Stem Cell Reports, 6*(4), 126–133. https://doi.org/10.1007/s40778-020-00179-x.

Cwik, B. (2020b). Revising, correcting, and transferring genes. *The American Journal of Bioethics, 20*(8), 7–18. 10.1080/15265161.2020.1783024.

Cyranoski, D. (2020). What CRISPR-baby prison sentences mean for research. *Nature, 577*(7789), 154–156. https://doi.org/10.1038/d41586-020-00001-y.

Dabrock, P. (2018). Who? What? How? Why? If you don't ask you'll never know: On criticism of the new uproar about germline editing – discourse analytical and socioethical metaperspectives. In M. Braun, H. Schickl, & P. Dabrock (Eds.), *Between Moral Hazard and Legal Uncertainty: Ethical, Legal and Societal Challenges of Human Genome Editing* (pp. 163–185). Springer VS. 10.1007/978-3-658-22660-2_11.

Daley, G. Q., Lovell-Badge, R., & Steffann, J. (2019). After the storm–a responsible path for genome editing. *The New England Journal of Medicine, 380*(10), 897–899. https://doi.org/10.1056/NEJMp1900504.

Daniels, N. (2009). Can anyone really be talking about ethically modifying human nature? In J. Savulescu & N. Bostrom (Eds.), *Human Enhancement* (pp. 25–42). Oxford University Press. https://doi.org/10.1093/oso/9780199299720.003.0002.

De Lecuona, I., Casadoa, M., Marfanyb, G., Lopez Baronia, M., & Escarrabilla, M. (2017). Gene editing in humans: Towards a global and inclusive debate for responsible research. *Yale Journal of Biology and Medicine, 90*(4), 673–681.

Deane-Drummond, C. (2019). Recovering practical wisdom as a guide for human flourishing: Navigating the CRISPR challenge. In E. Parens & J. Johnston (Eds.), *Human Flourishing in an Age of Gene Editing* (pp. 184–198). Oxford University Press. https://doi.org/10.1093/oso/9780190940362.003.0014.

Deltcheva, E., Chylinski, K., Sharma, C. M., Gonzales, K., Chao, Y., Pirzada, Z. A., Eckert, M. R., Vogel, J., & Charpentier, E. (2011). CRISPR RNA maturation by *trans*-encoded small RNA and host factor RNase III. *Nature, 471*(7340), 602–607. https://doi.org/10.1038/nature09886.

Dillon, R. S. (2021). Respect. In E. D. Zalta (Ed.), *The Stanford Encyclopedia of Philosophy* (Summer 2021 ed.). Retrieved September 29, 2024, from https://plato.stanford.edu/archives/sum2021/entries/respect.

Doudna, J. A. (2015). Genome-editing revolution: My whirlwind year with CRISPR. *Nature, 528*(7583), 469–471. https://doi.org/10.1038/528469a.

Doudna, J. A., & Charpentier, E. (2014). The new frontier of genome engineering with CRISPR-Cas9, *Science, 346*(6213). https://doi.org/10.1126/science.1258096.

Doudna, J. A., & Sternberg, S. (2017). *A Crack in Creation: The New Power to Control Evolution.* The Bodley Head.

Dunér, I. (2024). *Controlling Destiny: Julian Huxley's Post-Darwinan Evolutionism and the History of Transhumanism.* Lund University.

Duster, T. (1990). *Backdoor to Eugenics.* Routledge.

Dworkin, R. (1977). *Taking Rights Seriously.* Harvard University Press.

The Economist. (2015, May 2). *To the crack of doom: Scientists in China have just crossed one of biotechnology's red lines.* Retrieved September 29, 2024, from https://www.eco nomist.com/science-and-technology/2015/05/02/to-the-crack-of-doom.

Engelhardt, H. T. Jr. (1998). Human nature genetically re-engineered: Moral responsibilities to future generations. In E. Agius & S Busuttil (Eds.), *Germ-Line Intervention and Our Responsibilities to Future Generations* (pp. 51–63). Springer. 10.1007/978-94-011-5149-8_6.

European Academies Science Advisory Council. (2017). *Genome editing: Scientific opportunities, public interests and policy options in the European Union. EASAC policy report 31, March 2017.* Retrieved September 29, 2024, from https://easac.eu/fileadmin/PDF_s/reports_statements/Genome_Editing/EASAC_Report_31_on_Genome_Editing.pdf.

European Group on Ethics in Science and New Technologies. (2016). *EGE statement on gene editing.* Retrieved September 29, 2024, from https://research-and-innovation.ec.europa.eu/system/files/2018-10/gene_editing_ege_statement.pdf.

Evans, J. H. (2019). The dismal fate of flourishing in public policy bioethics: A sociological explanation. In E. Parens & J. Johnston (Eds.), *Human Flourishing in an Age of Gene Editing* (pp. 46–58). Oxford University Press. https://doi.org/10.1093/oso/978019 0940362.003.0004.

Evans, J. H. (2020). *The Human Gene Editing Debate.* Oxford University Press. https://doi.org/10.1093/oso/9780197519561.001.0001.

Evans, J. H. (2021). Setting ethical limits on human gene editing after the fall of the somatic/germline barrier. *Proceedings of the National Academy of Sciences, 118*(22), Article e2004837117. https://doi.org/10.1073/pnas.2004837117.

Evitt, N. H., Mascharak, S., & Altman, R. B. (2015). Human Germline CRISPR-cas modification: Toward a regulatory framework. *The American Journal of Bioethics, 15*(12), 25–29. 10.1080/15265161.2015.1104160.

Feinberg, J. (1980). The child's right to an open future. In W. Aikin & H. LaFollette (Eds.), *Whose Child? Children's Rights, Parental Authority, and State Power* (pp. 124–153). Rowman and Littlefield.

Fletcher, G. (Ed.). (2015). *The Routledge Handbook of Philosophy of Well-Being.* Routledge.

Fletcher, J. C., & Anderson, W. F. (1992). Germ-line gene therapy: A new stage of debate. *Law, Medicine, and Health Care, 20,* 26–39.

Foot, P. (1985). Utilitarianism and the virtues. *Mind, 94*(374), 196–209. https://doi.org/10.1093/mind/XCIV.374.196.

Fowler, G., Juengst, E. T., & Zimmerman, B. K. (1989). Germline gene therapy and the clinical ethos of medical genetics. *Theoretical Medicine, 10*(2), 151–165. https://doi.org/10.1007/BF00539880.

Fukuyama, F. (2003). *Our Posthuman Future: Consequences of the Biotechnology Revolution.* Profile Books.

Garland-Thomson, R. (2019). Welcoming the unexpected. In E. Parens & J. Johnston (Eds.), *Human Flourishing in the Age of Gene Editing* (pp. 15–28). Oxford University Press. https://doi.org/10.1093/oso/9780190940362.003.0002.

Garland-Thomson, R. (2020). How we got to CRISPR: The dilemma of being human. *Perspectives in Biology and Medicine, 63*(1), 28–43. https://doi.org/10.1353/pbm.2020.0002.

Gasiunas, G., Barrangou, R., Horvath, P., & Siksnys, V. (2012). Cas9-crRNA ribonucleoprotein complex mediates specific DNA cleavage for adaptive immunity in bacteria. *Proceedings of the National Academy of Sciences of the United States of America 109*(39). https://doi.org/10.1073/pnas.1208507109.

Gray, J., & Gorin, M. (2019). Some optimism about enhancement. *The American Journal of Bioethics, 19*(7), 26–28. 10.1080/15265161.2019.1618968.

Greely, H. T. (2019). CRISPR'd babies: Human germline genome editing in the 'He Jiankui affair.' *Journal of Law and the Biosciences, 6*(1), 111–183. https://doi.org/10.1093/jlb/lsz010.

Greely, H. T. (2021). *CRISPR People: The Science and Ethics of Editing Humans.* MIT Press.

Griffin, J. (1988). *Well-Being: Its Meaning.* Oxford University Press. 10.1093/0198248431.001.0001.

The Guardian. (2018, December 4). "Should we even consider this?" WHO starts work on gene editing ethics. https://www.theguardian.com/world/2018/dec/04/should-we-even-consider-this-who-starts-work-on-gene-editing-ethics.

The Guardian. (2019, January 22). *Second woman carrying gene-edited baby Chinese authorities confirm.* https://www.theguardian.com/science/2019/jan/22/second-woman-carrying-gene-edited-baby-chinese-authorities-confirm.

Gunderson, M. (2007). Seeking perfection: A Kantian look at human genetic engineering. *Theoretical Medicine and Bioethics, 28*(2), 87–102. https://doi.org/10.1007/s11017-007-9030-4.

Gunderson, M. (2008). Enhancing human rights: How the use of human rights treaties to prohibit genetic engineering weakens human rights. *Journal of Evolution and Technology, 18*(1), 27–34.

Guttinger, S. (2018). Trust in science: CRISPR-Cas9 and the ban on human germline editing. *Scientific Engineering Ethics, 24*(4), 1077–1096. https://doi.org/10.1007/s11948-017-9931-1.

Guttinger, S. (2020). Editing the reactive genome: Towards a postgenomic ethics of germline editing. *Journal of Applied Philosophy, 37*(1), 58–72. https://doi.org/10.1111/japp.12367.

Gyngell, C. A., & Savulescu, J. (2016). The medical case for gene editing. *Ethics in Biology, Engineering and Medicine: An International Journal, 6*(1–2), 57–66.

Gyngell, C., Bowman-Smart, H., & Savulescu, J. (2019). Moral reasons to edit the human genome: Picking up from the Nuffield report. *Journal of Medical Ethics, 45,* 514–523. https://doi.org/10.1136/medethics-2018-105084.

Gyngell, C., Douglas, T., & Savulescu, J. (2015, March 31). Editing the germline–A time for reason, not emotion. *Practical Ethics* [Blog]. Retrieved September 29, 2024, from http://blog.practicalethics.ox.ac.uk/2015/03/editing-the-germline-a-time-for-reason-not-emotion/.

Gyngell, C., Douglas, T., & Savulescu, J. (2017). The ethics of germline gene editing. *Journal of Applied Ethics, 34*(4), 498–513. https://doi.org/10.1111/japp.12249.

Habermas, J. (2003). *The Future of Human Nature.* Polity Press.

Hamilton, C. (2013). *Earthmasters: Playing God with the Climate.* Yale University Press.

Hansson, S. O. (2007). Philosophical problems in cost-benefit analysis. *Economics and Philosophy, 2323*(2), 163–183. https://doi.org/10.1017/S0266267107001356.

Harris, J. (1998). *Clones, Genes, and Immortality: Ethics and the Genetic Revolution.* Oxford University Press.

Harris, J. (2001). One principle and three fallacies of disability studies. *Journal of Medical Ethics, 27*(6), 383–387. https://doi.org/10.1136/jme.27.6.383.

Harris, J. (2007). *Enhancing Evolution: The Ethical Case for Making Better People.* Princeton University Press.

Harris, J. (2009). Enhancements are a moral obligation. In J. Savulescu & N. Bostrom (Eds.), *Human Enhancement* (pp. 131–154). Oxford University Press. https://doi.org/10.1093/oso/9780199299720.003.0007.

Harris, J. (2015a). Germline manipulation and our future worlds. *The American Journal of Bioethics, 15*(12), 30–34. 10.1080/15265161.2015.1104163.

Harris, J. (2015, December 2). Why human gene editing must not be stopped. *The Guardian.* https://www.theguardian.com/science/2015/dec/02/why-human-gene-editing-must-not-be-stopped.

Hauskeller, M. (2011). Human enhancement and the giftedness of life. *Philosophical Papers, 40*(1), 55–79. 10.1080/05568641.2011.560027.

Hauskeller, M. (2019). Editing the best of all possible worlds. In E. Parens & J. Johnston (Eds.), *Human Flourishing in an Age of Gene Editing* (pp. 61–71). Oxford University Press. https://doi.org/10.1093/oso/9780190940362.003.0005.

Hayenhjelm, M. (2018). Risk impositions, genuine losses, and reparability as a moral constraint. *Ethical Perspectives, 25*(3), 419–446. https://doi.org/10.2143/EP.25.3.3285424.

Hayenhjelm, M. (2024). The better option: Status quo vs. radical change. *Journal of Ethics, 1–19. https://doi.org/10.1007/s10892-024-09504-6*

Hayenhjelm, M., & Wolff, J. (2012). The moral problem of risk impositions: A survey of the literature. *European Journal of Philosophy, 20*(S1), E26–E51. https://doi.org/10.1111/j.1468-0378.2011.00482.x.

Herman, B. (2007). *Moral Literacy.* Harvard University Press.

Herman, B. (2021). *The Moral Habitat.* Oxford University Press.

Hill, T. (1992). *Dignity and Practical Reason in Kant's Moral Theory.* Cornell University Press.

Hill, T. (2014). Kantian perspectives on the rational basis of human dignity. In M. Düwell, J. Braarvig, R. Brownsword, & D. Mieth (Eds.), *The Cambridge Handbook of Human Dignity: Interdisciplinary Perspectives* (pp. 215–221). Cambridge University Press. https://doi.org/10.1017/CBO9780511979033.027.

Holland, A. (2016). The case against the case for Procreative Beneficence (PB). *Bioethics, 30*(7), 490–499. https://doi.org/10.1111/bioe.12253.

Holm, S. (2019). Let us assume that gene editing is safe-the role of safety arguments in the gene editing debate. *Cambridge Quarterly of Healthcare Ethics, 28*(1), 100–111. https://doi.org/10.1017/S0963180118000439.

Houser, K. (2019). China quietly confirms birth of third gene-edited baby. Retrieved September 30, 2024, from https://futurism.com/neoscope/china-confirms-birth-third-gene-edited-baby.

Howard, H. C. (2017, December 7). Gene editing–An international perspective. Presentation at SMER [Swedish National Council on Medical Ethic] seminar on ethics and new gene technologies: Smers etikdag 2017: Genombrott inom gentekniken – var finns etiken? Bankhallarna, Malmtorgsgatan 3, Stockholm. Retrieved September 30, 2024, from https://smer.se/calendar/smers-etikdag-2017-genombrott-inom-gentekniken-var-finns-etiken/.

Howard, H. C., Van El, C. G., Forzano, F., Radojkovic, D., Rial-Sebbag, E., De Wert, G., Borry, P., & Cornel, M. C [on behalf of the Public and Professional Policy Committee of the European Society of Human Genetics]. (2018). One small edit for humans, one giant edit for humankind? Points and questions to consider for a responsible way forward for gene editing in humans. *European Journal of Human Genetics, 26*(1), 1–11. https://doi.org/10.1038/s41431-017-0024-z.

Hunter, W., & Hasselbring, A. (2018). *CRISPR: Apocalypse.* AuthorHouse.

Hurlbut, J. B. (2015). Limits of responsibility: Genome editing, asilomar, and the politics of deliberation. *Hastings Center Report, 45*(5), 11–14. https://doi.org/10.1002/hast.484.

Hurlbut, J. B. (2020). Imperatives of governance: Human genome editing and the problem of progress. *Perspectives in Biology and Medicine, 63*(1), 177–194. https://doi.org/10.1353/pbm.2020.0013.

Hurlbut, J. B., Jasanoff, S., Saha, K., Ahmed, A., Appiah, A., Bartholet, E., Baylis, F., Bennett, G., Church, G., Cohen, I. G., Daley, G., Finneran, K., Hurlbut, W., Jaenisch, R., Lwoff, L., Kimes, J. P., Mills, P., Moses, J., Park, B. S., ... Woopen, C. (2018). Building capacity for a global genome editing observatory: Conceptual challenges. *Trends in Biotechnology, 36*(7), 639–641. https://doi.org/10.1016/j.tibtech.2018.04.009.

Häyry, M. (1994). Categorical objections to genetic engineering—A Critique. In A. Dyson & J. Harris (Eds.), *Ethics and Biotechnology* (pp. 202–215). Routledge.

Häyry, M. (2010). *Rationality and the Genetic Challenge: Making People Better?* Cambridge University Press. https://doi.org/10.1017/CBO9781139194679.

Jasanoff, S., & Hurlbut, J. B. (2018). A global observatory for gene editing. *Nature, 555*(7697), 435–437. https://doi.org/10.1038/d41586-018-03270-w.

Jasanoff, S., Hurlbut, J. B., & Saha, K. (2015). CRISPR democracy: Gene editing and the need for inclusive deliberation. *Issues in Science and Technology, 32*(1), 25–32.

Jiang, L., & Stevens, H. (2015). Chinese biotech versus international ethics? Accounting for the China-America CRISPR ethics divide. *BioSocieties, 10*, 483–488. https://doi.org/10.1057/biosoc.2015.34.

Jinek, M., Chylinski, K., Fonfara, I., Hauer, M., Doudna, J. A., & Charpentier, E. (2012). A programmable dual-RNA-guided DNA endonuclease in adaptive bacterial immunity. *Science, 337*(6069), 816–821. https://doi.org/10.1126/science.12258.

Jinek, M., East, A., Cheng, A., Lin, S., Ma, E., & Doudna, J. (2013). RNA-programmed genome editing in human cells. *eLife, 2*, e00471. https://doi.org/10.7554/eLife.00471.

Johnson, R., & Cureton, A. (2022). Kant's moral philosophy. In E. N. Zalta & U. Nodelman (Eds.), *The Stanford Encyclopedia of Philosophy* (Fall 2022 ed.). Retrieved September 30, 2024, from https://plato.stanford.edu/archives/fall2022/entries/kant-moral.

Juengst, E. T. (1998). What does enhancement mean? In E. Parens (Ed.), *Enhancing Human Traits: Ethical and Social Implications* (pp. 29–47). Georgetown University Press.

Juengst, E. T. (2009). What's taxonomy got to do with it? 'Species integrity', human rights, and science policy. In J. Savulescu & N. Bostrom (Eds.), *Human Enhancement* (pp. 42–58). Oxford University Press. https://doi.org/10.1093/oso/9780199299720.003.0003.

Juengst E. T. (2013). Subhuman, superhuman, and inhuman: Human nature and the enhanced athlete. In Tolleneer J., Sterckx S., & Bonte P. (Eds), *Athletic Enhancement, Human Nature and Ethics: Threats and Opportunities of Doping Technologies* (pp. 89–103). Springer. 10.1007/978-94-007-5101-9_5.

Juengst, E. T. (2017). Crowdsourcing the moral limits of human gene editing? *Hastings Center Report, 47*(3), 15–23. https://doi.org/10.1002/hast.701.

Kaiser, J. (2017, February 14). U.S. panel gives yellow light to human embryo editing. *Science.* https://www.sciencemag.org/news/2017/02/us-panel-gives-yellow-light-human-embryo-editing.

Kant, I. (2019). *Groundwork of the Metaphysics of Morals.* (C. Bennett, J. Saunders, J., & R. Stern, Transl.). Oxford University Press. (Original work published 1785).

Kass, L. (1972). New beginnings in life. In M. Hamilton (Ed.), *The New Genetics and the Future of Man* (pp. 15–63). Eerdmans.

Kass, L. R. (2008). Defending human dignity. In A. Schulman, & T. M. Merrill (Ed.), *Human Dignity and Bioethics: Essays Commissioned by the President's Council on Bioethics* (pp. 297–331). U.S. Independent Agencies and Commissions. http://hdl.handle.net/10822/559351.

Knapton, S. (2018, July 17). Designer babies on horizon as ethics council gives green light to genetically edited embryos. *The Telegraph.* https://www.telegraph.co.uk/science/2018/07/16/designer-babies-horizon-ethics-council-gives-green-light-genetically/.

Koplin, J. J., Gyngell, C., & Savulescu, J. (2019). Germline gene editing and the precautionary principle. *Bioethics, 34*(1), 49–59. https://doi.org/10.1111/bioe.12609.

Korsgaard, C. (1996). *Creating the Kingdom of Ends.* Cambridge University Press. https://doi.org/10.1017/CBO9781139174503.

Kozubek, J. (2016). *Modern Prometheus: Editing the Human Genome with CRISPR-Cas9.* Cambridge University Press. 10.1017/9781108597104.

Krimsky, S. (2015). Crossing the germline barrier: The three genome baby. *Ethics in Biology, Engineering & Medicine: An International Journal, 6*(3–4), 237–261. Retrieved September 30, 2024, from https://sites.tufts.edu/sheldonkrimsky/files/2018/05/pub2015CrossingtheGermlineBarrier.pdf.

Krimsky, S. (2019). Ten ways in which He Jiankui violated ethics. *Nature Biotechnology, 37*(1), 19–20. https://doi.org/10.1038/nbt.4337.

Lander, E. S. (2016). The heroes of CRISPR. *Cell, 164*(1–2), 18–28. https://doi.org/10.1016/j.cell.2015.12.041.

Lander, E. S., Baylis, F., Zhang, F., Charpentier, E., Berg, P., Bourgain, C., Friedrich, B., Joung, J. K., Li, J., Lie, D., Naldini, L., Nie, J.-B., Qui, R., Schoene-Seifert, B., Shao, F., Terry, S., Wei, W., & Winnacker, E.-L. (2019). Adopt a moratorium on heritable genome editing. *Nature, 567*(7747), 165–168. https://doi.org/10.1038/d41586-019-00726-5.

Lanphier, E., Urnov, F., Haecker, M., Werner, M., & Smolenski, J. (2015). Don't edit the human germline. *Nature, 519*(7544), 410–411. https://doi.org/10.1038/519410a.

Lappé, M. (1972). Moral obligations and the fallacies of "genetic control." *Theological Studies, 33*(3), 411–427. 10.1177/00405639720330.

Lappé, M. (1991). Ethical issues in manipulating the human germ line. *The Journal of Medicine and Philosophy: A Forum for Bioethics and Philosophy of Medicine, 16*(6), 621–639. https://doi.org/10.1093/jmp/16.6.621.

Larry, A., & Moore, M. (2021). Deontological ethics. In E. N. Zalta (Ed.), *The Stanford Encyclopedia of Philosophy* (Winter 2021 ed.). Retrieved September 30, 2024, from https://plato.stanford.edu/archives/win2021/entries/ethics-deontological.

Ledford, H. (2015). CRISPR, the disruptor. *Nature, 522*(7554), 20–24. https://doi.org/10.1038/522020a.

Ledford, H. (2016). The unsung heroes of CRISPR. *Nature, 535*(7612), 342–344. https://doi.org/10.1038/535342a.

Levin, S. B. (2017). Antiquity's missive to transhumanism. *Journal of Medicine and Philosophy: A Forum for Bioethics and Philosophy of Medicine, 42*(3), 278–303. https://doi.org/10.1093/jmp/jhx008.

Lewens, T. (2020). Blurring the germline: Genome editing and transgenerational epigenetic inheritance. *Bioethics, 34*(1), 7–15. https://doi.org/10.1111/bioe.12606.

Liang, P., Xu, Y., Zhang, X., Ding, C., Huang, R., Zhang, Z., Lv, J., Xiaowei, X., Chen, Y., Li, Y., Sun, Y., Bai, Y., Songyang, Z., Ma, W., Zhou, C., & Huang, J. (2015). CRISPR/Cas9-mediated gene editing in human tripronuclear zygotes. *Protein & Cell, 6*(5), 363–372. https://doi.org/10.1007/s13238-015-0153-5.

Lincoln, A. (1863). *The Gettysburg address.* Retrieved September 30, 2024, from http://www.abrahamlincolnonline.org/lincoln/speeches/gettysburg.htm.

Locke, J. (1988). *Locke: Two Treatises of Government* (P. Laslett, Ed.). Cambridge University Press. (Original work published 1689). https://doi.org/10.1017/CBO9780511810268.

Lynch, M. (2016). Mutation and human exceptionalism: Our future genetic load. *Genetics, 202*(3), 869–875. https://doi.org/10.1534/genetics.115.180471.

Ma, H., Marti-Gutierrez, N., Park, S.-W., Wu, J., Lee, Y., Suzuki, K., Koski, A., Ji, D., Hayama, T., Ahmed, R., Darby, H., Van Dyken, C., Li, Y., Kang, E., Park, A. R., Kim, D., Kim, S.-T., Gong, J., Gu, Y., ... Mitalipov, S. (2017). Correction of a pathogenic gene mutation in human embryos. *Nature, 548*(7668), 413–419. https://doi.org/10.1038/nature23305.

MacKellar, C., & Bechtel, C. (Eds.). (2016). *The Ethics of the New Eugenics.* Berghahn Books. 10.3167/9781782381204.

Mariscal, C., & Petropanagos, A. (2016). CRISPR as a driving force: The *Model T* of biotechnology. *Monash Bioethical Review, 34*(2), 101–116. https://doi.org/10.1007/s40592-016-0062-2.

Marks, L., & Camporesi, S. (2015, October 15). Join the debate around genome editing. *OpenDemocracy.* Retrieved September 30, 2024, from https://www.opendemocracy.net/en/join-debate-around-genome-editing/.

Mathews, D. J. H., Chan, S., Donovan, P. J., Douglas, T., Gyngell, G., Harris, J., Regenberg, A., & Lovell-Badge, R. (2015). CRISPR: A path through the thicket. *Nature, 527*(7577), 159–161. https://doi.org/10.1038/527159a.

Matthews-King, A. (2018, July 17). Designer babies: Picking traits for non-medical reasons could be 'morally permissible', says UK ethics group. *The Independent.* https://www.independent.co.uk/news/health/designer-babies-gene-editing-genetics-genome-nuffield-ethics-disease-a8449971.html.

McNamee, M. J., & Edwards, S. D. (2006). Transhumanism, medical technology and slippery slopes. *Journal of Medical Ethics, 32*(9), 513–518. https://doi.org/10.1136/jme.2005.013789.

Merriman, B. (2015). "Editing": A productive metaphor for regulating CRISPR. *American Journal of Bioethics, 15*(12), 62–64. 10.1080/15265161.2015.1103806.

Mertes, H., & Pennings, G. (2015). Modification of the embryo's genome: More useful in research than in the clinic. *The American Journal of Bioethics, 15*(12), 52–53. 10.1080/15265161.2015.1103813.

De Miguel Beriain, I. (2019a). Gene editing and the slippery slope argument: should we fix the enhancement/therapy distinction as the definitive boundary? *Science and Engineering Ethics, 25*(4), 1257–1258. https://doi.org/10.1007/s11948-018-0048-y.

De Miguel Beriain, I. (2019b). Should human germline editing be allowed? Some suggestions on the basis of the existing regulatory framework. *Bioethics, 33*(1), 105–111. https://doi.org/10.1111/bioe.12492.

Mill, J. S. (1998). *Utilitarianism* (R. Crisp, Ed.). Oxford University Press. (Original work published 1861).

Mill, J. S. (2008). *On Liberty and Other Essays*. Oxford University Press. (Original work published 1859).

Mintz, R. L., Loike, J. D., & Fischbach, R. L. (2019). Will CRISPR germline engineering close the door to an open future? *Science and Engineering Ethics, 25*(5), 1409–1423. https://doi.org/10.1007/s11948-018-0069-6.

Moore, G. E. (2005). *Ethics: and "The Nature of Moral Philosophy"* (W. H. Shaw, Ed.). Oxford University Press. (Original work published 1912). 10.1093/0199272018.001.0001.

More, M. (1990). Transhumanism: Towards a futurist philosophy. *Extropy: The Journal of Transhumanist Thought, 6*, 6–12.

Muller, H. J. (1950). Our load of mutations. *The American Journal of Human Genetics, 2*(2), 111–176.

Muller, H. J. (1959). The guidance of human evolution. *Perspectives in Biology and Medicine, 3*(1), 1–43. https://doi.org/10.1353/pbm.1959.0043.

Munson, R., & Davis, L. H. (1992). Germ-line gene therapy and the medical imperative. *Kennedy Institute of Ethics Journal, 2*(2), 37–158. https://doi.org/10.1353/ken.0.0091.

The National Academies of Sciences, Engineering, and Medicine (NASEM). (2015). *International Summit on Human Gene Editing: A Global Discussion*. National Academies Press. 10.17226/21913.

The National Academies of Sciences, Engineering, and Medicine (NASEM). (2017). *Human Genome Editing: Science, Ethics, and Governance*. National Academies Press. 10.17226/24623.

The National Academy of Medicine, The National Academy of Sciences, The Royal Society, & International Commission on the Clinical Use of Human Germline Genome Editing. (2020). *Heritable Human Genome Editing*. National Academies Press. 10.17226/25665.

Neuhaus, C. P. (2018). Should we edit the human germline? Is consensus possible or even desirable? *The Hastings Center* [Online Forum]. Retrieved September 30, 2024, from https://www.thehastingscenter.org/edit-human-germline-consensus-possible-even-desirable/.

Niu, Y., Shen, B., Cui, Y., Chen, Y., Wang, J., Wang, L., Kang, Y., Zhao, X., Si, W., Li, W., Xiang, A. P., Zhou, J., Guo, X., Bi, Y., Si, C., Hu, B., Dong, G., Wang, H., Zhou,

Z., … Sha, J. (2014). Generation of gene-modified cynomolgus monkey via Cas9/RNA-mediated gene targeting in one-cell embryos. *Cell, 156*(4), 836–843. https://doi.org/10.1016/j.cell.2014.01.027.

Nordlund, C. (2007). Endocrinology and expectations in 1930s America: Louis Berman's ideas on new creations in human beings. *The British Journal for the History of Science, 144*(1), 83–104. https://doi.org/10.1017/S0007087406009113.

Norman, C. (1983). Clerics urge ban on altering germline cells. *Science, 220*(4604), 1360–1361. https://doi.org/10.1126/science.65746.

Normile, D. (2018). Shock greets claim of CRISPR-edited babies. *Science, 362*(6418), 978–979. https://doi.org/10.1126/science.362.6418.97.

Nozick, R. (2006). *Anarchy, State, and Utopia.* Blackwell. (Original work published 1974).

Nuffield Council on Bioethics. (2016). *Genome editing: An ethical review.* Nuffield Council on Bioethics.

Nuffield Council on Bioethics. (2018). *Genome editing and human reproduction: Social and ethical issues.* Nuffield Council on Bioethics.

Nussbaum, M. C. (1989). Mortal immortals: Lucretius on death and the voice of nature. *Philosophy and Phenomenological Research, 50*(2), 303–351. 10.2307/2107963 .

Nussbaum, M. C. (2011). Creating capabilities: The human development approach. *Belknap Press.* https://doi.org/10.2307/j.ctt2jbt31.

O'Keefe, M., Perrault, S., Halpern, J., Ikemoto, L., Yarborough, M., & UC North Bioethics Collaboratory for Life & Health Sciences (2015). "Editing" genes: A case study about how language matters in bioethics. *The American Journal of Bioethics, 15*(12), 3–10. 10.1080/15265161.2015.1103804 .

O'Neill, O. (2002). *Autonomy and Trust in Bioethics.* Cambridge University Press. https://doi.org/10.1017/CBO9780511606250.

O'Neill, O. (2013). *Acting on Principle: An Essay on Kantian Ethics.* Cambridge University Press. https://doi.org/10.1017/CBO9781139565097.

Organizing Committee for the International Summit on Human Gene Editing. (2015, December 3). *On Human Gene Editing: International Summit Statement.* Retrieved September 30, 2024, from https://www.nationalacademies.org/news/2015/12/on-human-gene-editing-international-summit-statement.

Ormond, K. E., Mortlock, D. P., Scholes, D. T., Bombard, Y., Brody, L. C., Faucett, W. A., & Musunuru, K. (2017). Human germline genome editing. *The American Journal of Human Genetics, 101*(2), 167–176. https://doi.org/10.1016/j.ajhg.2017.06.012.

Parfit, D. (1986). *Reasons and Persons.* Oxford University Press. https://doi.org/10.1093/019824908X.001.0001.

Paul, D. B. (1987). "Our load of mutations" revisited. *Journal of the History of Biology, 20*(3), 321–335. https://www.jstor.org/stable/4331021.

Paul, D. B. (2005). Genetic engineering and eugenics: The uses of history. In H. W. Baille & T. K. Casey (Eds.), *Is Human Nature Obsolete? Genetics, Bioengineering, and the Future of the Human Condition.* MIT Press. https://doi.org/10.7551/mitpress/3977.003.0008.

Peters, T. (1995). "Playing god" and germline intervention. *The Journal of Medicine and Philosophy: A Forum for Bioethics and Philosophy of Medicine, 20*(4), 365–386. https://doi.org/10.1093/jmp/20.4.365.

Peters, T. (2007). Are we playing god with nanoenhancement? In F. Allhoff, P. Lin, J. H. Moor, & J. Weckert (Eds.), *Nanoethics: The Ethical and Social Implications of Nanotechnology* (pp. 173–183). Wiley.

Peters, T. (2017). Should CRISPR scientists play god? *Religions, 8*(61), 1–11. https://doi.org/10.3390/rel8040061.

Peters, T. (2018). Playing god with Frankenstein. *Theology and Science, 16*(2), 145–150. 10.1080/14746700.2018.1455264.

Porter, A. (2017). Bioethics and transhumanism. *The Journal of Medicine and Philosophy: A Forum for Bioethics and Philosophy of Medicine, 42*(3), 237–260. https://doi.org/10.1093/jmp/jhx001.

Powell, R. (2015). In genes we trust: germline engineering, eugenics, and the future of the human genome. *The Journal of Medicine and Philosophy: A Forum for Bioethics and Philosophy of Medicine, 40*(6), 669–695. https://doi.org/10.1093/jmp/jhv025.

Powell, R., & Buchanan, A. (2011). Breaking evolution's chains: The prospect of deliberate genetic modification in humans. *The Journal of Medicine and Philosophy: A Forum for Bioethics and Philosophy of Medicine, 36*(1), 6–27. https://doi.org/10.1093/jmp/jhx001.

President's Commission for the Study of Ethical Problems in Medicine and Biomedical and Behavioral Research. (1982). *Splicing life: A report on the social and ethical issues of genetic engineering with human beings.* Library of Congress. Retrieved October 3, 2024, from http://hdl.handle.net/10822/548744.

Primc, N. (2018). Germline modifications as a severe intervention into human nature. In M. Braun, H. Schickl, & P. Dabrock (Eds.), *Between Moral Hazard and Legal Uncertainty: Ethical, Legal and Societal Challenges of Human Genome Editing* (pp. 99–110). Springer VS. 10.1007/978-3-658-22660-2_7.

Primc, N. (2020). Do we have a right to an unmanipulated genome? The human genome as the common heritage of mankind. *Bioethics, 34*(1), 41–48. https://doi.org/10.1111/bioe.12608.

Pugh, J., Kahane, G., & Savulescu, J. (2013). Cohen's conservatism and human enhancement. *Journal of Ethics, 17*(4), 331–354. https://doi.org/10.1007/s10892-013-9151-0.

Qiu, R. (2016). Debating ethical issues in genome editing technology. *Asian Bioethics Review, 8*(4), 307–326. https://doi.org/10.1353/asb.2016.0026.

Quigley, M., & Harris, J. (2009). To fail to enhance is to disable. In D. C. Ralston & J. H. Ho (Eds.), *Philosophical Reflections on Disability* (pp. 123–131). Springer. 10.1007/978-90-481-2477-0_7.

Rahner, K. (1968). Experiment: man. *Theology Digest, 16*, 57–69.

Ramsey, P. (1970). *Fabricated Man: The Ethics of Genetic Control.* Yale University Press.

Ranisch, R. (2020). Germline genome editing versus preimplantation genetic diagnosis: Is there a case in favour of germline interventions? *Bioethics, 34*(1), 60–69. https://doi.org/10.1111/bioe.12635.

Ranisch, R., & Ehni, H.-J. (2020). Fading the lines? Bioethics of germline editing. *Bioethics, 34*(1), 3–6. https://doi.org/10.1111/bioe.12709.

Rawls, J. (1988). The priority of right and ideas of the good. *Philosophy & Public Affairs, 17*(4), 251–276. https://www.jstor.org/stable/2265400.

Raz, J. (1986). *The Morality of Freedom.* Oxford University Press. 10.1093/0198248075.001.0001 .

Reardon, S. (2015a, November 30). Human-genome editing summit to sample global attitudes. *Nature.* https://doi.org/10.1038/nature.2015.18879.

Reardon, S. (2015b, April 29). NIH reiterates ban on editing human embryo DNA. *Nature.* https://doi.org/10.1038/nature.2015.17452.

Regalado, A. (2019, February 21). China's CRISPR twins might have had their brains inadvertently enhanced. *MIT Technology Review.* Retrieved October 1, 2024, from https://www.technologyreview.com/2019/02/21/137309/the-crispr-twins-had-their-brains-altered/.

Regulation (EU) No 536/2014 of the European Parliament and of the Council of 16 April 2014 on clinical trials on medicinal products for human use, and repealing Directive 2001/20/EC. Retrieved October 1, 2024, from http://data.europa.eu/eli/reg/2014/536/oj.

Resnik, D. B. (1994). Debunking the slippery slope argument against human germ-line gene therapy. *The Journal of Medicine and Philosophy: A Forum for Bioethics and Philosophy of Medicine, 19*(1), 23–40. https://doi.org/10.1093/jmp/19.1.23.

Resnik, D. B., & Langer, P. J. (2001). Human germline gene therapy reconsidered. *Human Gene Therapy, 12*(11), 1449–1458. 10.1089/104303401750298607.

Resnik, D. B., & Vorhaus, D. B. (2006). Genetic modification and genetic determinism. *Philosophy, Ethics, and Humanities in Medicine, 1*(9). 10.1186/1747-5341-1-9.

Rixen, S. (2018). Genome editing and the law: Some remarks on current legal challenges of CRISPR-Cas9. In M. Braun, H. Schickl, & P. Dabrock (Eds.), *Between Moral Hazard and Legal Uncertainty: Ethical, Legal and Societal Challenges of Human Genome Editing* (pp. 17–30). Springer VS. 10.1007/978-3-658-22660-2_2.

Roll-Hansen, N. (2017). Some thoughts on genetics and politics: The historical misrepresentation of scandinavian eugenics and sterilization. In H. I. Petermann, P. S. Harper, & S. Doetz (Eds.), *History of Human Genetics: Aspects of Its Development and Global Perspectives* (pp. 167–187). Springer. 10.1007/978-3-319-51783-4_11.

The Royal Swedish Academy of Sciences (2020). *Genetic scissors: A tool for rewriting the code of life.* Retrieved October 1, 2024, from https://www.nobelprize.org/uploads/2020/10/popular-chemistryprize2020.pdf.

Rubeis, G. (2018). Human germline genome editing in the clinical context: The case of disease prevention. In M. Braun, H. Schickl, & P. Dabrock (Eds.), *Between Moral Hazard and Legal Uncertainty: Ethical, Legal and Societal Challenges of Human Genome Editing* (pp. 149–160). Springer VS. 10.1007/978-3-658-22660-2_10.

Sagoff, M. (2005). Nature and human nature. In H. W. Baille & T. K. Casey (Eds.), *Is Human Nature Obsolete? Genetics, Bioengineering, and the Future of the Human Condition* (pp. 67–98). MIT Press. https://doi.org/10.7551/mitpress/3977.003.0006.

Sample, I. (2018, July 7). Genetically modified babies given go ahead by UK ethics body. *The Guardian.* https://www.theguardian.com/science/2018/jul/17/genetically-modified-babies-given-go-ahead-by-uk-ethics-body.

Sandel, M. J. (2004). The case against perfection. *The Atlantic, 293*(3). https://www.theatlantic.com/magazine/archive/2004/04/the-case-against-perfection/302927/.

Sandel, M. J. (2007). *The Case Against Perfection: Ethics in the Age of Genetic Engineering.* The Belknap Press of Harvard University Press.

Sandel, M. J. (2009). The case against perfection: What's wrong with designer children, bionic athletes, and genetic engineering? In J. Savulescu & N. Bostrom (Eds.), *Human*

Enhancement (pp. 71–89). Oxford University Press. https://doi.org/10.1093/oso/978019 9299720.003.0005.

Sarewitz, D. (2015). CRISPR: Science can't solve it. *Nature, 522*(7557), 413–414. https:// doi.org/10.1038/522413a.

Sataline, S. (2018, November 27). 'Of course it's not ethical': Shock at gene-edited baby claims. *The Guardian.* https://www.theguardian.com/science/2018/nov/27/he-jiankui-chi nese-gene-edited-baby-claims-scientists-shocked-global-outcry.

Sataline, S., & Sample, I. (2018, November 28). Scientist in China defends human embryo gene editing. *The Guardian.* https://www.theguardian.com/science/2018/nov/28/scient ist-in-china-defends-human-embryo-gene-editing.

Savulescu, J. (2001). Procreative beneficence: Why we should select the best children. *Bioethics, 15*(5–6), 413–426. 10.1111/1467-8519.00251.

Savulescu, J. (2005). New breeds of humans: The moral obligation to enhance. *Reproductive BioMedicine Online, 10*(Supplement 1: Ethics, Law and Moral Philosophy of Reproductive Biomedicine), 36–39. https://doi.org/10.1016/S1472-6483(10)62202-X.

Savulescu, J. (2006). Justice, fairness, and enhancement. *The Annals of the New York Academy of Sciences, 1093*, 321–338. https://doi.org/10.1196/annals.1382.021.

Savulescu, J. (2007). In defence of procreative beneficence. *Journal of Medical Ethics, 33*(5), 284–288. https://doi.org/10.1136/jme.2006.018184.

Savulescu, J. (2008). Procreative beneficence: reasons to not have disabled children. In L. Skene & J. Thompson (Eds.), *The Sorting Society: The Ethics of Genetic Screening and Therapy* (pp. 51–68). Cambridge University Press. https://doi.org/10.1017/CBO978051 1545573.006.

Savulescu, J. (2009). The human prejudice and the moral status of enhanced beings: What do we owe the gods? In J. Savulescu & N. Bostrom (Eds.), *Human Enhancement* (pp. 211–247). Oxford University Press. https://doi.org/10.1093/oso/9780199299720.003.0011.

Savulescu, J. (2014). Commentary: The Nature of the Moral Obligation to Select the Best Children. In A. Akabayashi (Ed.), *Future of Bioethics: International Dialogues* (pp. 170–182). Oxford University Press. https://doi.org/10.1093/acprof:oso/9780199682676.003.0020.

Savulescu, J. (2019). Rational freedom and six mistakes of a bioconservative. *The American Journal of Bioethics, 19*(7), 1–5. 10.1080/15265161.2019.1626642.

Savulescu, J., & Bostrom, N. (Eds.). (2009). *Human Enhancement.* Oxford University Press. https://doi.org/10.1093/oso/9780199299720.001.0001.

Savulescu, J., & Gyngell, C. (2015). The medical case for gene editing. *Ethics in Biology, Engineering & Medicine: An International Journal, 6*(1–2), 57–66. https://doi.org/10.1615/ethicsbiologyengmed.2015014314.

Savulescu, J., & Kahane, G. (2009). The moral obligation to create children with the best chance of the best life. *Bioethics, 23*(5), 274–290. https://doi.org/10.1111/j.1467-8519.2008.00687.x.

Savulescu, J., Pugh, J., Douglas, T., & Gyngell, C. (2015). The moral imperative to continue gene editing research on human embryos. *Protein & Cell, 6*(7), 476–479. https://doi.org/10.1007/s13238-015-0184-y.

Scanlon, T. (1998). *What We Owe to Each Other.* Harvard University Press.

Scheffler, S. (Ed.). (1988). *Consequentialism and Its Critics.* Oxford University Press.

Schultz-Bergin, M. (2018). Is CRISPR an ethical game changer? *Journal of Agricultural and Environmental Ethics, 31*(2), 219–238. https://doi.org/10.1007/s10806-018-9721-z.

Scientific American. (2016, February 4). *The embarrassing, destructive fight over biotech's big breakthrough.* https://www.scientificamerican.com/article/the-embarrassing-destructive-fight-over-biotech-s-big-breakthrough/.

Sen, A., & Williams, B. (Eds.). (1982). *Utilitarianism and Beyond.* Cambridge University Press. https://doi.org/10.1017/CBO9780511611964.

Sidgwick, H. (1907). *The Methods of Ethics* (7th ed.). Macmillan. (Original work published 1874).

Simonstein, F. (2019). Gene editing, enhancing and women's role. *Science and Engineering Ethics, 25*(4), 1007–1016. https://doi.org/10.1007/s11948-017-9875-5.

Singer, P. (1972). Famine, affluence, and morality. *Philosophy and Public Affairs, 1*(3), 229–243. https://www.jstor.org/stable/2265052.

Singer, P. (2009). Parental choice and human improvement. In J. Savulescu & N. Bostrom (Eds.), *Human Enhancement* (pp. 277–289). Oxford University Press. https://doi.org/10.1093/oso/9780199299720.003.0013.

Singer, P. (2011). *Practical Ethics* (3rd ed.). Cambridge University Press.

Singer, P. (2015). *The Most Good You Can Do: How Effective Altruism is Changing Ideas About Living Ethically.* Yale University Press.

Sinnott-Armstrong, W. (2021). Consequentialism. In E. N. Zalta (Ed.), *The Stanford Encyclopedia of Philosophy* (Fall 2021 ed.). Retrieved October 2, 2024, from https://plato.stanford.edu/archives/fall2021/entries/consequentialism.

Slovic, P. (Ed.). (2000). *The Perception of Risk.* Earthscan. 10.4324/9781315661773.

Slovic, P., Fischhoff, B., & Lichtenstein, S. (2000). Facts and fears: Understanding perceived risk. In Slovic, P. (Eds.), *The Perception of Risk.* Earthscan.

Smart, J. J. C., & Williams, B. (1973). *Utilitarianism: For and Against.* Cambridge University Press. Retrieved October 2, 2024, from https://www.utilitarianism.com/utilitarianism-for-and-against.pdf.

Southern University of Science and Technology. (2018). Southern University of Science and Technology statement on the genetic editing of human embryos conducted by Dr. Jiankui HE.

Sparrow, R. (2011). A not-so-new eugenics: Harris and Savulescu on human enhancement. *Hastings Center Report, 41*(1), 32–42. https://doi.org/10.1002/j.1552-146X.2011.tb00098.x.

Sparrow, R. (2012). A child's right to a decent future? Regulating human genetic enhancement in multicultural societies. *Asian Bioethics Review, 4*(4), 355–373. https://muse.jhu.edu/article/494968.

Sparrow, R. (2015). Enhancement and obsolescence: Avoiding an 'enhanced rat race.' *Kennedy Institute of Ethics Journal, 25*(3), 231–260. https://doi.org/10.1353/ken.2015.0015.

Sparrow, R. (2019). Yesterday's child: How gene editing for enhancement will produce obsolescence—and why it matters. *The American Journal of Bioethics, 19*(7), 6–15. 10.1080/15265161.2019.1618943.

Sternberg, S. H., & Doudna, J. A. (2015). Expanding the biologist's toolkit with CRISPR-Cas9. *Molecular Cell, 58*(4), 568–574. https://doi.org/10.1016/j.molcel.2015.02.032.

Sufian, S., & Garland-Thomson, R. (2021, February 16). The dark side of CRISPR: Its potential ability to "fix" people at the genetic level is a threat to those who are judged by society to be biologically inferior. *Scientific American.* https://www.scientificamerican.com/art icle/the-dark-side-of-crispr/.

Sugarman, J. (2015). Ethics and germline gene editing. *EMBO Reports, 16*(8), 879–880. https://doi.org/10.15252/embr.201540879.

Sulmasy, D. P. (2008). Dignity and bioethics: History, theory, and selected applications. In A. Schulman & T. M. Merrill (Eds.), *Human Dignity and Bioethics: Essays Commissioned by the President's Council on Bioethics* (pp. 469–501). U.S. Independent Agencies and Commissions. http://hdl.handle.net/10822/559351.

Sykora, P., & Caplan, A. (2017a). The Council of Europe should not reaffirm the ban on germline genome editing in humans. *EMBO Reports, 18*(11), 1871–1872. https://doi.org/ 10.15252/embr.201745246.

Sykora, P., & Caplan, A. (2017b). Germline gene therapy is compatible with human dignity. *EMBO Reports, 18*(12), 2086. https://doi.org/10.15252/embr.201745378.

Thomson, J. J. (1986). *Rights, Restitution, and Risk: Essays in Moral Theory.* Harvard University Press.

Thomson, J. J. (1992). *The Realm of Rights.* Harvard University Press.

Thrasher, A., Baltimore, D., Pei, D., Lander, E. S., Winnacker, E-L., Baylis, F., Daley, G. Q., Doudna, J. A., Berg, P., Ossorio, P., Zhou, Q., & Lovell-Badge, R. (2016). On Human gene editing: International summit statement by organizing committee. *Issues in Science and Technology, 32*(3), 55–56. https://issues.org/on-human-gene-editing-international-summit-statement-by-the-organizing-committee/.

Turney, J. (1998). *Frankenstein's Footsteps: Science, Genetics and Popular Culture.* Yale University Press.

UNESCO (1997). *Universal declaration on the human genome and human rights,* 11 November 1997, Part A. Article 1. Retrieved October 3, 2024, from https://www.unesco.org/en/ legal-affairs/universal-declaration-human-genome-and-human-rights?hub=387.

United Nations. (1948). *Universal declaration of human rights.* Retrieved October 3, 2024, from https://www.un.org/en/about-us/universal-declaration-of-human-rights.

The U.S. Declaration of Independence. (1776). Retrieved October 3, 2024, from https:// www.archives.gov/founding-docs/declaration-transcript.

Vallentyne, P. (1987). The teleological/deontological distinction. *The Journal of Value Inquiry, 21,* 21–32. https://doi.org/10.1007/BF00135526.

Vogel, G. (2015). Embryo engineering alarm. *Science, 347*(6228), 1301. https://doi.org/10. 1126/science.347.6228.130.

Walton, D. (2016). The slippery slope argument in the ethical debate on genetic engineering of humans. *Science and Engineering Ethics, 23*(6), 1507–1528. https://doi.org/10.1007/ s11948-016-9861-3.

Weckert, J. (2016). Playing God: What is the problem? In S. Clarke, J. Savulescu, T. Coady, A. Giubilini, & S. Sanyal (Eds.), *The Ethics of Human Enhancement: Understanding the Debate* (pp. 87–99). Oxford University Press. https://doi.org/10.1093/acprof:oso/978019 8754855.003.0006.

De Wert, G., Heindryckx, B., Pennings, G., Clarke, A., Eichenlaub-Ritter, U., van El, C. G., Forzano, F., Goddijn, M., Howard, H. C., Radojkovic, D., Rial-Sebbag, E., Dondorp, W., Tarlatzis, B. C., Cornel, M. C., & European Society of Human Genetics and the

European Society of Human Reproduction and Embryology. (2018). Responsible innovation in human germline gene editing. Background document to the recommendations of ESHG and ESHRE. *European Journal of Human Genetics*, *26*(4), 450–470. https://doi.org/10.1038/s41431-017-0077-z.

De Wert, G., Pennings, G., Clarke, A., Eichenlaub-Ritter, U., Van El, C. G., Forzano, F., Goddijn, M., Heindryckx, B., Howard, H. C., Radojkovic, D., Rial-Sebbag, E., Tarlatzis, B. C., Cornel, M. C., & European Society of Human Genetics and the European Society of Human Reproduction and Embryology. (2018). Human germline gene editing: Recommendations of ESHG and ESHRE. *European Journal of Human Genetics*, *26*(4), 445–449. https://doi.org/10.1038/s41431-017-0076-0.

Westerlund, K. (2004). Det normala och naturliga: Om kulturella normers betydelse i mötet med barnlöshet. In C. Nordlund (Ed.), *Livsföreställningar: Kultur, samhälle och biovetenskap* (pp. 61–74). Royal Skyttean Society.

Wirth, M. (2018). Transition and care: Theological concepts of dynamic creation and the ethics of genome editing. In M. Braun, H. Schickl, & P. Dabrock (Eds.), *Between Moral Hazard and Legal Uncertainty: Ethical, Legal and Societal Challenges of Human Genome Editing* (pp. 129–148). Springer VS. 10.1007/978-3-658-22660-2_9.

Wolf, S. (1982). Moral saints. *The Journal of Philosophy, 79*(8), 419–439. 10.2307/2026228.

Wolinetz, C. D., & Collins, F. S. (2019). NIH supports call for moratorium on clinical uses of germline gene editing. *Nature, 567*(7747), 175. https://doi.org/10.1038/d41586-019-008 14-6.

Yong, E. (2018, December 3). The CRISPR baby scandal gets worse by the day. *The Atlantic*. https://www.theatlantic.com/science/archive/2018/12/15-worrying-things-about-crispr-babies-scandal/577234/.

Zhang, L., & Zhou, Q. (2014). CRISPR/Cas9 technology: A revolutionary approach for genome engineering. *Science China Life Sciences, 57*(6), 639–640. https://doi.org/10.1007/s11427-014-4670-x.

Printed in the United States
by Baker & Taylor Publisher Services